D1305956

DECISION MAKING IN

Pulmonary Medicine

Medical Titles in the Clinical Decision Making™ Series

Consulting Editor
Ben Eiseman, M.D.

DECISION MAKING IN
Pulmonary Medicine

Joel B. Karlinsky, M.D.

Associate Professor of Medicine
Boston University School of Medicine
Instructor, Tufts University School of Medicine
Chief, Pulmonary Outpatient Clinic
Assistant Chief, Medical Service
Department of Veterans Affairs Medical Center
Boston, Massachusetts

Joseph Lau, M.D.

Assistant Professor of Medicine
Tufts University School of Medicine
Staff Physician
Department of Veterans Affairs Medical Center
Boston, Massachusetts

Ronald H. Goldstein, M.D.

Associate Professor of Medicine
Boston University School of Medicine
Chief, Bronchoscopy Service
Department of Veterans Affairs Medical Center
Boston, Massachusetts

B.C. Decker • Philadelphia

Publisher

B.C. Decker
320 Walnut Street
Suite 400
Philadelphia, Pennsylvania 19106

Sales and Distribution

United States and Puerto Rico
Mosby-Year Book Inc.
11830 Westline Industrial Drive
Saint Louis, Missouri 63146

Canada
Mosby-Year Book Limited
5240 Finch Avenue E., Unit 1
Scarborough, Ontario M1S 5A2

Australia
McGraw-Hill Book Company Australia Pty. Ltd.
4 Barcoo Street
Roseville East 2069
New South Wales, Australia

Brazil
Editora McGraw-Hill do Brasil, Ltda.
rua Tabapua, 1.105, Itaim-Bibi
Sao Paulo, S.P. Brasil

Colombia
Interamericana/McGraw-Hill de Colombia, S.A.
Carrera 17, No. 33-71
(Apartado Postal, A.A., 6131)
Bogota, D.E., Colombia

Europe, United Kingdom, Middle East and Africa
Wolfe Publishing Limited
Brook House
2–16 Torrington Place
London WC1E 7LT England

Hong Kong and China
McGraw-Hill Book Company
Suite 618, Ocean Centre
5 Canton Road
Tsimshatsui, Kowloon
Hong Kong

India
Tata McGraw-Hill Publishing Company, Ltd.
12/4 Asaf Ali Road, 3rd Floor
New Delhi 110002, India

Indonesia
Mr. Wong Fin Fah
P.O. Box 122/JAT
Jakarta, 1300 Indonesia

Japan
Igaku-Shoin Ltd.
Tokyo International P.O. Box 5063
1-28-36 Hongo, Bunkyo-ku,
Tokyo 113, Japan

Korea
Mr. Don-Gap Choi
C.P.O. Box 10583
Seoul, Korea

Malaysia
Mr. Lim Tao Slong
No. 8 Jalan SS 7/6B
Kelana Jaya
47301 Petaling Jaya
Selangor, Malaysia

Mexico
Interamericana/McGraw-Hill de Mexico, S.A. de C.V.
Cedro 512, Colonia Atlampa
(Apartado Postal 26370)
06450 Mexico, D.F., Mexico

New Zealand
McGraw-Hill Book Co. New Zealand Ltd.
5 Joval Place, Wiri
Manukau City, New Zealand

Portugal
Editora McGraw-Hill de Portugal, Ltda.
Rua Rosa Damasceno 11A–B
1900 Lisboa, Portugal

Singapore and Southeast Asia
McGraw-Hill Book Co.
21 Neythal Road
Jurong, Singapore 2262

South Africa
Libriger Book Distributors
Warehouse Number 8
"Die Ou Looiery"
Tannery Road
Hamilton, Bloemfontein 9300

Spain
McGraw-Hill/Interamericana de Espana, S.A.
Manuel Ferrero, 13
28020 Madrid, Spain

Taiwan
Mr. George Lim
P.O. Box 87–601
Taipei, Taiwan

Thailand
Mr. Vitit Lim
632/5 Phaholyothin Road
Sapan Kwai
Bangkok 10400
Thailand

Venezuela
Editorial Interamericana de Venezuela, C.A.
2da. calle Bello Monte
Local G-2
Caracas, Venezuela

NOTICE

The authors and publisher have made every effort to ensure that the patient care recommended herein, including choice of drugs and drug dosages, is in accord with the accepted standards and practice at the time of publication. However, since research and regulation constantly change clinical standards, the reader is urged to check the product information sheet included in the package of each drug, which includes recommended doses, warnings, and contraindications. This is particularly important with new or infrequently used drugs.

Decision Making in Pulmonary Medicine ISBN 1–55664–164–8

Library of Congress catalog card number: 90–83570

10 9 8 7 6 5 4 3 2 1

To my parents, Jean and Nathan, for their love, support, and encouragement. — J.B.K.

To my loving parents, who made it all possible. — J.L.

To Andrea, my wife, to Cassie, my daughter, and to Elsie, my mother, for their love. — R.H.G.

FOREWORD

The past 50 years have witnessed a phenomenal growth in knowledge of pulmonary diseases. Most of our present knowledge of lung function in health and disease has developed during this period. Thoracic imaging has been greatly improved by the development of several new methods: the use of the gamma camera following the administration of radionuclides; ultrasonography; and, most recently and of most importance, computed axial tomographic scanning. Information on the fine structure, biochemistry, cell biology, molecular biology, and immunology of the lungs has exploded during the latter half of this century. For example, everything we know about surfactants has been developed during this period. The fiberoptic bronchoscope has largely replaced the rigid bronchoscope, and lung cytology, transbronchoscopic biopsy, and open lung biopsy have come of age. Innumerable published studies have correlated clinical information and lung structure, function, and imaging, and the basic sciences in lung diseases. Since the large amount of information derived from the patient's history and physical examination continues to be of great importance during this period, the clinician has been provided with ever-expanding knowledge and data bases for the diagnosis and treatment of patients. The high cost of many of the newer diagnostic techniques requires their informed use if medical care resources are not to be wasted.

The last quarter century has also seen the development of the academic and professional discipline of decision analysis. In his recent monograph, Holtzman traces the history of and provides a clear exposition on the theory and practice of this discipline.[1] He defines decision analysis as a discipline comprising the philosophy, theory, methodology, and professional practice necessary for formally making important decisions. The intent is to assist in making difficult decisions by applying decision theory—a formal decision method—to real decisions. Decision analysis is meant to focus the decision-maker's attention on important issues and away from unimportant ones, in order to provide a simpler and more effective formulation of the decision at hand, and ultimately, to lead to a more effective decision.

Holtzman points out that decision analysis has as yet had limited use in medical decision making. The high cost of the technique, the difficulties in measuring an individual's preferences over a wide range of medical outcomes, and the high stakes involved in many medical decisions stand in the way of its widespread use.

Decision Making in Pulmonary Medicine, written by two experts on pulmonology (JBK and RHG) and an expert on decision analysis (JL), is not based on decision theory. It attempts rather to codify the approach to decision making in pulmonary medicine by utilizing algorithms based on the clinical experience of the authors and the published literature. An algorithm is a set of rules for solving a problem in a finite number of steps.[2] The book focuses more on diagnosis than on therapy because of limitations of space and because therapy is frequently straightforward once the diagnosis is established. Also because of limitations of space, there is little consideration of the role that a patient's attitudes, preferences, and varying circumstances have in patient management.

It is apparent, given the lack of objective outcome data for many diagnostic and therapeutic approaches, that there will not be unanimity of opinion of all experts in pulmonology on the particular steps chosen by the authors of this book in algorithms. However, the algorithms, presented both in diagrammatic form and in text, provide a rapidly available expert opinion on the conditions and disorders considered in the book. Many of the algorithms represent a first attempt to use this format to identify the steps used by physicians expert in their field in establishing a diagnosis and treating patients with pulmonary disease.

These algorithms will be useful to practicing physicians, nurses, and other clinicians as well as to those interested in quality assurance activities and in health care research. *Decision Making in Pulmonary Medicine* will help clinicians to systematize the ways in which they think about patients with pulmonary disease and in which they use the powerful new tools available for patient care at the close of the twentieth century. It will also be helpful in carrying out focused reviews of the records of pulmonary patients and in developing instruments for carrying out analyses of process and outcomes in the management of patients with pulmonary disease.

Gordon L. Snider, M.D.

References

1. Holtzman S. Intelligent decision systems. Reading MA: Addison-Wesley Publishing Company, Inc., 1989.
2. The Random House Dictionary. Stein J, ed. New York: Ballantine Books, 1980.

PREFACE

The purpose of this book is to guide physicians in making clinical judgments regarding pulmonary problems. Most cases selected for inclusion in this book are commonly encountered; some are unusual and will rarely be seen. Although this volume incorporates the clinical algorithm approach to solving pulmonary problems, every patient is unique, and every problem is unique to a particular patient. No clinical algorithm can take into account the myriad of physical, social, and psychological variations among patients. Therefore only the major issues that we have found to be of importance in our own practice of pulmonary medicine have been emphasized.

We remind the reader, as have many others in this series, that laboratory tests and procedures are no substitute for a conscientious and thorough history and physical examination. We believe that attention to the patient's wishes, combined with a systematic approach to clinical problems (the algorithm) and tempered by the unique characteristics of each patient, all as practiced by a caring physician, results in the best medicine.

Finally, we would like to thank the Pulmonary Center at the Boston University School of Medicine and the Division of Clinical Decision Making at Tufts University School of Medicine and the Department of Veterans Affairs Medical Center in Boston for their efforts on our behalf with respect to this book. We would also like to thank Brian Decker for giving us the opportunity to contribute this volume. Finally, we especially give great thanks to Mary Mansor and Vicki Hoenigke, our editors at B.C. Decker, for their unfailing good-humored encouragement, persistence, helpful comments, and focused criticism.

Joel B. Karlinsky, M.D.
Joseph Lau, M.D.
Ronald H. Goldstein, M.D.

CONTENTS

INTRODUCTION

The cases in this volume have been analyzed using the clinical algorithm technique. Each algorithm is presented as a series of steps, with branches placed at key decision points, representing a logical progression of clinical thinking focused on diagnosis and therapy. Branch points are especially important in these algorithms because they signify the stages at which the physician's judgment enters into the decision-making process. Although there is room for disagreement regarding the steps at which we have chosen to place specific branch points, each algorithm is a distillation of our clinical thinking and experience, tempered by consideration of current information from the literature. The reader should view these algorithms as a general guide systematically and logically organized to be applied to a specific patient problem, but which can be altered as circumstances demand. In particular, the branch points may vary, depending on the individual patient. Also, individual practice patterns depend on the availability of procedures and laboratory tests; not all procedures and tests used in these algorithms are universally available. All algorithms in this book have been reviewed by all the authors and therefore reflect the compromises that they made.

GENERAL APPROACHES TO PULMONARY DYSFUNCTION

Acute Dyspnea
Chronic Dyspnea
Cough
Chest Pain

Hemoptysis
Pleural Effusion
Atelectasis

ACUTE DYSPNEA

Dyspnea is a sensation of shortness of breath. Organic causes include diseases that result in increased airway resistance or decreased lung compliance. Nonorganic causes of shortness of breath such as hyperventilation syndrome should be excluded prior to institution of diagnostic measures. Acute dyspnea signifies the occurrence of a sudden cardiopulmonary event, acute decompensation of chronic cardiopulmonary diseases, or a compensatory respiratory response to acute metabolic acidosis. Causes of acute dyspnea include pneumonia, asthma, spontaneous pneumothorax, pulmonary edema, pulmonary embolism, upper airway obstruction, adult respiratory distress syndrome, and acute myocardial infarction. The approach to patients with acute dyspnea is first to identify and treat promptly immediate life-threatening conditions. Patients with acute respiratory failure or impending cardiopulmonary arrest should be immediately intubated and placed on controlled or assisted ventilation prior to the diagnostic evaluation.

A. The history and physical examination, along with routine laboratory tests, arterial blood gas analysis, electrocardiography, and chest x-ray examination should determine the cause of acute dyspnea. Due to delays and time lags in obtaining results of laboratory tests and chest films, a presumptive diagnosis must be made on the basis of the history and physical examination alone. Bilateral rales throughout most of the lung in a patient with history of cardiac disease or acute chest pain suggest pulmonary edema; wheezing is the hallmark of asthma; and stridor indicates upper airway obstruction. Obtain electrocardiograms early in the evaluation of patients with acute dyspnea to identify acute myocardial infarction and arrhythmias. Electrocardiograms sometimes suggest other causes of dyspnea such as pulmonary embolism (right heart strain pattern) and pericarditis with tamponade (electrical alternans).

B. The arterial blood gas analysis is extremely important in the early evaluation of acute dyspnea and is helpful in determining the severity of hypoxemia or acidosis. The alveolar-arterial oxygen tension gradient ($D(A-a)O_2$) is the difference between calculated alveolar oxygen tension and the measured arterial oxygen tension, and normally is less than 10 to 15 mm Hg. Patients with diffusion defects or ventilation-perfusion mismatch (shunting) have an elevated $D(A-a)O_2$. The $D(A-a)O_2$ remains normal for patients with alveolar hypoventilation.

C. Patients with anemia are dyspneic owing to decreased oxygen carrying capacity. An elevated white blood cell count further supports the diagnosis of pneumonia in patients with fever and pulmonary infiltrates. Diabetic ketoacidosis is a common cause of metabolic acidosis. Arterial blood gas pH and measurement of anion gap provide evidence of metabolic acidosis. Compensatory hyperventilation occurs to correct blood pH. The degree of dyspnea depends on the severity of acidosis and patient's pulmonary reserve.

D. Chest films are necessary to confirm or diagnose most of the remaining causes of acute dyspnea.

E. In patients with a high clinical suspicion of pulmonary embolism, perform a perfusion lung scan and/or pulmonary angiography.

References

Burki NK. Dyspnea. Lung 1987; 165:269.

Cherniack NS, Altose MD. Mechanisms of dyspnea. Clin Chest Med 1987; 8:207.

Cockcroft A, Adams L, Guz A. Assessment of breathlessness. Q J Med 1989; 72:669.

Sivraprasad R, Payne CB Jr. Nonpulmonary causes of dyspnea. Radiol Clin North Am 1984; 22:463.

Stark RD. Dyspnoea: assessment and pharmacological manipulation. Eur Respir J 1988; 1:280.

Patient with ACUTE DYSPNEA

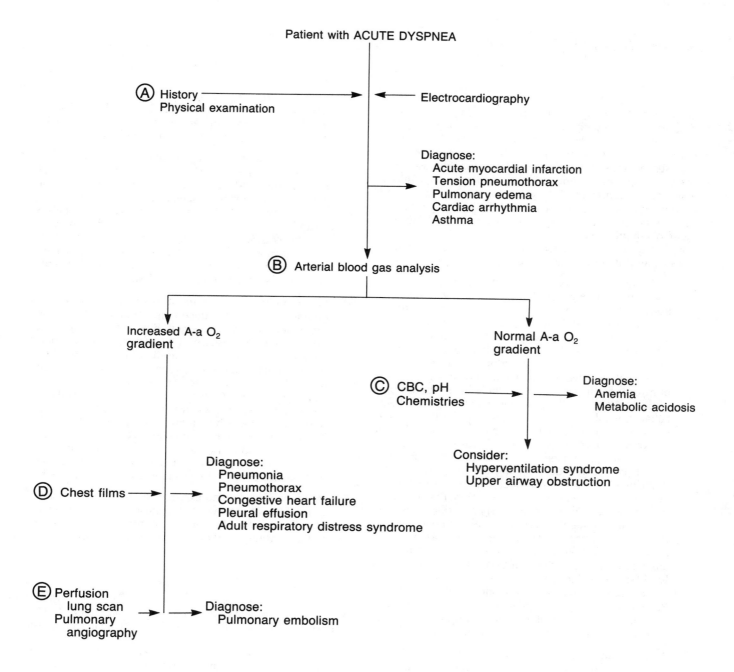

A History ——— Electrocardiography
Physical examination

Diagnose:
    Acute myocardial infarction
    Tension pneumothorax
    Pulmonary edema
    Cardiac arrhythmia
    Asthma

B Arterial blood gas analysis

Increased A-a O_2 gradient

Normal A-a O_2 gradient

C CBC, pH
Chemistries

Diagnose:
    Anemia
    Metabolic acidosis

Consider:
    Hyperventilation syndrome
    Upper airway obstruction

Diagnose:
    Pneumonia
    Pneumothorax
    Congestive heart failure
    Pleural effusion
    Adult respiratory distress syndrome

D Chest films

E Perfusion
    lung scan
    Pulmonary
    angiography

Diagnose:
    Pulmonary embolism

CHRONIC DYSPNEA

Concomitant cardiac and pulmonary etiologies of chronic dyspnea frequently occur. Chronic dyspnea may be caused by obstructive lung diseases, including chronic bronchitis, chronic bronchial asthma, and emphysema. Restrictive lung diseases include sarcoidosis, scleroderma lung disease, rheumatoid lung disease, lymphangitic carcinomatosis, histiocytosis X, pneumoconiosis, kyphoscoliosis, thoracoplasty, pulmonary alveolar proteinosis, and desquamative interstitial pneumonia. Pulmonary hypertension is an additional cause of chronic dyspnea. Nonpulmonary etiologies include congestive heart failure, ischemic heart disease, anemia, obesity, and upper airway obstruction.

A. A detailed history of the patient's symptoms includes questions regarding their duration, associated symptoms, exertional symptoms, orthopnea, paroxysmal nocturnal dyspnea, cough, and sputum production. In many cases, the history provides clear answers to the etiology. Patients with a history of cigarette smoking, chronic sputum production, and gradual development of dyspnea are more likely to have obstructive lung disease. A history of myocardial infarction or ischemic heart disease predisposes patients to the development of congestive heart failure. Carefully review the occupational history; chronic exposures to asbestos, coal dust, and other mineral dusts are known causes of pulmonary fibrosis and dyspnea. Patients with psychogenic causes of chronic dyspnea frequently complain of deep sighing and an inability to take deep breaths. This is not a specific finding, and psychogenic dyspnea is a diagnosis of exclusion. Physical signs provide additional evidence of a specific diagnosis. Emphysematous patients characteristically appear thin and asthenic, with barrel-shaped chests. Decreased breath sounds and hyper-resonance is found on pulmonary examination. Patients with chronic bronchitis are more likely to be stocky and may appear cyanotic; rhonchi and wheezing are found on auscultation in these patients. Patients with congestive heart failure have the typical findings of end-inspiratory rales, peripheral edema, elevated venous pressure, and cardiac gallops.

B. Anemia can be readily detected with routine blood counts. Use the arterial blood gas (ABG) determination to assess the severity of hypoxemia, and to a lesser extent the chronicity of dyspnea; it will also provide a baseline for future comparisons and is helpful in distinguishing chronic bronchitis from emphysema.

C. Chest films identify obvious lung diseases as well as document the heart size and the presence of pleural effusion. The findings of bullae, hyperinflation, and decreased pulmonary vascular markings are consistent with emphysema. Diffuse parenchymal and pleural fibrosis and interstitial markings may be seen in patients with restrictive diseases. The echocardiogram diagnoses cardiac dysfunction and valvular heart diseases. A hypokinetic left ventricle with low ejection fraction strongly implicates the heart as the cause of dyspnea.

D. Obtain pulmonary function tests in patients when the etiology of dyspnea is uncertain. Spirometry and measurement of lung volumes help differentiate obstructive from restrictive disease. Obstructive diseases have reduced flow rates, decreased vital capacity (VC), reduced ratio of forced expiratory volume to vital capacity (FEV/FVC%), and increased expiratory time. The total lung capacity (TLC), functional residual capacity (FRC), and residual volume (RV) are increased in emphysema. Restrictive diseases have reduced TLC, FRC, RV, and VC. The FEV_1 is reduced, but the FEV/FVC% may have normal or above-normal values. Additional diagnostic workup is indicated in patients found to have a restrictive lung disease and possible pulmonary vascular involvement.

E. Pulmonary or cardiac exercise testing should be performed in patients whose diagnoses remain uncertain after the above evaluation, in order to exclude exercise-induced asthma and/or ischemic heart disease.

References

Killian KJ. Assessment of dyspnoea. Eur Respir J 1988; 1:195.

Mahler DA. Dyspnea: diagnosis and management. Clin Chest Med 1987; 8:215.

Wasserman K, Casaburi R. Dyspnea: physiological and pathophysiological mechanisms. Ann Rev Med 1988; 39:503.

Patient with CHRONIC DYSPNEA

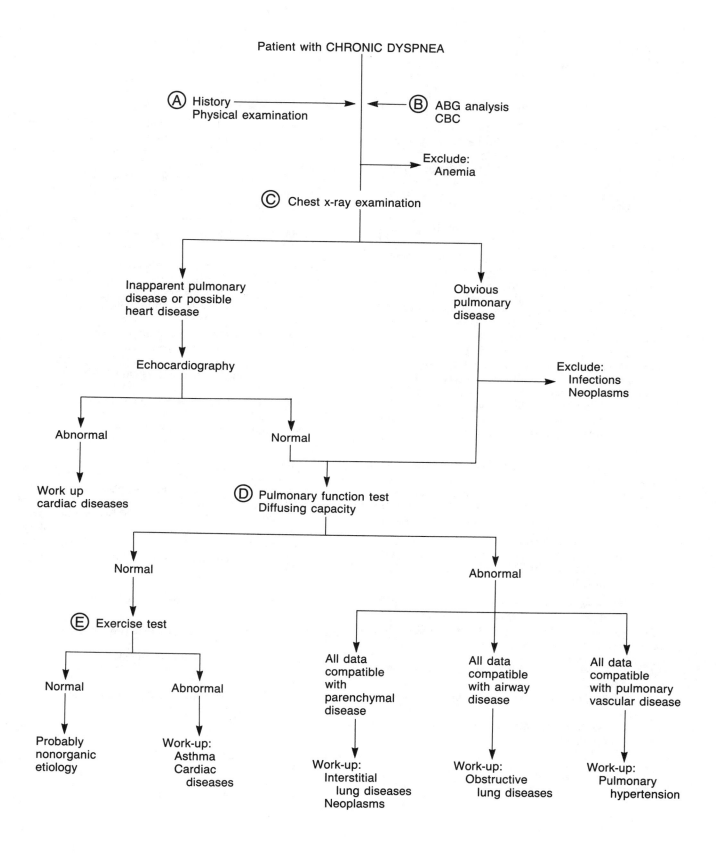

(A) History
Physical examination

(B) ABG analysis
CBC

Exclude:
Anemia

(C) Chest x-ray examination

Inapparent pulmonary disease or possible heart disease

Obvious pulmonary disease

Echocardiography

Exclude:
Infections
Neoplasms

Abnormal

Normal

Work up cardiac diseases

(D) Pulmonary function test
Diffusing capacity

Normal

Abnormal

(E) Exercise test

Normal

Abnormal

All data compatible with parenchymal disease

All data compatible with airway disease

All data compatible with pulmonary vascular disease

Probably nonorganic etiology

Work-up:
Asthma
Cardiac diseases

Work-up:
Interstitial lung diseases
Neoplasms

Work-up:
Obstructive lung diseases

Work-up:
Pulmonary hypertension

COUGH

Coughing, which is the result of a complex series of physiologic reflexes, protects the lungs against aspiration. A cough is produced after stimulation of cough receptors in the airways and transmission of afferent impulses to the cough center in the medulla. Persistent cough is a sign of respiratory disease and should not be treated symptomatically until specific etiologies have been excluded.

A. The history is of prime importance and should be obtained in detail, including a vocal history. Patients usually complain of cough accompanied by mucus production; examine closely any sputum produced. Mucoid sputum produced in the early morning usually indicates chronic bronchitis, whereas thick, dark green or yellow sputum indicates an infective process. Cough accompanied by a feeling of mucus dripping in the back of the throat suggests sinus disease, and any associated wheezing suggests asthma. Cough accompanied by hemoptysis and other constitutional symptoms suggests a diagnosis of neoplasm. Rule out environmental dust or noxious fume exposures and allergies. The physical examination includes a full examination of the mouth, throat, pharynx, and, if the history warrants, the larynx. Perform pulmonary function tests (PFTs) using bronchodilators in order to detect occult asthmatic disease.

B. If the cough is acute, having been present over days to several weeks, rule out reversible, inflammatory, or allergic conditions. If the cough is chronic, having been present over weeks to months, seriously consider neoplastic, inflammatory, and immunologic etiologies.

C. Vocal change or hoarseness in a patient with a chronic or nonproductive cough points toward a pharyngeal or laryngeal cause. Refer these patients for an otolaryngologic examination.

D. Obtain a chest film in all patients who have cough that is new and/or who do not have a clearly defined upper airway abnormality to explain it. A normal chest film excludes pneumonias, cystic fibrosis, congestive heart failure, emphysema, restrictive parenchymal diseases, and pleural effusions. It does not exclude airway hyperresponsiveness, sinus problems, foreign bodies, pericarditis, pulmonary hypertension, pulmonary embolic disease, or endobronchial tumor. A chest film that reveals pathology initiates the appropriate work-up to make a specific diagnosis.

E. Follow a negative chest film with bronchoscopy to rule out foreign-body aspiration and endobronchial neoplastic disease. If pulmonary spirometry and lung volume measurements are consistent with restrictive lung disease, obtain transbronchoscopic lung biopsies to rule out sarcoidosis. A positive diagnosis resulting from bronchoscopy dictates further specific treatment. A negative bronchoscopy in a patient with a chronic cough, negative sputum examination, no upper airway pathology, and a negative chest film indicates symptomatic treatment.

F. The use of symptomatic treatment does not necessarily depend on the presence of signs or symptoms of airway obstruction. If such signs are present, try bronchodilators by metered-dose inhalers and a short course of corticosteroids. If improvement occurs, and the patient has airway hypersensitivity, use maintenance aerosolized bronchodilators and aerosolized steroids. If no improvement occurs, rule out sinusitis (sinus films, computed tomograms of the head) and low-grade occult aspiration (barium swallow) as etiologies of cough. If no diagnosis is made, perform a methacholine challenge test to rule out asthma. Treat patients with asthma with a short course of bronchodilators and perform pulmonary function tests, repeated in 6 weeks.

G. Treat an acute cough in the presence of symptoms and signs of upper respiratory infection (URI) with the appropriate antibiotic, cough suppressants at night, and expectorants as necessary. If the infection remits and the cough remains (becomes chronic), rule out other etiologies. Postviral cough occurring after upper respiratory infections may require oral as well as aerosolized steroid therapy for a prolonged period of time.

References

Irwin RS, Rosen MJ. Cough: a comprehensive review. Arch Intern Med 1977; 137:1186.

Loudon RG, Shaw GB. Mechanisms of cough in normal subjects and in patients with obstructive airway disease. Am Rev Respir Dis 1967; 96:666.

Poe RH, Israel RH, Utell MJ, Hall WJ. Chronic cough: bronchoscopy or pulmonary function testing. Am Rev Respir Dis 1982; 126:160.

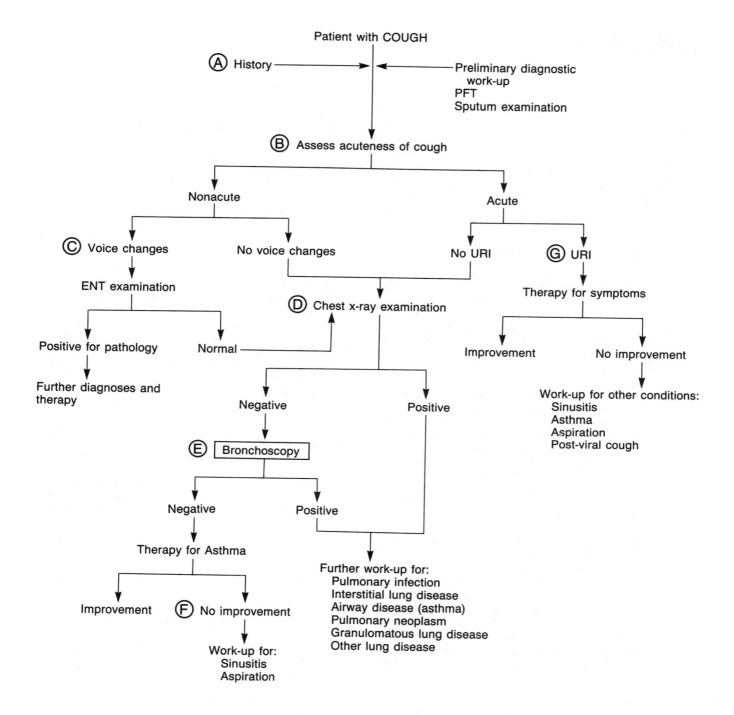

Patient with COUGH

(A) History — Preliminary diagnostic work-up
PFT
Sputum examination

(B) Assess acuteness of cough

Nonacute

Acute

(C) Voice changes

No voice changes

No URI

(G) URI

ENT examination

(D) Chest x-ray examination

Therapy for symptoms

Positive for pathology

Normal

Improvement

No improvement

Further diagnoses and therapy

Negative

Positive

Work-up for other conditions:
Sinusitis
Asthma
Aspiration
Post-viral cough

(E) Bronchoscopy

Negative

Positive

Therapy for Asthma

Further work-up for:
Pulmonary infection
Interstitial lung disease
Airway disease (asthma)
Pulmonary neoplasm
Granulomatous lung disease
Other lung disease

Improvement

(F) No improvement

Work-up for:
Sinusitis
Aspiration

CHEST PAIN

Chest pain is a symptomatic manifestation of many diseases, ranging from life-threatening conditions such as acute myocardial infarction, aortic dissection, pulmonary embolism, and tension pneumothorax, to more benign conditions such as esophagitis, Tietze's syndrome, and herpes zoster. Chest pain may originate from any of the organs within and surrounding the thorax and its vicinity, including musculoskeletal structures, heart, blood vessels, lung, neck, esophagus, and upper abdominal organs. Chest pain may be acute, chronic, or recurrent in nature. Acute chest pain should be considered a medical emergency and evaluated promptly.

A. A complete and thorough history is the most important aspect of the evaluation of chest pain. Although the history alone is seldom diagnostic, it helps to differentiate among the many potential etiologies of the pain. Characterization of the chest pain includes location, quality, intensity, duration, and radiation, as well as any associated symptoms, precipitating causes, and accentuating and relieving factors. In the presence of two or more concurrent diseases, more than one pattern of chest pain may be identified. Because of its prevalence and seriousness, chest pain due to myocardial ischemia or infarction must always be considered and excluded. Chest pain associated with ischemic heart disease is frequently exertional and typically described as heavy, substernal, and radiating to the left arm or neck. Suspect myocardial infarction when the duration of the chest pain exceeds 30 minutes. Pain of esophageal origin is often substernal and difficult to distinguish from that of cardiac ischemia. Chest pain resulting from aortic dissection is commonly described as being severe, tearing, and radiating to the back. Abnormal physical findings are present in many conditions associated with chest pain, although they are mostly nonspecific. The dermatomal distribution of painful skin lesions is pathognomonic for herpes zoster. Suspect rib fractures in the setting of chest wall injury and tenderness. Percussion and auscultation may identify the presence of a pneumothorax or a pneumonia; mediastinal crunch may be present in patients with pneumomediastinum. Patients with mitral valve prolapse may have atypical chest pain; a mid-systolic click and late-systolic murmur may be present on auscultation.

B. After reviewing the history and performing an examination, obtain an electrocardiogram when ischemic heart disease is suspected. Although many patients with acute myocardial infarction have a diagnostic electrocardiogram, a normal electrocardiogram does not exclude acute myocardial infarction when the history is compatible with the diagnosis. Abnormal electrocardiographic findings may also be present in patients with pericarditis and pulmonary embolism.

C. The chest film is neither a sensitive nor a specific diagnostic tool in the evaluation of chest pain; its role is to confirm clinical suspicion of pneumonia, pneumothorax, or rib fractures, or to detect the presence of tumors. A widened mediastinum and a left-sided pleural effusion noted on a chest film suggest the possibility of aortic dissection; perform a chest CT scan, aortography, or ultrasonography to confirm the diagnosis.

D. Additional evaluation is needed if the diagnosis is not established by the history, physical examination, electrocardiography, and chest x-ray examination. Pulmonary embolism may be present in patients with acute pleuritic chest pain associated with dyspnea. Obtain the arterial blood gas to assess the degree of hypoxemia; a perfusion lung scan and pulmonary arteriography confirm the diagnosis. Noninvasive cardiac procedures such as an exercise test or thallium stress test are indicated for patients with undiagnosed, atypical chest pain. Cardiac catheterization is indicated for those with high clinical suspicion of coronary artery disease. Chest pain due to esophageal origin often mimics that of cardiac origin. Between 10 and 30 percent of patients undergoing cardiac catheterization have normal coronary arteries or insignificant stenosis, and approximately 30 percent of these patients are believed to have esophageal diseases. Perform esophagogastroscopy, esophageal manometry, and provocative tests when ischemic heart disease is sufficiently excluded. Echocardiography may be used to diagnose mitral valve prolapse, especially in young patients with atypical chest pain. Bony metastases causing pain, which may not be seen on chest or rib films, may be confirmed with a bone scan.

References

Chambers CE, Leaman DM. Management of acute chest pain syndrome. Crit Care Clin 1989; 5:415.

Donat WE. Chest pain: cardiac and noncardiac causes. Clin Chest Med 1987; 8:241.

Fam AG. Approach to musculoskeletal chest wall pain. Prim Care 1988; 15:767.

Lin A, Warfield CA. Differentiating causes of chest pain. Hosp Pract 1989; 24:43–44, 47–48, 50–53.

Magarian GJ, Hickam DH. Noncardiac causes of angina-like chest pain. Prog Cardiovasc Dis 1986; 29:65.

Rustgi AK, Chopra S. Chest pain of esophageal origin. J Gen Intern Med 1989; 4:151.

Rutledge JC, Amsterdam EA. Differential diagnosis and clinical approach to the patient with acute chest pain. Cardiol Clin 1984; 2:257.

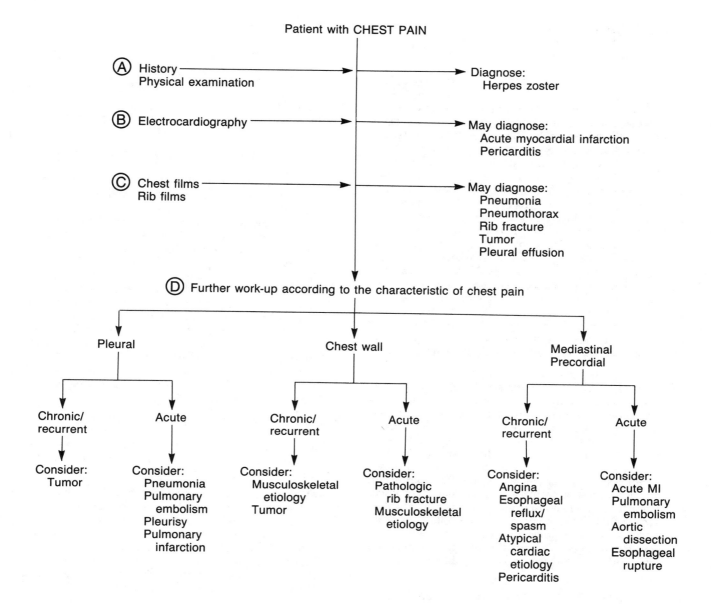

Patient with CHEST PAIN

Ⓐ History —————→ Diagnose:
Physical examination   Herpes zoster

Ⓑ Electrocardiography —————→ May diagnose:
                            Acute myocardial infarction
                            Pericarditis

Ⓒ Chest films —————→ May diagnose:
Rib films   Pneumonia
                       Pneumothorax
                       Rib fracture
                       Tumor
                       Pleural effusion

Ⓓ Further work-up according to the characteristic of chest pain

Pleural

Chronic/recurrent
Consider:
Tumor

Acute
Consider:
Pneumonia
Pulmonary embolism
Pleurisy
Pulmonary infarction

Chest wall

Chronic/recurrent
Consider:
Musculoskeletal etiology
Tumor

Acute
Consider:
Pathologic rib fracture
Musculoskeletal etiology

Mediastinal Precordial

Chronic/recurrent
Consider:
Angina
Esophageal reflux/spasm
Atypical cardiac etiology
Pericarditis

Acute
Consider:
Acute MI
Pulmonary embolism
Aortic dissection
Esophageal rupture

HEMOPTYSIS

Hemoptysis is the expectoration of blood or bloody sputum. It is a manifestation of an underlying disease process rather than a specific disease entity. The causes of hemoptysis are many and include bronchogenic carcinoma, bronchitis, tuberculosis, inflammatory diseases, autoimmune diseases, bronchiectasis, pulmonary sequestration, idiopathic pulmonary hemosiderosis, pulmonary embolism, pulmonary infarction, pneumonia, lung abscesses, lung cysts, fungal infection, parasitic infections, bronchial adenoma, broncholiths eroding into blood vessels, mitral stenosis, endometriosis, and arteriovenous malformation. The etiology of all hemoptysis must be investigated unless its cause is clearly known. Hemoptysis may range from a small amount of blood-streaked sputum to a large amount that results in asphyxiation and exsanguination. The severity of the hemoptysis is not correlated with any specific diagnosis, although bronchitis and pneumonia are unlikely to be the cause of massive hemoptysis. Fatal hemorrhages are more likely to be found in patients with septic pulmonary infarction and tuberculosis.

A. The history is often suggestive of the diagnosis. Hemoptysis, accompanied by dyspnea and acute pleuritic chest pain, suggests pulmonary embolism with infarction or pneumonia. Patients with bronchiectasis often have recurrent episodes of hemoptysis and purulent sputum. Weight loss, night sweats, cough, and fever suggest active pulmonary tuberculosis. The diagnosis of carcinoma must be considered in cigarette smokers. Recurrent hemoptysis in otherwise young healthy nonsmoking females suggests bronchial adenoma. Pulmonary auscultation findings are nonspecific although they may allow localization of the hemorrhagic site. Clubbing of the fingers suggests a chronic underlying pulmonary process. A history of rheumatic heart disease and findings of congestive heart failure and a diastolic rumble suggest mitral stenosis.

B. Order arterial blood gas (ABG) and coagulation studies in addition to routine blood counts and chemistries. Sputum stains and cultures are used to diagnose infectious processes. Sputum examination for ova and parasites is appropriate in patients with a history of recent travel to or residence in endemic areas. Routine urinalysis and renal function tests may provide clues to the presence of Goodpasture's syndrome. Chest x-ray examination may demonstrate an underlying pulmonary process as well as help to localize the site of hemorrhage. Cardiac ultrasonography is indicated when mitral stenosis is suspected.

C. A careful history may exclude hematemesis masquerading as hemoptysis. Perform an otolaryngoscopic examination on patients suspected of nasopharyngeal hemorrhage. Hemoptysis, which occurs in up to one-third of patients with pulmonary embolism, is usually minor and self-limiting. Anticoagulation is not contraindicated in this setting unless the hemoptysis is massive.

D. The management of hemoptysis depends on the severity of the hemorrhage. Patients with massive hemoptysis and those with significant underlying diseases should be hospitalized and monitored in the intensive care unit. Massive hemoptysis is generally defined as loss of more than 600 ml of blood over a 24-hour period. Since massive hemoptysis is life-threatening, immediate therapeutic and diagnostic measures must be taken. Protection of the airway of the uninvolved lung to prevent asphyxiation may sometimes be accomplished by having the patient lie on the involved side. Endotracheal tube intubation is usually indicated, and balloon catheters have been used to occlude segmental or lobar bronchi that lead to an identified source. Perform early bronchoscopy to establish the etiology and to locate the bleeding site. Use codeine to diminish coughing paroxysms that may trigger rebleeding. Identify and treat infections and bleeding disorders. Many cases of hemoptysis improve with supportive therapy and specific treatment of the underlying disease.

E. Patients without significant underlying diseases and only blood-streaked sputum may be treated and investigated as outpatients. Patients with continued hemoptysis, abnormal chest films, and smoking history should undergo bronchoscopic evaluation.

F. Mortality exceeds 70 percent for those with blood loss exceeding 600 ml over 4 hours. Consider surgery for those patients with uncontrolled massive hemoptysis. Arteriography with embolization is an alternative for those who cannot tolerate surgery because of poor pulmonary reserve, diffuse or bilateral lesions, or when underlying diseases preclude the surgical option. A significant complication of embolization is spinal cord infarction, caused because the anterior spinal arteries may originate from the bronchial arteries, particularly on the right side.

References

Bobrowitz ID, Ramakrishna S, Shim YS. Comparison of medical vs surgical treatment of major hemoptysis. Arch Intern Med 1983; 143:1343.

Conlan AA, Hurwitz SS, Krige L, Nicolaou N, Pool R. Massive hemoptysis: review of 123 cases. J Thorac Cardiovasc Surg 1983; 85:120.

Garzon AA, Gourin A. Surgical management of massive hemoptysis: a ten-year experience. Ann Surg 1978; 187:267.

Ingbar D. A systematic workup for hemoptysis. Contemp Intern Med 1989; Jul/Aug:60.

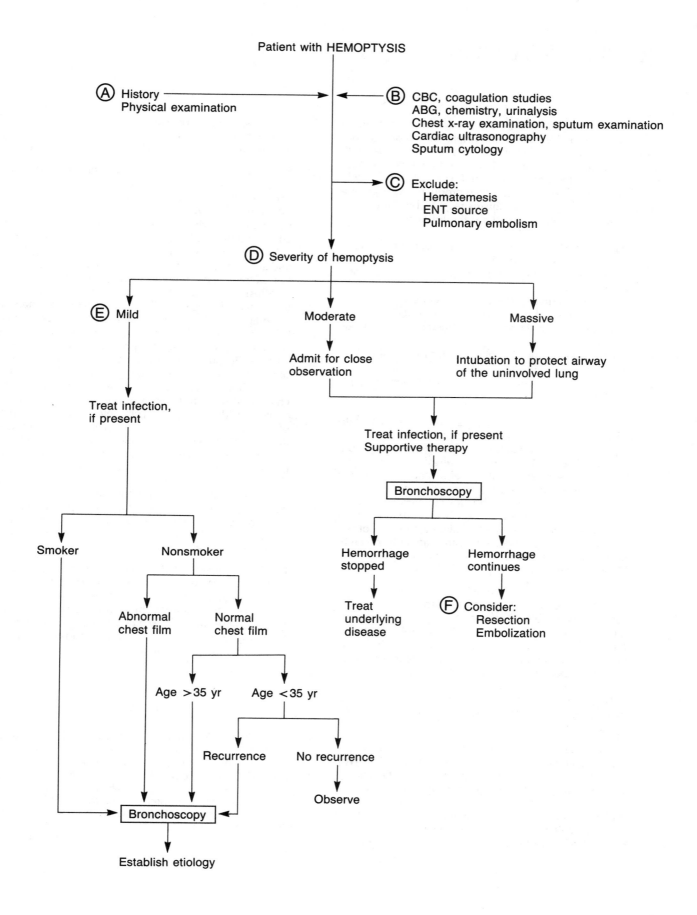

Patient with HEMOPTYSIS

(A) History ———→   ←——— (B) CBC, coagulation studies
Physical examination   ABG, chemistry, urinalysis
                                     Chest x-ray examination, sputum examination
                                     Cardiac ultrasonography
                                     Sputum cytology

(C) Exclude:
    Hematemesis
    ENT source
    Pulmonary embolism

(D) Severity of hemoptysis

(E) Mild   Moderate   Massive

                      Admit for close   Intubation to protect airway
                      observation   of the uninvolved lung

Treat infection,
if present

                      Treat infection, if present
                      Supportive therapy

                      | Bronchoscopy |

Smoker   Nonsmoker   Hemorrhage   Hemorrhage
                      stopped   continues

Abnormal   Normal   Treat   (F) Consider:
chest film chest film underlying   Resection
                      disease   Embolization

          Age >35 yr   Age <35 yr

                    Recurrence   No recurrence

                                    Observe

          | Bronchoscopy |

Establish etiology

PLEURAL EFFUSION

The pleural cavity of a healthy person contains less than 20 ml of fluid. Normal pleural fluid is clear and colorless, containing less than 1.5 g of proteins/100 ml and 1,500 cells/microliter; it is composed of mesothelial cells; monocytes, lymphocytes, and a few granulocytes. Approximately 50 ml of pleural fluid is necessary to produce a radiographically evident effusion. Mechanisms responsible for the formation of pleural effusion include the following:

1. Increased hydrostatic pressure in the pulmonary capillaries (congestive heart failure).
2. Decreased oncotic pressure (cirrhosis, nephrotic syndrome).
3. Decreased pleural space pressure (atelectasis).
4. Increased permeability of the capillaries due to inflammatory process (infections, neoplasms, and immunologic diseases).
5. Obstruction of the lymphatics (tumors, pulmonary fibrosis).
6. Influx of extrapulmonary fluids into the pleural space (ascites).

A. Awareness of the underlying disease provides insight into the nature of the pleural effusion. Effusions associated with congestive heart failure are usually right-sided, but may be bilateral. Parapneumonic effusions occur in approximately 40 percent of bacterial pneumonias as a result of inflammatory pleural reaction or empyema. Pleural effusion sometimes heralds the presence of neoplasms. Physical examination generally reveals dullness to percussion and diminished fremitus and breath sounds over the effusion, but pleural effusion cannot be differentiated from localized pleural thickening or lobar consolidation on the basis of physical findings.

B. The measurement of serum albumin is useful to assess the role of oncotic pressure in the formation of the effusion, and white blood cell counts and sputum evaluation help to diagnose infections. Perform tuberculin skin testing to detect parenchymal or pleural tuberculosis, and measure rheumatoid factors and antinuclear antibodies in those suspected of having autoimmune diseases. Order lateral decubitus chest films to demonstrate the mobility of the fluid. Ultrasonography differentiates thickened pleura and localizes loculated effusion for thoracentesis.

C. Pleural effusions associated with ascites due to congestive heart failure, cirrhosis, and nephrotic syndrome typically are bilateral and are transudates. Diagnostic thoracentesis generally is not necessary in these conditions unless infection or additional diseases are suspected. However, patients symptomatic from large effusions will benefit from therapeutic thoracentesis. Removal of more than 1 L of pleural fluid may cause hypotension due to decreased intravascular volume, and a sudden reduction of pleural pressure during lung expansion may precipitate unilateral pulmonary edema.

D. Prior to performing the thoracentesis, obtain lateral decubitus chest films to demonstrate the mobility of the fluid, and use ultrasonography to localize loculations. Carefully insert the thoracentesis needle just superior to the rib to avoid injuring the neurovascular bundle. Routine analysis of the fluid includes protein, LDH, glucose, and cell counts. Obtain simultaneous serum protein, LDH, and glucose in order to determine the effusion-to-serum ratio. Order microbiologic stains (Gram stain, acid-fast bacillus) and cultures (bacterial, fungal, mycobacterial) for suspected infections. Pleural fluid pH helps establish the diagnosis of empyema, pancreatitis-related pleural effusion, or ruptured esophagus (Boerhave's syndrome). Amylase levels help diagnose pleural effusion due to pancreatitis. In suspected malignancies or tuberculosis, pleural biopsy increases the diagnostic yield. Unless the pleural fluid is grossly purulent, bloody, or chylous, the characterization of the effusion into transudate and exudate provides the first step in determining the nature of the fluid. A transudative effusion is defined as pleural fluid protein of less than 3 g/100 ml and a pleural fluid-to-serum protein ratio of less than 0.5, pleural fluid LDH of less than 200 IU/L, and a pleural fluid-to-serum LDH ratio of less than 0.6. Empyema, parapneumonic effusion, tuberculous effusion, rheumatoid and lupus effusion all have a pH that is often less than 7.3. Ruptured esophagus produces effusions with a pH in the range of 6. A low pleural fluid pH is also sometimes found in patients with malignant effusion.

E. Exudative effusions are caused by a variety of disease conditions such as infection, malignancy, inflammation, and a number of extrapulmonary causes. Laboratory tests should be able to identify most of these conditions. Infectious causes must be excluded. Order chest computed tomography for patients without a diagnosis in order to exclude pulmonary neoplasms.

References

Henschke CI, Davis SD, Romano PM, Yankelevitz DF. The pathogenesis, radiologic evaluation, and therapy of pleural effusions. Radiol Clin North Am 1989; 27:1241.

Houston MC. Pleural fluid pH: diagnostic, therapeutic, and prognostic value. Am J Surg 1987; 154:333.

Light RW. Pleural effusion. Med Clin North Am 1977; 61:1339.

Rosa UW. Pleural effusion: How to avoid a diagnostic stalemate. Postgrad Med 1984; 75:253.

Sahn SA. The pleura. Am Rev Respir Dis 1988; 138:184.

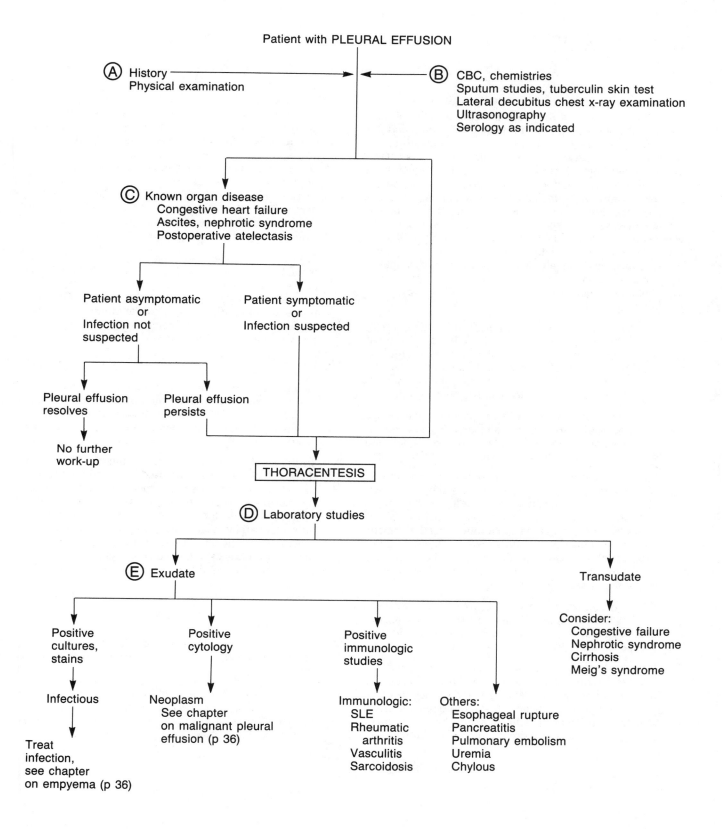

Patient with PLEURAL EFFUSION

(A) History
Physical examination

(B) CBC, chemistries
Sputum studies, tuberculin skin test
Lateral decubitus chest x-ray examination
Ultrasonography
Serology as indicated

(C) Known organ disease
Congestive heart failure
Ascites, nephrotic syndrome
Postoperative atelectasis

Patient asymptomatic
or
Infection not
suspected

Patient symptomatic
or
Infection suspected

Pleural effusion
resolves

Pleural effusion
persists

No further
work-up

THORACENTESIS

(D) Laboratory studies

(E) Exudate

Transudate

Positive
cultures,
stains

Positive
cytology

Positive
immunologic
studies

Consider:
Congestive failure
Nephrotic syndrome
Cirrhosis
Meig's syndrome

Infectious

Neoplasm
See chapter
on malignant pleural
effusion (p 36)

Immunologic:
SLE
Rheumatic
arthritis
Vasculitis
Sarcoidosis

Others:
Esophageal rupture
Pancreatitis
Pulmonary embolism
Uremia
Chylous

Treat
infection,
see chapter
on empyema (p 36)

ATELECTASIS

Physiologic factors that influence the collapsibility of lung include: alveolar size, pleural pressure distribution, and the integrity of surfactant. Clinical factors that predispose non-ventilated individuals toward the development of atelectasis include increasing age, obesity, loss of thoracic cage muscle tone, elevated intra-abdominal pressure, cardiomegaly or pleural effusion, post-surgical (anesthetic effects), obstructing bronchial lesions or mucus, and inflammatory parenchymal disease with effects on collateral ventilation. In ventilated individuals, low tidal volume settings and high inspired oxygen concentrations must also be considered. Atelectasis occurs through one of four mechanisms operating alone or in combination. These include resorption, passive collapse, adhesive collapse of small airways, and cicatrization.

A. The history and physical examination provide information about the process causing the atelectasis. If lobar atelectasis is present, the physical examination may reveal shift of the trachea toward the side of the atelectasis, and auscultation may reveal bronchial breath sounds and/or rales over the atelectatic segment of lung.

B. The chest film usually reveals the presence and degree of atelectasis. In some cases, a chest CT scan is necessary to define the anatomy of atelectasis completely and may reveal a central obstructing lesion (Golden's S sign).

C. Postoperative atelectasis is commonly found after thoracic or abdominal procedures and is caused by neuromuscular depression secondary to anesthesia, increased secretions, and pain. The atelectasis is usually localized to basilar segments of lung and reverses after the immediate postoperative period. Treatment with bronchodilators, CPAP, and physical therapy may be necessary. Bronchoscopy is rarely indicated and should not be done routinely for secretion removal.

D. If the atelectasis is acute and platelike, it may be caused by obesity, neuromuscular disease, pulmonary embolus, acute asthma, or a new rib fracture. These conditions should be excluded.

E. If the atelectasis is acute and lobar in extent, foreign-body aspiration and inflammatory and neoplastic disease must be ruled out, although the latter is much less likely. If cytologic examination of sputum does not reveal malignant cells or infectious agents, perform bronchoscopy to rule out these conditions definitively.

F. If atelectasis is acute and associated with sputum cytologies that are positive for malignancy, or if atelectasis is chronic and lobar, exophytic neoplastic disease becomes much more likely. Other diagnostic considerations include large adenopathies caused by neoplastic or granulomatous diseases and intrabronchial mucous casts. Patients with chronic lobar atelectasis should undergo CT to rule out neoplastic disease and should undergo bronchoscopy whether or not neoplastic disease is found.

G. Bronchoscopy is useful in visualizing obstructing lesions of the bronchus and in obtaining cellular material for diagnosis. In the special case of right middle lobe atelectasis, bronchoscopy is usually within normal limits and no lesions or predisposing factors are found (right middle lobe syndrome). If a foreign body is found, it may often be removed during the bronchoscopy.

H. If the atelectasis is chronic and platelike, the diagnostic considerations are similar to those for acute platelike atelectasis; however, pulmonary function tests should be done to determine whether the restrictive lung disease is present. A restrictive pattern, along with the appropriate history, indicates the diagnosis of neuromuscular disease (e.g., myasthenia gravis) or interstitial lung disease.

I. Treatment of atelectasis depends on the underlying conditions. If the atelectasis is caused by an obstructing neoplasm, the treatment should focus on therapy of the neoplasm—surgical resection and radiotherapy, with or without laser resection, as a primary option. If the atelectasis is caused by inflammatory disease, bronchodilators, mucolytic agents, and physical therapy are important therapeutic choices. If the atelectasis is caused by neuromuscular disease, the use of steroids or more specific therapy is employed.

References

Fraser RG, Pare JA, Pare PDP, Fraser RS, Genereux GP. Diagnosis of diseases of the chest. Philadelphia: WB Saunders, 1988:472.

Marini JJ, Pierson DJ, Hudson LD. Acute lobar atelectasis: a prospective comparison of fiberoptic bronchoscopy and respiratory therapy. Am Rev Resp Dis 1979; 119:971.

Naidich DP, Zerhouni EA, Siegelman SS. Computed tomography of the thorax. New York: Raven Press, 1984:111.

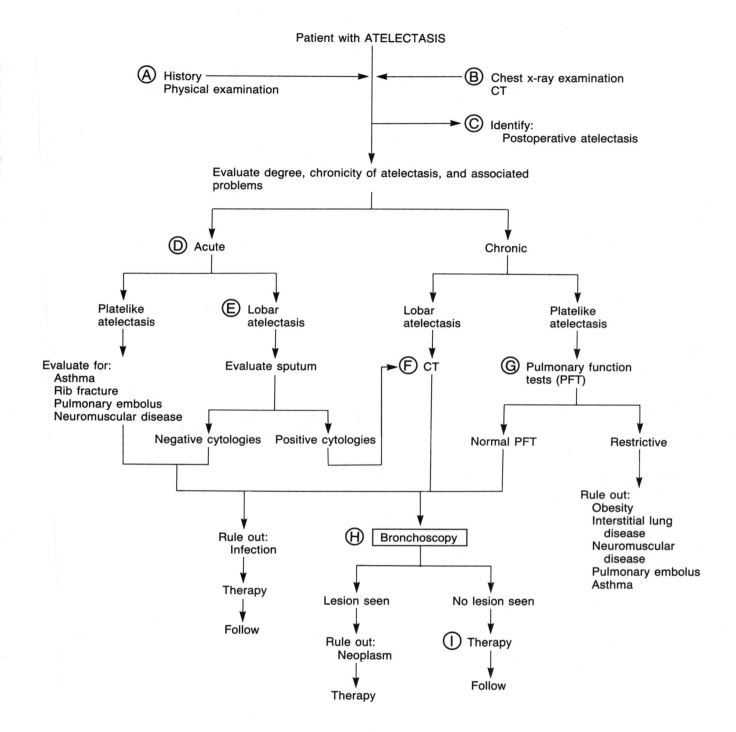

Patient with ATELECTASIS

Ⓐ History — Physical examination

Ⓑ Chest x-ray examination CT

Ⓒ Identify:
Postoperative atelectasis

Evaluate degree, chronicity of atelectasis, and associated problems

Ⓓ Acute

Chronic

Platelike atelectasis

Ⓔ Lobar atelectasis

Lobar atelectasis

Platelike atelectasis

Evaluate for:
Asthma
Rib fracture
Pulmonary embolus
Neuromuscular disease

Evaluate sputum

Ⓕ CT

Ⓖ Pulmonary function tests (PFT)

Negative cytologies

Positive cytologies

Normal PFT

Restrictive

Rule out:
Infection

Ⓗ Bronchoscopy

Rule out:
Obesity
Interstitial lung disease
Neuromuscular disease
Pulmonary embolus
Asthma

Therapy

Lesion seen

No lesion seen

Follow

Rule out:
Neoplasm

Ⓘ Therapy

Therapy

Follow

PULMONARY PHYSIOLOGY

Pulmonary Function Testing
Pulmonary Exercise Testing
Preoperative Pulmonary Evaluation

PULMONARY FUNCTION TESTING

Pulmonary function testing measures the mechanical ability of the respiratory system and cannot be used to make a specific clinical diagnosis. It can be used to differentiate primary airway problems from primary parenchymal or respiratory muscle problems. Pulmonary function data should be used in concert with the information obtained from the history and physical examination to confirm a suspected pulmonary diagnosis, to determine the extent of lung disease, or to follow the course of a pulmonary illness and the effect of therapy. The indications for pulmonary function testing are (1) to differentiate airway processes from parenchymal processes; (2) to assess bronchoresponsiveness; (3) to confirm the diagnosis of neuromuscular disease; (4) to evaluate function prior to general anesthesia; (5) to follow the effects of therapy (e.g., corticosteroids, bleomycin); and (6) to assess the degree of pulmonary impairment for legal or insurance reasons. Patients who cannot cooperate or follow instructions are not suitable candidates for testing, nor are patients who have extremely limited pulmonary function ($FEV_1 < 500$ ml), since results will be unreliable. Routine pulmonary function testing consists of measurements of flow (forced vital capacity, FEV_1, maximal midexpiratory flow rate, flow-volume loop) before and after inhalation of bronchodilators, measurements of lung volumetric compartments (vital capacity, functional residual capacity, residual volume, expiratory reserve volume, total lung capacity), a measurement of gas (carbon monoxide) diffusion (diffusing capacity, DLCO), and a measurement of total respiratory ability (maximal voluntary ventilation). Supplementary studies include measurement of maximal inspiratory (Pi_{max}) and expiratory (Pe_{max}) pressures, and placement of esophageal and gastric balloons to measure transdiaphragmatic pressures and static lung compliance. Balloon studies are not performed routinely since they are uncomfortable and are necessary only in the unusual individual with complex respiratory muscle problems or when lung compliance must be evaluated.

A. The history, physical examination, and chest x-ray examination provide information that leads to a tentative diagnosis of a primary airway disease, a primary parenchymal process, or a primary neuromuscular problem. Further diagnostic clinical evaluation requires pulmonary function testing. Patients with lung disease who require lung resectional surgery or other procedures associated with general anesthesia need a preoperative pulmonary evaluation.

B. Simple spirometry distinguishes patients with primarily obstructive physiologies (decreased forced vital capacity, FEV_1 percent < 75 percent of predicted value) from those with primarily restrictive physiologies (decreased FVC, normal FEV_1 percent). The pattern on a flow-volume curve may substantiate this distinction and also aid in the diagnosis of possible upper airway obstruction. Reduced flow rates in the mid- to low-lung volume range will help establish the diagnosis of small airways disease.

C. Lung volumes must be measured to confirm the diagnosis of either obstructive or restrictive disease. In the case of obstructive disease, vital capacity may be reduced, but residual volume and the residual volume/total lung capacity ratio are increased. If wheezing is present, repeat spirometry after inhalation of a beta-agonist. If flow improvement occurs (> 20 percent), a diagnosis of reversible bronchospasm may be made. In the absence of wheezing, but if occult bronchospasm is clinically suspected, perform a methacholine challenge to induce bronchospasm, and repeat the spirometry. In the absence of bronchospasm, emphysema is the likely diagnosis. The diffusing capacity is reduced in patients with emphysema.

D. All lung volumes are reduced in patients with a restrictive process. A reduced diffusing capacity is also found in patients with restriction due to parenchymal disease and in patients with severe anemia, but it is not found in patients who have restriction due to obesity or due to neuromuscular disease but who have otherwise normal lungs.

E. Patients with a restrictive process and a normal DL should have Pi_{max} and Pe_{max} measured. Reduced inspiratory pressures indicate possible diaphragmatic weakness due to partial paralysis, hypothyroidism, or muscle enzyme deficiencies. Placement of esophageal and gastric balloons to measure transdiaphragmatic pressure throughout the respiratory cycle or other diagnostic procedures may be necessary to confirm these diagnoses. Reduced expiratory pressures may indicate respiratory accessory muscle weakness or a lack of effort. Full exercise testing may be indicated to further test the respiratory muscles.

References

Celli BR. Clinical and physiologic evaluation of respiratory muscle function. Clin Chest Med 1989; 10:199.

Gardner RM, Crapo RO, Nelson SB. Spirometry and flow-volume curves. Clin Chest Med 1989; 10:145.

Ries A. Measurement of lung volumes. Clin Chest Med 1989; 10:177.

PULMONARY FUNCTION TESTING

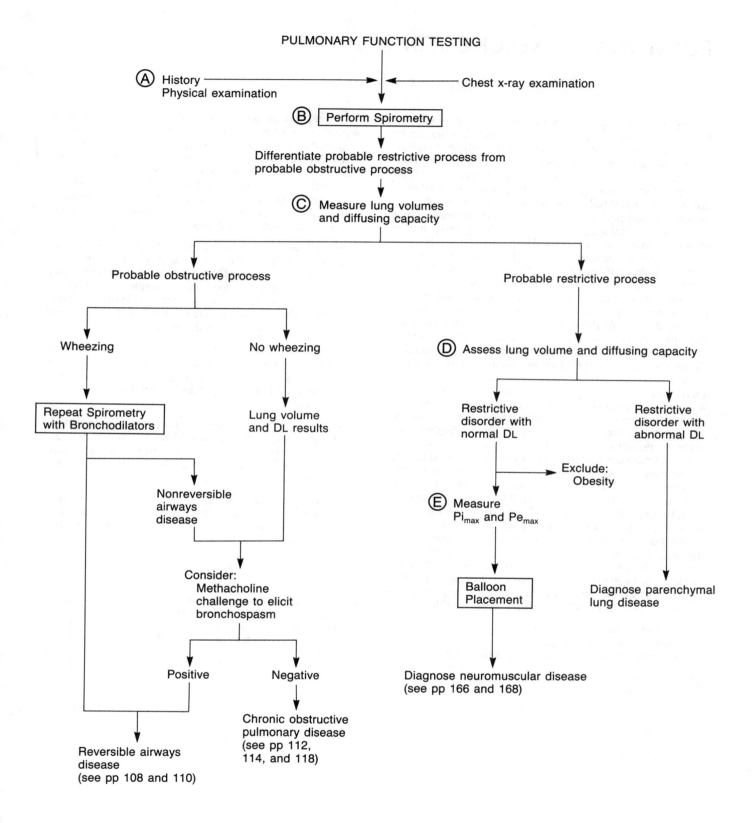

PULMONARY EXERCISE TESTING

During exercise, both the cardiac and pulmonary systems become stressed while attempting to meet the increased metabolic demands of active muscles. The ability to generate an adequate supply of oxygen and fuel to respiratory muscles and to remove waste products of muscle metabolism requires efficient operation of the lung and chest wall musculature, a normal pulmonary circulation with matching of ventilation and perfusion within the lungs, normal cardiac function, a normal systemic circulation, adequate quantities of hemoglobin, and normal regulatory mechanisms. Pulmonary exercise testing is necessary to (1) evaluate patients with marginal pulmonary function for thoracic surgery; (2) distinguish cardiac from pulmonary causes of dyspnea; (3) establish the degree of pulmonary impairment for legal reasons; (4) evaluate function of respiratory muscles; and (5) as a part of a pulmonary rehabilitation or sports medicine program. Patients must be able to follow instructions and be free of certain cardiac and vascular conditions (exercise-induced arrhythmias, exercise-induced angina, aortic stenosis, peripheral vascular disease). Exercise is usually performed at increasing power outputs until limiting symptoms are reached. The electrocardiogram and oxygen saturation are continuously monitored. Every 30 to 60 seconds, minute ventilation ($\dot{V}E$), oxygen consumption, CO_2 production, tidal volume, respiratory rate, and inspiratory time are measured. The maximum oxygen consumption is recorded. At the end of the exercise period, alveolar ($\dot{V}A$) and dead space ($\dot{V}D$) ventilation are calculated. The anaerobic threshold occurs at the point at which the minute ventilation and oxygen consumption begin to decrease with increasing workload. It is measured as the oxygen consumption at that point divided by the body weight and varies depending on the patient's age and sex. It normally occurs at 49 to 63 percent of maximal oxygen consumption. Other variables of importance include the oxygen uptake–work rate relationship, ventilatory equivalents for oxygen and carbon dioxide, and arterial to end-tidal oxygen and carbon dioxide rest-exercise differences.

A. Patients selected for exercise testing should give a complete history and undergo physical examination and pre-exercise routine pulmonary function testing.

B. Testing may be performed in patients who require lung resectional surgery if they have marginal pulmonary function. If exercise testing reveals a low anaerobic threshold (<15 ml oxygen consumption per kg per min), the patient is at a very high risk for developing postoperative complications. The anaerobic threshold may improve after patients undergo a supervised exercise program. If the heart rate cannot increase appropriately with exercise and is limiting, patients may have cardiac disease.

C. Patients with airflow obstruction exhibit increases in carbon dioxide production associated with large increases in minute ventilation. Dead space ventilation is high and alveolar ventilation low. The anaerobic threshold is reduced, inspiratory time is short, and expiratory time is long. The maximal inspiratory pressure (Pi_{max}) may be reduced in patients with severe emphysema.

D. Patients with interstitial disease exhibit increases in minute ventilation related to increases in both alveolar and dead space ventilation. Oxygen desaturation is commonly found. The Pi_{max} may be reduced in these individuals.

E. Patients with vascular disease have increases in carbon dioxide production associated with low cardiac outputs, pulmonary hypertension, and low anaerobic thresholds. Often large increases in minute ventilation, alveolar ventilation, and dead space ventilation are noted.

F. Patients with diseases of respiratory muscles exhibit reduced Pi_{max} with a normal breathing pattern, and carbon dioxide production and minute ventilation may be only slightly reduced.

References

Loke J, ed. Symposium on exercise: physiology and clinical applications. Clin Chest Med 1984; 5:3.

Wasserman K, Hansen JE, Sue DY, Whipp BJ. Principles of exercise testing and interpretation. Philadelphia: Lea and Febiger, 1986.

PULMONARY EXERCISE TESTING

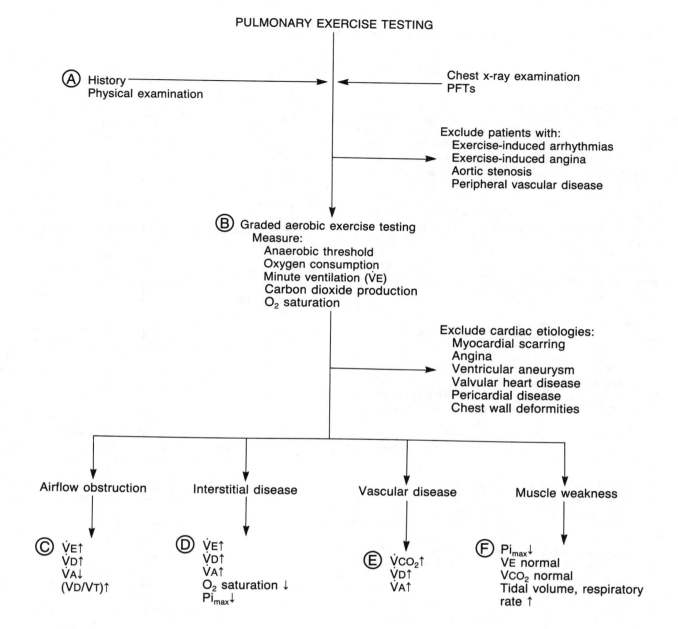

A History — Physical examination

Chest x-ray examination
PFTs

Exclude patients with:
    Exercise-induced arrhythmias
    Exercise-induced angina
    Aortic stenosis
    Peripheral vascular disease

B Graded aerobic exercise testing
   Measure:
      Anaerobic threshold
      Oxygen consumption
      Minute ventilation ($\dot{V}E$)
      Carbon dioxide production
      O_2 saturation

Exclude cardiac etiologies:
    Myocardial scarring
    Angina
    Ventricular aneurysm
    Valvular heart disease
    Pericardial disease
    Chest wall deformities

Airflow obstruction

Interstitial disease

Vascular disease

Muscle weakness

C $\dot{V}E\uparrow$
$V_D\uparrow$
$V_A\downarrow$
$(V_D/V_T)\uparrow$

D $\dot{V}E\uparrow$
$V_D\uparrow$
$V_A\uparrow$
O_2 saturation $\downarrow$
$Pi_{max}\downarrow$

E $\dot{V}CO_2\uparrow$
$V_D\uparrow$
$V_A\uparrow$

F $Pi_{max}\downarrow$
VE normal
VCO_2 normal
Tidal volume, respiratory
rate $\uparrow$

PREOPERATIVE PULMONARY EVALUATION

Pulmonary complications are significant causes of postoperative surgical morbidity and mortality. Infections and atelectasis are the major postoperative pulmonary complications, and upper abdominal and thoracic operations have the highest rates of these complications. Patients with abnormal pulmonary functions have also been found to be at increased risk for these complications. Conditions that predispose patients to infectious complications include diminished cough, atelectasis, and decreased mucociliary clearance of foreign particles. Postoperative pain, decreased spontaneous deep breaths, diaphragmatic dysfunction, and splinting are the primary problems responsible for the development of atelectasis. Preoperative pulmonary evaluation should be performed to identify patients at increased risk of postoperative pulmonary complications and those patients who are not suitable candidates for lung resection. Appropriate preoperative therapeutic measures and cessation of smoking should be instituted for those found to be at increased risk.

A. Preoperative pulmonary assessment includes a history of cigarette smoking and cardiopulmonary diseases, recent cough and sputum production, and signs and symptoms of cardiopulmonary diseases. Notation of wheezes, rhonchi, and decreased breath sounds on physical examination identifies patients with active and chronic pulmonary diseases. Obtain chest films and pulmonary function tests in these patients to confirm the history and clinical findings.

B. Patients undergoing lung resection must have a preoperative evaluation to estimate postresectional lung function. A preoperative pulmonary function test with spirometry is the most popular method of evaluation. Test patients with a marginal FEV_1 on spirometry with a regional ventilation or perfusion lung scan for a more accurate determination of the predicted postoperative FEV_1. Most authorities use a predicted postoperative FEV_1 of 800 ml as a minimum criterion for surgery. In patients judged to be candidates for lung resection, an arterial blood gas (ABG) determination should be done before surgery.

C. For patients undergoing abdominal surgery and non-lung–resection thoracic surgery, additional risks for postoperative pulmonary complications include older age, obesity, a history or findings of cardiopulmonary dis-

eases, and a history of smoking. These patients require spirometry to determine their pulmonary functions. In those found to have pulmonary function abnormalities (forced vital capacity [FVC] less than 75 percent of that predicted, an FEV_1/FVC ratio of less than 70 percent, and maximal expiratory flow rate of less than 200 L/min), an ABG determination should be done.

D. Obtain ABGs for all patients being evaluated for lung resection and those with abnormal spirometric results being evaluated for abdominal or non-lung–resection thoracic surgery. Patients with hypercapnia ($PCO_2 > 50$ mm Hg) or hypoxemia ($PaO_2 < 60$ mm Hg) have increased postoperative pulmonary complications. However, in some patients with lung cancer, the PaO_2 may actually improve after resection of nonventilated section of the lung.

E. Prophylactic treatment of those at risk helps reduce the incidence of postoperative pulmonary complications. Forty-eight to 72 hours before surgery, start treatment with antibiotics, bronchodilators, and chest physiotherapy for those with significant sputum production.

F. Smoking cessation for 8 weeks or more before surgery has been found to reduce postoperative pulmonary complications by at least one-half; shorter periods of smoking cessation have not been found to be effective. Other preoperative measures that reduce postoperative pulmonary complications include teaching deep breathing (to be used postoperatively) and coughing, mobilization of secretions, early ambulation, and avoidance of excessive narcotics for pain control.

References

Azarow KS, Molloy M, Seyfer AE, Graeber GM. Preoperative evaluation and general preparation for chest-wall operations. Surg Clin North Am 1989; 69:899.

Jackson CV. Preoperative pulmonary evaluation. Arch Intern Med 1988; 148:2120.

Keating HJ III. Preoperative considerations in the geriatric patient. Med Clin North Am 1987; 71:569.

Tisi GM. Preoperative identification and evaluation of the patient with lung disease. Med Clin North Am 1987; 71:399.

PREOPERATIVE PULMONARY EVALUATION

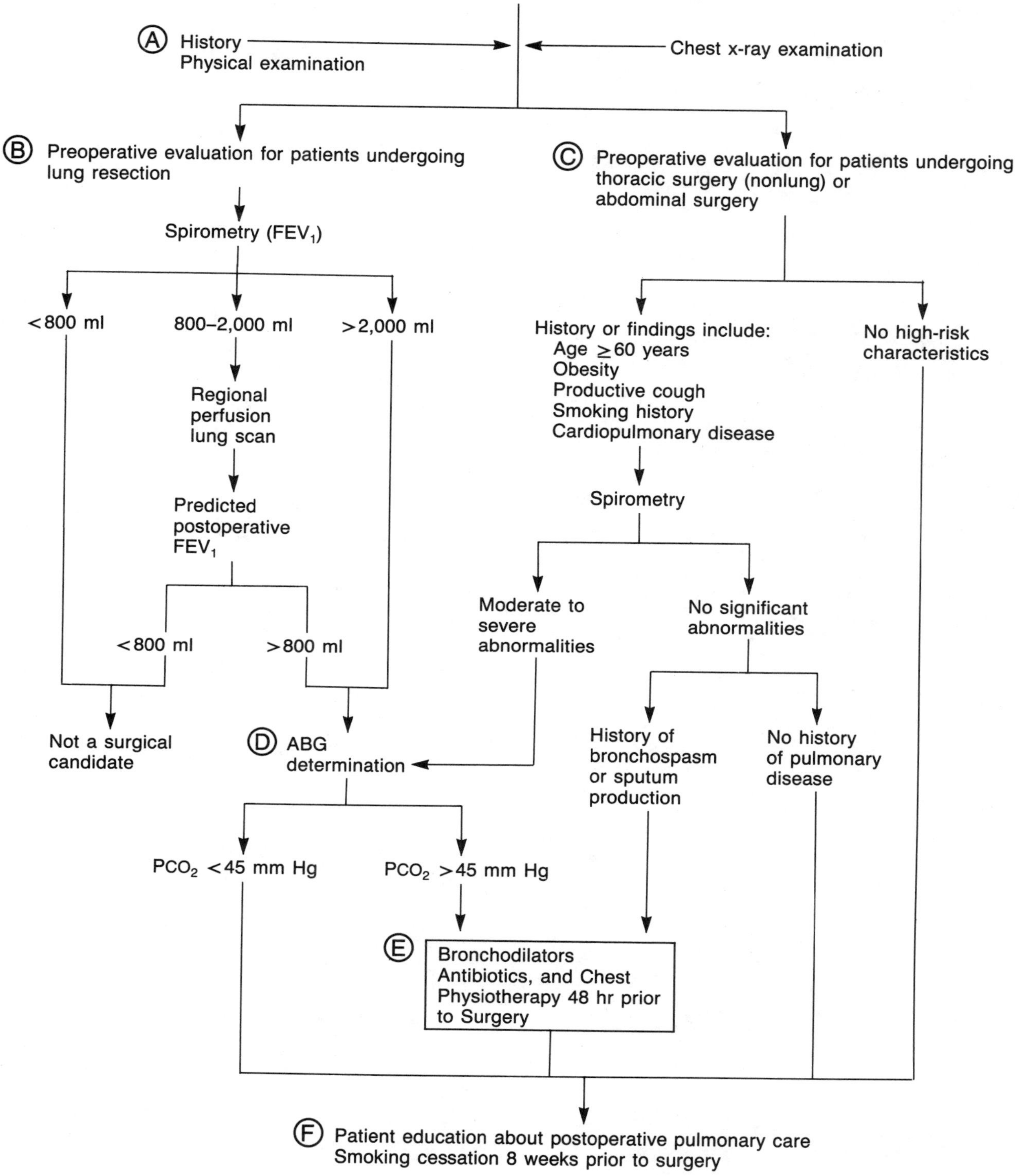

(A) History —————————— ←———————— Chest x-ray examination
Physical examination

(B) Preoperative evaluation for patients undergoing lung resection

Spirometry (FEV_1)

- <800 ml
- 800–2,000 ml
- >2,000 ml

Regional perfusion lung scan

Predicted postoperative FEV_1

- <800 ml
- >800 ml

Not a surgical candidate

(D) ABG determination

PCO_2 <45 mm Hg

PCO_2 >45 mm Hg

(C) Preoperative evaluation for patients undergoing thoracic surgery (nonlung) or abdominal surgery

History or findings include:
Age ≥60 years
Obesity
Productive cough
Smoking history
Cardiopulmonary disease

No high-risk characteristics

Spirometry

Moderate to severe abnormalities

No significant abnormalities

History of bronchospasm or sputum production

No history of pulmonary disease

(E) Bronchodilators Antibiotics, and Chest Physiotherapy 48 hr prior to Surgery

(F) Patient education about postoperative pulmonary care
Smoking cessation 8 weeks prior to surgery

23

NEOPLASTIC AND NEOPLASTIC-RELATED DISEASES OF THE LUNG

Solitary Pulmonary Nodule
Mediastinal Adenopathy
Carcinoid
Pulmonary Involvement in Hodgkin's Disease
Lymphangitic Metastasis
Malignant Pleural Effusion

Mesothelioma
Pancoast Tumor
Carcinoma In Situ
Superior Vena Cava Syndrome
Multiple Pulmonary Nodules
Radiation Pneumonitis

SOLITARY PULMONARY NODULE

Solitary pulmonary nodule is defined as an isolated, round intrapulmonary lesion less than 6 cm in diameter. It is usually discovered incidentally on a chest film of an asymptomatic patient. The probability of malignancy depends on a number of risk factors, including the age and sex of the patient, the presence of a smoking history, and the size of the nodule. Approximately 10 percent of the solitary pulmonary nodules in the general community and up to 40 percent in clinical settings are malignant.

A. In addition to the history and physical examination, a preliminary diagnostic work-up with tuberculin skin testing, sputum cytology, and sputum stains and culture for fungi and acid-fast organisms may reveal the etiology of the lesion. The diagnostic process should not be delayed while one is waiting for mycobacterial culture results. A negative sputum cytology does not exclude malignancy, since this test has only a 20 percent sensitivity for the detection of cancer.

B. Lung cancers have reported doubling times between 37 and 465 days. Stability of the lesion on the chest film over the previous 2-year period probably signifies a benign lesion.

C. Calcification within a nodule, especially among low-risk patients, increases the likelihood that the nodule is benign; only approximately 1 in 100 calcified nodules is malignant. "Popcorn" calcification is pathognomonic for hamartoma, which represents approximately 5 percent of all solitary nodules. Histoplasmosis often presents with concentric calcifications. Other benign calcific nodular patterns include uniform density calcification and central calcification. Eccentrically calcified nodules should raise the suspicion of malignancy, since these are often associated with scar carcinoma.

D. The probability of cancer can be estimated from various risk factors (Table 1). High-risk patients—typically those with a smoking history and large lesions, and who are older than 35 years of age—should undergo further diagnostic tests whether their pulmonary nodules are calcified or not. In the absence of previous chest films for comparison, a small (2-cm or less) uncalcified lesion in a patient younger than 35 years of age without a smoking history is likely benign. Invasive procedures in this low-risk setting are not indicated, but follow-up chest films at quarterly intervals should be performed for 1 year to establish the stability of the lesion. Calcified lesions in low-risk patients need no further follow-up, although some authorities perform a chest film 3 months later to establish stability definitively.

E. Order chest CT scans to identify possible additional nodules not seen on chest films and to evaluate the mediastinum for evidence of adenopathy. Additional nodules seen on the chest CT scan indicate metastatic cancer and the need for a more detailed evaluation. Investigate mediastinal adenopathy with mediastinoscopy.

F. Flexible fiberoptic bronchoscopy with washing, brushing, and bronchial and transbronchial biopsy may determine the etiology of the pulmonary nodule. The sensitivity of the procedure for diagnosing cancer increases with the size of the nodules, from approximately 25 percent for nodules less than 2 cm to better than 50 percent for 4-cm nodules. Some authorities bypass bronchoscopy and proceed directly to thoracotomy if the chest CT scan does not reveal adenopathy.

G. Percutaneous-needle aspiration of large peripheral lesions in the lung may increase the overall diagnostic yield for cancer detection. This procedure is performed in selected patients where the risk of morbidity is low.

H. Patients diagnosed with, or suspected of having, primary pulmonary malignancy undergo a metastatic work-up and preoperative evaluation prior to thoracotomy. Such a metastatic work-up might include stool guaiac, acid phosphatase, and head CT. Patients judged not to be candidates for thoracotomy and resection should be considered for either curative or palliative radiotherapy.

TABLE 1 Likelihood Ratio for Malignancy in Solitary Pulmonary Nodule in Men*

Diameter of Nodule (cm)	LCA**	Patient's Age (yr)	LCA	Smoking History (cigarettes/day)	LCA
<1.5	0.1	<35	0.1	0	0.15
1.5–2.2	0.5	36–44	0.3	1–9	0.3
2.3–3.2	1.7	45–49	0.7	10–20	1.0
3.3–4.2	4.3	50–59	1.5	21–40	2.0
4.3–5.2	6.6	60–69	2.1	>40	3.9
5.3–6.0	29.4	70–83	5.7		

*Data from Cummings SR, Lillington GA, Richard RJ. Estimating the probability of malignancy in solitary pulmonary nodules. Am Rev Resp Dis 1986; 134:449.

**LCA = likelihood ratio of cancer.

References

Cummings SR, Lillington GA, Richard RJ. Estimating the probability of malignancy in solitary pulmonary nodules. Am Rev Resp Dis 1986; 134:449.

Inouye SK, Sox HC. Standard and computed tomography in the evaluation of neoplasms of the chest. Ann Int Med 1986; 105:906.

Lillington GA. The solitary pulmonary nodule—1974. Am Rev Resp Dis 1974; 110:699.

Wallace JM, Deutsch AL. Flexible fiberoptic bronchoscopy and percutaneous needle lung aspiration for evaluating the solitary pulmonary nodule. Chest 1982; 8:665.

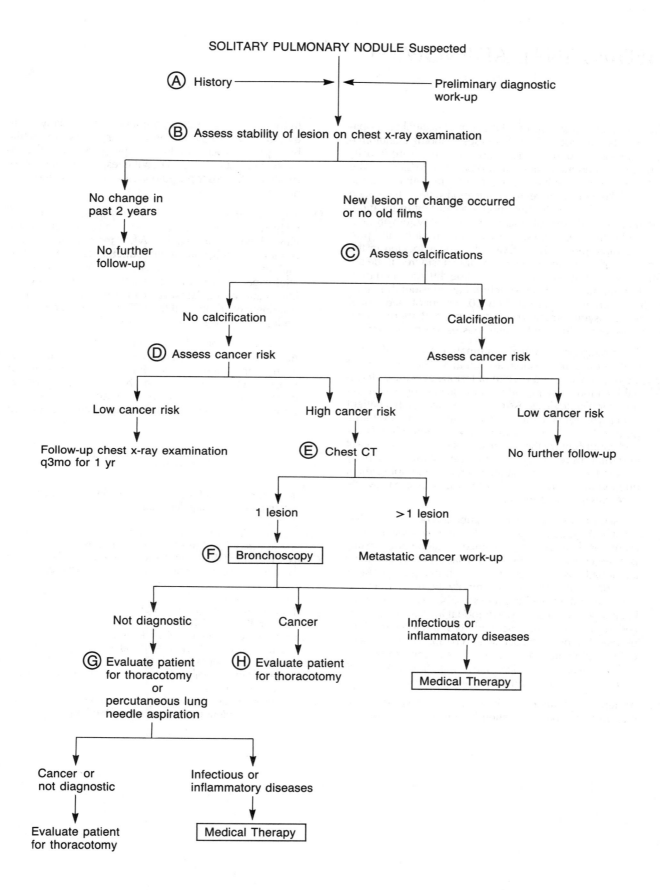

SOLITARY PULMONARY NODULE Suspected

(A) History ← → Preliminary diagnostic work-up

(B) Assess stability of lesion on chest x-ray examination

No change in past 2 years → No further follow-up

New lesion or change occurred or no old films → (C) Assess calcifications

No calcification → (D) Assess cancer risk

Calcification → Assess cancer risk

Low cancer risk → Follow-up chest x-ray examination q3mo for 1 yr

High cancer risk → (E) Chest CT

Low cancer risk → No further follow-up

1 lesion → (F) Bronchoscopy

>1 lesion → Metastatic cancer work-up

Not diagnostic → (G) Evaluate patient for thoracotomy or percutaneous lung needle aspiration

Cancer → (H) Evaluate patient for thoracotomy

Infectious or inflammatory diseases → Medical Therapy

Cancer or not diagnostic → Evaluate patient for thoracotomy

Infectious or inflammatory diseases → Medical Therapy

27

MEDIASTINAL ADENOPATHY

The differential diagnosis of hilar and mediastinal adenopathy consists of a wide variety of diseases including granulomatous diseases such as tuberculosis and sarcoidosis, lymphomas, and metastatic carcinomas. The location of the nodes within the mediastinum is helpful in delineating the differential diagnosis. Several classification systems have been devised to define mediastinal nodes according to location. The simplest and probably the most practical system arbitrarily divides the mediastinum into anterior, middle, and posterior compartments. The prevascular nodes located in the superior aspect of the mediastinum are considered to be anterior nodes. Mediastinal nodes must be differentiated from mediastinal masses. This distinction has considerable diagnostic importance. Approximately 50 percent of mediastinal masses are asymptomatic at presentation, and approximately 50 percent of the mediastinal masses are malignant.

A. The history and physical examination are useful in the evaluation of mediastinal adenopathy. The detection of adenopathy or the presence of lesions at extramediastinal locations may provide a more accessible site to biopsy for histologic assessment. For example, in a patient with asymptomatic hilar adenopathy, a careful examination of the skin may yield nodules which when biopsied could confirm the diagnosis of sarcoidosis. The onset of symptoms resulting from mediastinal involvement by nonHodgkin's lymphoma usually relates to impingement upon vital structures such as the superior vena cava by an enlarging mass lesion.

B. Chest CT readily defines the distribution of nodal involvement in the mediastinum. The location of nodal involvement has diagnostic significance. Bilateral adenopathy is more consistent with sarcoidosis, whereas unilateral adenopathy is more consistent with malignancy. Anterior adenopathy is more commonly the result of malignant rather than benign processes, but exceptions have been reported. Similarly, extranodal involvement is suggestive of malignancy, particularly non-Hodgkin's lymphoma. The presence of calcified lymph nodes suggests old granulomatous disease such as histoplasmosis. Finally, the scan differentiates fatty infiltration of the mediastinum from true mediastinal adenopathy.

C. When pulmonary parenchymal lesions are present, the diagnosis can be established by transbronchial biopsy.

In the case of sarcoidosis, the lesions are usually located diffusely throughout the lung, and a transbronchial biopsy with or without fluoroscopic guidance will often yield diagnostic tissue. When the lesions are nodular or localized, fluoroscopic guidance will increase the diagnostic yield.

D. Patients with sarcoidosis commonly present with isolated hilar adenopathy or hilar adenopathy associated with parenchymal abnormalities. When the hilar adenopathy is associated with pulmonary function test (PFT) abnormalities associated with sarcoidosis (decreased forced vital capacity or diffusing capacity for carbon monoxide), a transbronchial biopsy can often provide tissue for histologic verification. If the PFTs are normal, the lymph nodes themselves can be biopsied.

E. When transbronchial biopsy yields only nondiagnostic tissue or when the parenchyma is normal, mediastinoscopy offers a direct but invasive diagnostic approach. Most mediastinal lymph nodes can be biopsied by the cervical mediastinal approach; some anterior nodes require the more extensive left anterior approach.

References

Bein ME, Putman CE, McCloud TC, Mink JH. A reevaluation of intrathoracic lymphadenopathy in sarcoid. AJR 1978; 131:409.

Berkmen YM, Javors BR. Anterior mediastinal lymphadenopathy in sarcoidosis. Am J Roentgenol 1976; 127:983.

Chang CH, Zinn TW. Roentgen recognition of enlarged hilar lymph nodes: an anatomical review. Radiology 1976; 120:291.

Levitt LJ, Aisenberg AC, Harris NL, Linggood RM, Poppema S. Primary non-Hodgkin's lymphoma of the mediastinum. Cancer 1982; 50:2486.

Lichtenstein AK, Levine A, Taylor CR, et al. Mediastinal lymphoma in adults. Am J Med 1980; 68:508.

McCloud TC, Kalisher L, Stark P, Greene R. Intrathoracic lymph node metastases from extrathoracic neoplasms. Am J Roentgenol 1978; 131:403.

Winterbauer RH, Belic N, Moores KD. A clinical interpretation of bilateral adenopathy. Ann Intern Med 1973; 78:65.

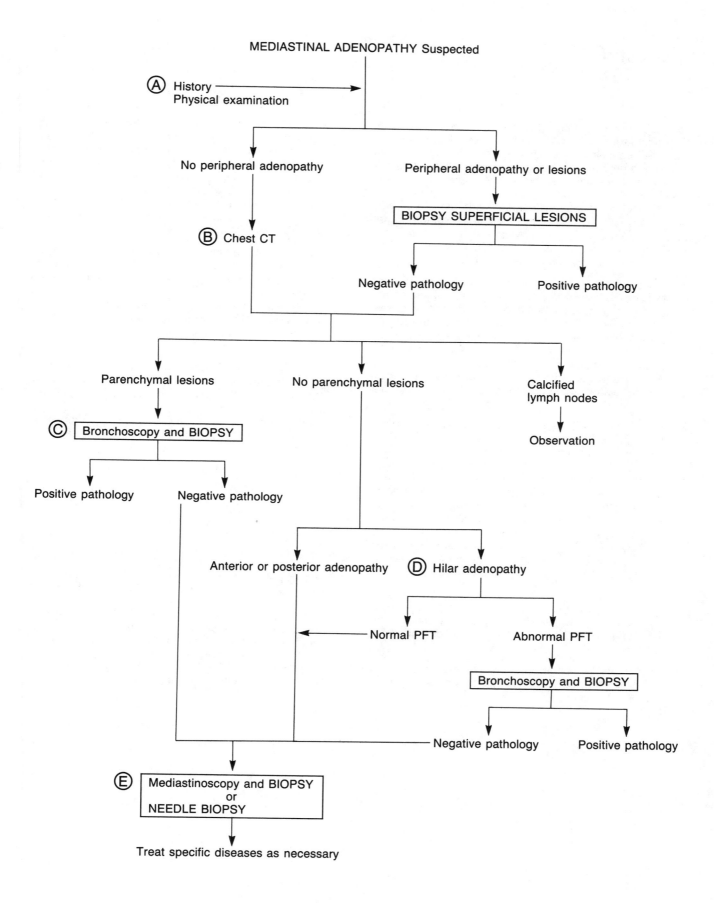

MEDIASTINAL ADENOPATHY Suspected

(A) History
Physical examination

No peripheral adenopathy

Peripheral adenopathy or lesions

BIOPSY SUPERFICIAL LESIONS

(B) Chest CT

Negative pathology

Positive pathology

Parenchymal lesions

No parenchymal lesions

Calcified
lymph nodes

(C) Bronchoscopy and BIOPSY

Observation

Positive pathology

Negative pathology

Anterior or posterior adenopathy

(D) Hilar adenopathy

Normal PFT

Abnormal PFT

Bronchoscopy and BIOPSY

Negative pathology

Positive pathology

(E) Mediastinoscopy and BIOPSY
or
NEEDLE BIOPSY

Treat specific diseases as necessary

CARCINOID

Carcinoid tumors comprise less than 5 percent of all bronchial neoplasms and are thought to arise from neurosecretory cells located in the bronchial mucosa. They arise in both central and peripheral locations in lung. Unlike carcinoids of the gastrointestinal tract, they rarely produce measurable quantities of 5-hydroxyindoleacetic acid (5-HIAA) and therefore rarely give rise to the carcinoid syndrome. Neoplasms are found equally in men and women, and most tumors are found in middle-aged patients. Metastasis or local spread is unusual but may occur. Consequently, this tumor has a better prognosis than bronchogenic carcinoma.

A. Patients present with a variety of nonspecific symptoms ranging from mild cough to significant wheezing not responsive to bronchodilator therapy. Patients may have hemoptysis, and if large, centrally located tumors are present, they may present with a postobstructive pneumonitis. Peripherally located carcinoids are asymptomatic and are usually discovered during routine chest x-ray examination performed for other reasons. Significant weight loss or other constitutional symptoms may not be present.

B. The physical examination may be unremarkable or may be significant for the presence of a single, localized wheeze on forced expiration. Clubbing is not a feature of this syndrome. The laboratory examination is also usually not remarkable. If episodic flushing, bronchospasm, and diarrhea are present, assess the urine for the presence of 5-HIAA which, if found, suggests the diagnosis. Oxygenation of arterial blood may be normal, depending on the presence or absence of associated pneumonia. Pulmonary function may also be normal, and examination of sputum is unrevealing. The diagnosis cannot be made from sputum cytologies.

C. If a new peripheral lesion is seen on the chest x-ray examination, CT of the thorax should be performed to ensure that other, smaller lesions are not present. If the lesion is solitary, the case reduces to that of solitary pulmonary nodule.

D. A fiberoptic bronchoscopy should be performed to rule out the presence of a small central lesion not visualized on the CT scan.

E. If the patient has a negative PPD and pulmonary functions permit, have the peripheral lesion removed surgically. If the patient has a positive tuberculin skin test, sputums should be obtained for mycobacterial culture. The patient may be begun on a trial of INH for 6 weeks and the radiologic response of the lesion measured to rule out the possibility of tuberculous tuberculoma. If the lesion remains the same size or grows, proceed with surgical removal.

F. If the patient presents with a central intrabronchial lesion and postobstructive pneumonia, treat the pneumonia prior to further work-up. Once the pneumonia has cleared, perform flexible fiberoptic bronchoscopy. Do not biopsy lesions resembling bronchial carcinoid (exophytic, polypoid, cherry red) through this instrument, because the chance of significant bleeding is high, and control of bleeding is difficult.

G. The patient may undergo bronchoscopy using a rigid instrument in the operating room. Frozen sections suggest the diagnosis, and surgical removal can then be done. Lobectomy is the operation of choice. Bronchial and mediastinal nodes are usually tumor-free, and adjuvant radiotherapy or chemotherapy is rarely necessary.

References

Hurt R, Bates M. Carcinoid tumors of the bronchus: a 33 year experience. Thorax 1984; 39:617.

Naidich DR, McCauley DI, Siegelman SS. Computed tomography of bronchial adenomas. J Comput Assist Tomogr 1982; 6:725.

Scully RE, Mark EJ, McNeely BU. Case records of the Massachusetts General Hospital, Case 5-1986 (bronchial carcinoid). N Engl J Med 1986; 314:368.

Wilkins EW Jr, Grillo HC, Moncure AC, Scannell JG. Changing times in the surgical management of bronchopulmonary carcinoid tumor. Ann Thorac Surg 1984; 38:339.

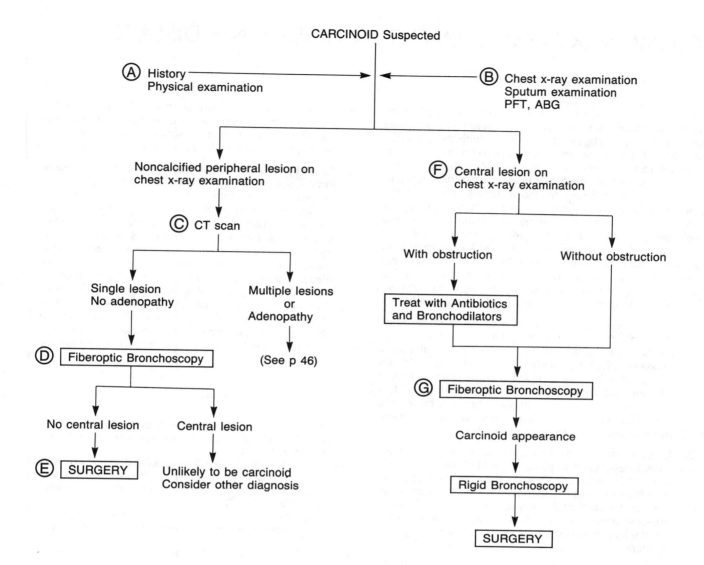

CARCINOID Suspected

Ⓐ History —
Physical examination

Ⓑ Chest x-ray examination
Sputum examination
PFT, ABG

Noncalcified peripheral lesion on
chest x-ray examination

Ⓒ CT scan

Single lesion
No adenopathy

Multiple lesions
or
Adenopathy

(See p 46)

Ⓓ Fiberoptic Bronchoscopy

No central lesion

Central lesion

Ⓔ SURGERY

Unlikely to be carcinoid
Consider other diagnosis

Ⓕ Central lesion on
chest x-ray examination

With obstruction

Without obstruction

Treat with Antibiotics
and Bronchodilators

Ⓖ Fiberoptic Bronchoscopy

Carcinoid appearance

Rigid Bronchoscopy

SURGERY

PULMONARY INVOLVEMENT IN HODGKIN'S DISEASE

Hodgkin's disease frequently involves the mediastinal lymph nodes and lung parenchyma. The frequency of pulmonary involvement in Hodgkin's disease varies with the particular cell type. Parenchymal involvement is common in patients with the mixed cellularity subtype (40 percent) and uncommon in patients with the lymphocyte predominant subtype. In patients not previously treated with radiation or chemotherapy, hilar adenopathy may occur with or without lung involvement. The most common presentation is markedly enlarged superior mediastinal nodes. Isolated involvement of the posterior nodes and paracardiac nodes is uncommon. Approximately 12 percent of patients with untreated Hodgkin's disease have pulmonary lesions that are accompanied by hilar or mediastinal adenopathy. Pulmonary involvement may also present as an extension from bulky central nodes.

A. The history and physical examination are of limited value in the diagnosis of pulmonary Hodgkin's disease. The key problem is differentiating infection from pulmonary invasion by malignant cells. This is particularly difficult in patients who have received chemotherapy. Cough is the only pulmonary symptom consistently present in Hodgkin's disease. Hemoptysis is rarely a presenting complaint. Occasionally, superior vena cava syndrome or laryngeal nerve paralysis is present.

B. CT of the chest is required to delineate the extent of disease. Parenchymal involvement in Hodgkin's disease in untreated patients usually takes the form of direct extension from mediastinal adenopathy. Compression of airways by enlarged nodes may result in lobar collapse or postobstructive pneumonia. In addition, localized interstitial edema may occur from compression of lymphatic drainage.

C. Pleural effusion may result from obstruction of lymphatic drainage. However, chylous effusions are more common in non-Hodgkin's lymphoma. In contrast to bronchogenic cancer, pleural metastatic disease is less common. Less than 10 percent of patients with Hodgkin's disease and pleural effusion have positive fluid cytologies. Treatment of the effusion usually involves radiation to the mediastinum rather than chemical pleural sclerosis.

D. The presence of mediastinal adenopathy is commonly found in Hodgkin's disease and may be the initial finding. The reappearance of adenopathy may indicate recurrence of disease and the need for further treatment.

E. Parenchymal involvement in treated patients with Hodgkin's disease has a variable presentation and includes single or multiple nodules with or without cavitation. The borders of the nodules may be sharp or irregular. In patients with advanced disease, the diagnostic possibilities include opportunistic infections such as aspergillosis. The initial diagnostic evaluation consists of sputum examination followed by bronchoscopy, if necessary. If the infiltrate worsens, open-lung biopsy may be indicated to establish the diagnosis when diagnosis cannot be established by less invasive procedures. The treatment regimens for Hodgkin's disease consist of radiation and/or chemotherapy, depending on the presence or absence of symptoms, extent of disease, and previous therapy and response.

References

Costello P, Mauch P. Radiographic features of recurrent intrathoracic Hodgkin's disease following radiation therapy. AJR 1979; 133:201.

Filly R, Blank N, Castellino RA. Radiographic distribution of intrathoracic disease in previously untreated patients with Hodgkin's disease and non-Hodgkin's lymphoma. Radiology 1976; 120:277.

Harper PG, Fisher C, McLennan K, Souhami RL. Presentation of Hodgkin's disease as endobronchial lesions. Cancer 1984; 53:147.

McDonald JB. Lung involvement in Hodgkin's disease. Thorax 1977; 32:664.

North NB, Fuller LM, Hagenmeister FB, et al. Importance of initial mediastinal adenopathy in Hodgkin's disease. AJR 1982; 138:229.

Strickland B. Intra-thoracic Hodgkin's disease. Br J Radiol 1967; 40:930.

Whitcolm ME, Schwarz MI, Keller AR, Flannery EP, Blom J. Hodgkin's disease of the lung. Am Rev Respir Dis 1972; 106:79.

ABNORMAL CHEST FILM IN A PATIENT WITH KNOWN HODGKIN'S DISEASE

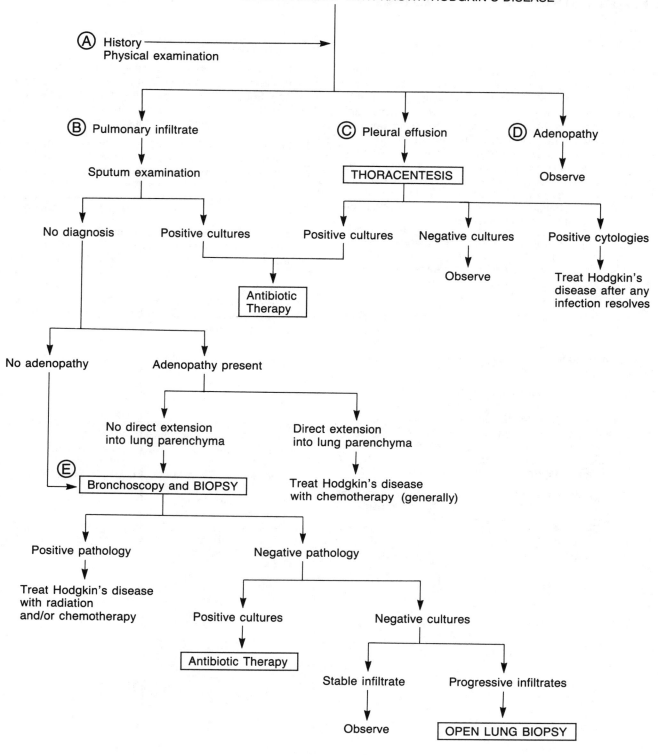

LYMPHANGITIC METASTASIS

A. The spread of a primary neoplasm to the lymphatic and peribronchovascular and interlobular connective tissue is common. Neoplastic metastasis usually occurs first by the tumor embolizing to small pulmonary arteries and later extending through vessel walls to invade adjacent interstitium and lymphatics. The most common neoplasms that spread by this route are primary breast, lung, gastrointestinal, ovarian, and cervical cancers. Patients present with rapidly progressive dyspnea and usually experience a rapid downhill course. The PO_2 of arterial blood is substantially decreased and does not greatly improve with the addition of oxygen.

B. The chest film usually demonstrates a coarse linear or reticular pattern. Kerley B lines may be seen. If invasion of lymphatics is due to a primary neoplasm located outside the chest, there will be no evidence of a primary pulmonary tumor visible on the chest film.

C. If patients present with dyspnea but the results of the chest x-ray examination are normal, it is important to perform routine pulmonary function tests (spirometry, lung volumes, diffusing capacity) to determine the cause of the dyspnea.

D. If the pulmonary function tests reveal restriction, perform CT to document the presence or absence of interstitial lung disease. If no interstitial disease can be documented and the patient remains symptomatic, other organ systems may be involved and other diagnoses should be considered, such as congestive heart failure, chronic small pulmonary emboli, and emphysema.

E. If the patient has interstitial infiltrates, rule out infectious and cardiogenic etiologies, using the history, physical examination, and basic laboratory data.

F. If the patient has a history of malignancy and has a reticulonodular or interstitial pattern on the chest film, the likely diagnosis is metastatic carcinomatosis. Confirmation of this diagnosis, if necessary, is forthcoming only from histologic diagnosis of pulmonary tissue. Tissue in small amounts may be obtained using fiberoptic bronchoscopy with transbronchial biopsies.

G. However, if the material obtained from bronchoscopy is insufficient for diagnosis or is negative, an open procedure is necessary to make the diagnosis. If the patient has a neoplasm that is treatable, and making a diagnosis of lymphangitic metastasis would influence the therapeutic decision, then tissue should be obtained.

H. Treatment of this disorder is symptomatic. Give the patient a short course of diuretic therapy on an empiric basis to be sure that mild left ventricular failure is not a component. Administer oxygen at high-flow rates as well as narcotics in small doses to reduce the dyspnea. If the primary neoplasm is sensitive to chemotherapeutic agents, these should be tried, assuming a relatively good performance status.

References

Crow J, Slavin G, Kreel L. Pulmonary metastasis. A pathologic and radiologic study. Cancer 1981; 47:2595.

Friedmann G, Bohndorf K, Kruger J. Radiology of pulmonary metastases. Comparison of imaging techniques with operative findings. Thorac Cardiovas Surg 34 Spec. No. 2, 1986; 120.

Trapnel DH. Radiological appearance of lymphangitis carcinomatosa of the lung. Thorax 1964; 19:251.

Yang S-P, Lin C-C. Lymphangitic carcinomatosis of the lungs. The clinical significance of its roentgenologic classification. Chest 1972; 62:179.

Patient with LYMPHANGITIC METASTASIS

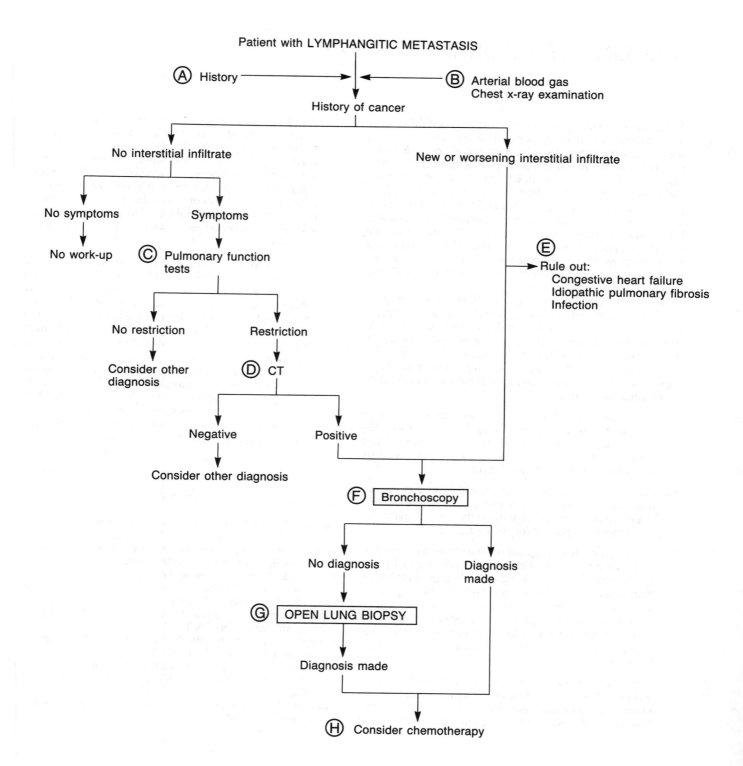

MALIGNANT PLEURAL EFFUSION

The diagnosis of malignant pleural effusion is established by the demonstration of malignant cells in the pleural fluid. In some cases, the diagnosis is suspected early on. For example, in a patient with known unresectable lung cancer, effusions may occur from a variety of etiologies including malignant seeding of the pleural space, obstruction of lymphatic drainage, postobstructive pneumonia, and others. In other cases, pleural effusion is the presenting sign. Lung and breast cancer are common malignancies that cause pleural effusion, and ovarian and gastric malignancies, although less common, frequently cause effusions. Malignant effusions are usually exudates, but the character of the fluid is variable; it may be clear or serosanguinous in appearance. The cell counts and differential of the pleural fluid can vary widely. The effusions may have a low pH and glucose levels without evidence of infection. Certain malignant effusions, such as that resulting from a mesothelioma, are associated with pain and the presence of a pleural-based mass lesion. Other effusions present with dyspnea on exertion. The quantity of pleural fluid that induces symptoms depends upon the state of the underlying lung.

A. Pleural fluid should be sent for cytologic examination whenever a diagnostic thoracentesis is performed. Recent studies have shown that cytologic examination of pleural fluid is more likely to yield a positive diagnosis of malignancy than pleural biopsy.

B. When the cytology results are negative, further evaluation should include a pleural biopsy. If the biopsy fails to yield a positive cytology, drain the pleural space dry and follow the patient for recurrence.

C. The treatment for malignant pleural effusion depends in part on the cell type. In general, the primary malignancy should be aggressively treated when possible rather than treating the effusions themselves. This is particularly the case when the primary malignancy is a lymphoma. The initial approach is to remove all the fluid in symptomatic patients and observe for recurrence. Rapidly reaccumulating effusions require further treatments.

D. Chemical sclerosis of the pleural cavity has been used with variable success. Pleural instillation of tetracycline often results in pleural adhesion and reduced accumulation of fluid. This procedure requires a chest tube, and the pleural space must be dry prior to instillation. The patient is rotated to increase the surface area exposed to the sclerosing agent. Chemical sclerosis using tetracycline or quinacrine is associated with pain and fever, although tetracycline may have fewer side effects. Other agents such as talc have no clear advantage over tetracycline. The instillation of *Corynebacterium* has generated interest because of the ability of this material to induce a fibrosed, thickened pleura and possible immunologic reactions.

E. Pleuroperitoneal shunting involves the placement of a catheter that is similar or identical to the Denver peritoneal-venous shunt. Fluid is shunted from the pleural space to the subhepatic space or to the pelvic area. This treatment has been used in the treatment of chylothorax as well. The problems associated with shunts include infection, tumor implantation into the abdominal cavity, and migration of one of the catheter limbs. Pleurectomy is a definitive treatment for malignant pleural effusions. It is associated with a high incidence of complications (approximately 20 percent) which include empyema and persistent bronchopleural fistulas. It should be reserved for those patients with a reasonable expectation of prolonged survival.

References

Chernow B, Sahn SA. Carcinomatous involvement of the pleura. Am J Med 1977; 63:695.

Felletti R, Ravazzoni C. Intrapleural *Corynebacterium parvum* for malignant pleural effusion. Thorax 1983; 38:22.

Hickman JA, Jones MC. Treatment of neoplastic pleural effusions with local instillations of quinacrine (mepacrine) hydrochloride. Thorax 1970; 25:226.

Leff A, Hopewell PC, Costello J. Pleural effusion from malignancy. Ann Intern Med 1978; 88:532.

Martini N, Bains MS, Beattie EJ. Indications for pleurectomy in malignant effusion. Cancer 1975; 35:734.

Millar JW, Hunter AM, Horne NW. Intrapleural immunotherapy with *Corynebacterium parvum* in recurrent malignant pleural effusion. Thorax 1979; 35:856.

Wallach HW. Intrapleural tetracycline for malignant pleural effusion. Chest 1975; 68:510.

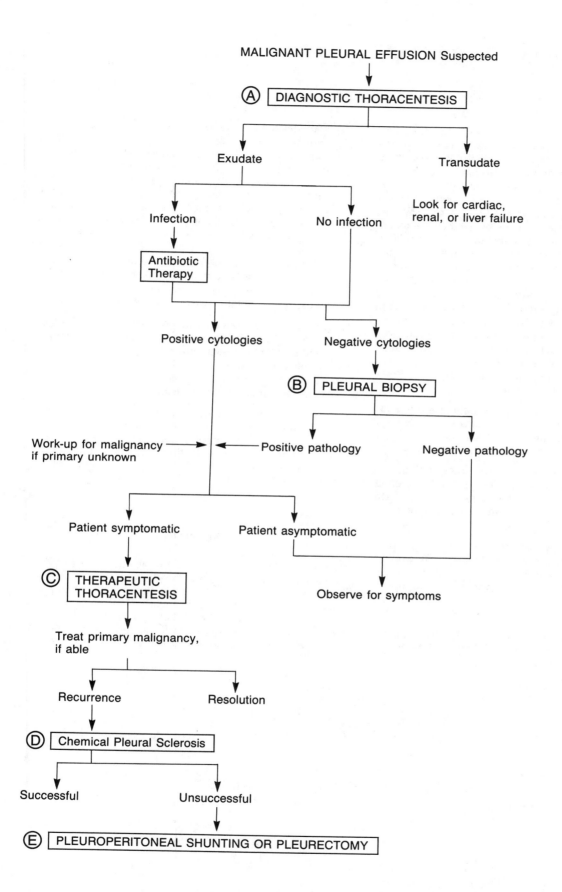

MALIGNANT PLEURAL EFFUSION Suspected

Ⓐ DIAGNOSTIC THORACENTESIS

Exudate — Transudate → Look for cardiac, renal, or liver failure

Infection → Antibiotic Therapy

No infection

Positive cytologies

Negative cytologies → Ⓑ PLEURAL BIOPSY

Positive pathology — Negative pathology

Work-up for malignancy if primary unknown

Patient symptomatic

Patient asymptomatic → Observe for symptoms

Ⓒ THERAPEUTIC THORACENTESIS

Treat primary malignancy, if able

Recurrence — Resolution

Ⓓ Chemical Pleural Sclerosis

Successful — Unsuccessful

Ⓔ PLEUROPERITONEAL SHUNTING OR PLEURECTOMY

MESOTHELIOMA

A. Mesothelioma usually occurs in males during their fifth to sixth decades. If the mesothelioma is diffuse and malignant, patients complain of persistent chest pain, dyspnea, weight loss, and may also have fever. Patients also give a history of remote asbestos exposure. The physical examination reveals clubbing and hypertrophic pulmonary osteoarthropathy of the hands, feet, or distal tibia and fibula. Hypoglycemia may be seen if the mesothelioma is of the fibrous variety and is large and localized. The chest pain is usually dull and aching rather than pleuritic and may be the initial presenting symptom. Cytologic examination of the sputum may rule out bronchogenic carcinoma that may have metastasized to the pleura; however, this examination will not be positive in patients who have mesothelioma. Gram stain of the sputum rules out infectious etiologies of pleural-based masses (empyema) such as aerobic or anaerobic lung infections. The complete data base serves to rule out primary carcinomas in extrathoracic locations that may have metastasized to the pleura.

B. The chest film usually demonstrates either a single circumscribed round pleural-based mass or multiple lobulated densities overlying visceral and parietal pleura. Pleural plaques and effusion may also be present.

C. The CT appearance of malignant mesothelioma is pathognomonic and is characterized by circumferential envelopment of the lung by a lumpy pleural process. The lung eventually becomes shrunken due to complete encasement by the tumor mass.

D. Perform bronchoscopy in all patients who have a positive sputum cytology and the roentgenographic findings described above in order to rule out bronchogenic carcinoma. This diagnosis is much more likely in the setting of remote asbestos exposure if the patient has a history of smoking.

E. A diagnostic thoracentesis should always be performed if pleural fluid is present. The pleural fluid associated with malignant mesothelioma is usually thick, due to the presence of hyaluronic acid and blood. Routine cytologic examination of pleural fluid almost always yields positive results for malignancy but will not distinguish between malignant mesothelioma and metastatic primary lung adenocarcinoma or other metastatic extrathoracic carcinoma; lack of mucicarmine staining suggests mesothelioma. If a cytologic diagnosis of malignancy can be made, however, it is usually not necessary to obtain an exact diagnosis, since significant pleural extension or metastases from intrathoracic or extrathoracic neoplasms imply incurable disease. If the patient is otherwise a candidate and wishes experimental therapy, then it may be necessary to obtain tissue for a precise diagnosis.

F. If pleural fluid is not present, performance of a minithoracotomy should be considered to obtain tissue for exact diagnosis. Minithoracotomy may be accomplished with minimal morbidity by marking the chest wall over the lesion using CT guidance. Tissue may then be obtained through a small 2-inch incision.

G. Experimental treatments should be carried out at a center that specializes in this type of neoplasm. Regimens usually consist of surgical removal of the tumor and adjacent chest wall and adjuvant radiation therapy and chemotherapy.

References

England DM, Hochholzer L, McCarthy MJ. Localized benign and malignant fibrous tumors of the pleura. A clinicopathologic review of 223 cases. Am J Surg Pathol 1989; 13:640.

Kannerstein M, Churg J, McCaughey WTE. Asbestos and mesothelioma: a review. Pathol Ann 1978; 13:81.

Selikoff IJ, Churg J, Hammond FC. Relations between exposure to asbestos and mesothelioma. N Engl J Med 1965; 272:560.

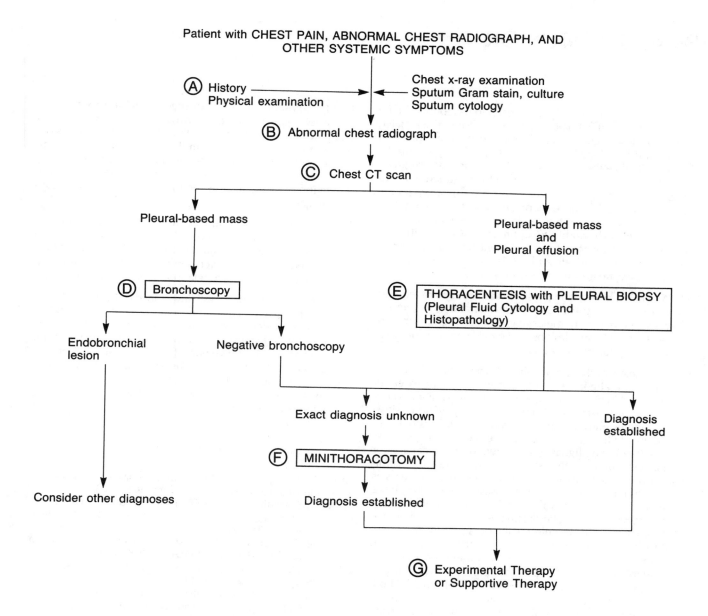

Patient with CHEST PAIN, ABNORMAL CHEST RADIOGRAPH, AND OTHER SYSTEMIC SYMPTOMS

(A) History — Physical examination

Chest x-ray examination
Sputum Gram stain, culture
Sputum cytology

(B) Abnormal chest radiograph

(C) Chest CT scan

Pleural-based mass

Pleural-based mass and Pleural effusion

(D) Bronchoscopy

(E) THORACENTESIS with PLEURAL BIOPSY (Pleural Fluid Cytology and Histopathology)

Endobronchial lesion

Negative bronchoscopy

Exact diagnosis unknown

Diagnosis established

Consider other diagnoses

(F) MINITHORACOTOMY

Diagnosis established

(G) Experimental Therapy or Supportive Therapy

PANCOAST TUMOR

Pancoast tumors are bronchogenic carcinomas located in the superior sulcus at the thoracic inlet. The tumors are associated with a syndrome consisting of shoulder pain, atrophy and pain of muscles of the hand, Horner's syndrome, and rib destruction. Unlike the case of other bronchogenic malignancies, the use of preoperative radiation to the superior sulcus prolongs survival. Patients with chest wall involvement are treated with moderate doses of preoperative irradiation (3,000 cGy). Treatment with high-dose preoperative radiation is associated with high morbidity and mortality. In the absence of chest wall involvement the treatment remains controversial. Some cases of localized lesions without chest wall involvement are treated with resection alone.

A. A detailed history and physical examination are required to diagnose the Pancoast syndrome and to detect the presence of distant metastatic lesions. The presence of possible metastatic lesions may provide an accessible site to biopsy for histologic confirmation.

B. Diagnostic evaluation involves the histologic documentation of malignancy and determination of the extent of disease. No treatment is begun before malignancy is confirmed histologically. Bronchoscopy may yield positive cytologies even though the tumor is peripherally located. In addition, a bronchoscopic evaluation helps assess whether the malignancy is limited to the apical area or has extended to other structures. The chest CT examination is necessary to evaluate mediastinal structures as well as the extent of chest wall invasion. Invasion of bone in areas contiguous with the primary tumor does not affect survival but does indicate the need for preoperative irradiation. The variable results obtained for treatment in different studies likely reflect variations in patient populations and extent of disease. Careful staging is important in order to exclude patients with distant metastases. Extensive local involvement of vertebral bodies, invasion of the subclavian artery, or significant involvement of mediastinal nodes are contraindications to surgery.

C. These tumors are often accessible to needle biopsy for diagnostic purposes. The lesions are usually located adjacent to the chest wall, which reduces the likelihood of pneumothorax. Only a limited number of patients require thoracotomy to establish the diagnosis.

D. The presence of nodal or mediastinal involvement severely reduces the long-term survival. The presence of mediastinal nodes greater than 1 cm in diameter as determined by chest CT indicates the need for mediastinoscopy to assess whether the nodes contain tumor. This procedure may also provide histologic documentation of malignancy when the bronchoscopy was nondiagnostic.

E. The presence of contralateral nodal involvement or extension of malignant cells through the capsule of the node are contraindications to surgery. Minimal ipsilateral, intranodal involvement is a relative contraindication and must be considered in relation to the individual patient.

F. Patients with chest wall invasion can be treated with preoperative radiation and surgery. The proper selection of these patients ensures reasonable results. Exclude patients with extensive chest wall invasion, such as those with vascular involvement, from aggressive therapy. In patients who are not candidates for surgery, radiation can be used for palliation. In these patients, the results of treatment are poor, and radiation alone does not prolong survival.

References

Attar S, Miller JE, Satterfield J, et al. Pancoast's tumor: irradiation or surgery. Ann Thorac Surg 1978; 28:578.

Hilaris BS, Martini N, Wong GY, Dattatreyudu N. Treatment of superior sulcus tumor (Pancoast tumor). Surgical treatment of lung carcinoma. Surg Clin North Am 1987; 67:965.

Pancoast HK. Importance of careful roentgen-ray investigation of apical chest tumors. JAMA 1924; 83:1407.

Paulson DL. Carcinoma of the superior pulmonary sulcus. J Thorac Cardiovasc Surg 1975; 70:1095.

Shahian DM, Neptune WB, Ellis FH. Pancoast tumors: improved survival with preoperative and postoperative radiation. Ann Thorac Surg 1987; 43:32.

Stanford W, Barnes RP, Tucker AR. Influence of staging in superior sulcus Pancoast tumors of the lung. Ann Thorac Surg 1979; 29:406.

Webb WR, Jeffery JD, Godwin JD. Thoracic computed tomography in superior sulcus tumors. J Comput Assist Tomogr 1981; 5:361.

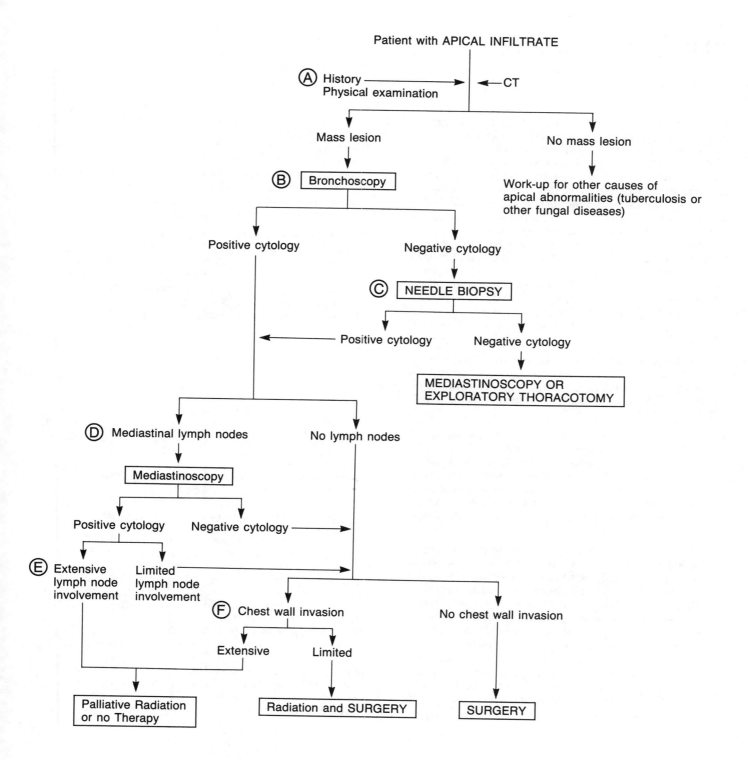

Patient with APICAL INFILTRATE

(A) History ——————→ | ←— CT
Physical examination

Mass lesion   No mass lesion

(B) Bronchoscopy

Positive cytology   Negative cytology   Work-up for other causes of
                                                    apical abnormalities (tuberculosis or
                                                    other fungal diseases)

                           (C) NEEDLE BIOPSY

                    Positive cytology   Negative cytology

                                         MEDIASTINOSCOPY OR
                                         EXPLORATORY THORACOTOMY

(D) Mediastinal lymph nodes   No lymph nodes

    Mediastinoscopy

Positive cytology   Negative cytology

(E) Extensive   Limited
lymph node   lymph node
involvement   involvement
                          (F) Chest wall invasion   No chest wall invasion

                        Extensive   Limited

Palliative Radiation   Radiation and SURGERY   SURGERY
or no Therapy

CARCINOMA IN SITU

The diagnosis of carcinoma in situ is an uncommon clinical event. Carcinoma in situ refers to the situation where certain epithelial cells have become malignant but have not invaded the subepithelial layers. This lesion is not visible on the chest film. It is occasionally detected as part of a experimental screening program for lung cancer. It is also discovered when a sputum cytology examination is performed during a routine physical examination or for pulmonary symptoms that may later turn out to be unrelated to the carcinoma. However, it should be noted that screening for lung cancer by repeated sputum cytologies is not considered to be cost effective. The approach described here evaluates the problem of positive sputum cytologies in a patient with a normal chest film. Whether the tumor is in situ or frankly invasive does not alter the diagnostic evaluation. Most of the malignancies in this group are squamous cell type and are frequently multicentric.

A. The abnormal cells may originate at any location in the tracheobronchial tree, including the upper airway. An otolaryngologic evaluation excludes upper airway pathology prior to embarking on a diagnostic work-up for pulmonary pathology.

B. Chest CT is indicated to evaluate the mediastinal nodes and to detect pulmonary masses not seen on the chest film. These include small peripheral lesions as well as larger lesions that are obscured by mediastinal structures. Small lesions require further evaluation by bronchoscopy or needle biopsy. The particular diagnostic evaluation that is selected depends on the skills available at the institution.

C. The presence of positive cytologies in the absence of radiographic evidence of a lesion requires a comprehensive bronchoscopic evaluation. If a lesion is present it should be brushed and biopsied. Questionable or subtle abnormalities should be considered potentially significant and biopsied. In the absence of a observable lesion, obtain brushing and washing samples from each lobe and analyze them separately. The presence of positive samples obtained from one lobe suggests evidence for minimally invasive malignancy or carcinoma in situ. Negative cytologies from a bronchoscopic evaluation indicate the need for an esophagoscopy to exclude a gastrointestinal malignancy.

D. In patients with negative bronchoscopic examinations, perform repeat studies after 3 months. If bronchoscopy yields a positive result, do at least two additional repeat procedures to determine whether the positive results can reproducibly be obtained from one location. Biopsies of the suspected area provide definitive evidence of location. Some centers attempt to increase the accuracy of localization using hematoporphyrin derivatives.

E. The decision to resect when positive cytologies are repeatedly obtained from one lobe without biopsy-proven malignancy is an extremely difficult judgment, which depends, in part, on the age of the patient and the overall pulmonary function. Several approaches are currently under investigation including photoradiation therapy with hematoporphyrin derivatives.

References

Hayata Y, Kato H, Konaka C, et al. Photoradiation therapy with hematoporphyrin derivative in early and stage I lung cancer. Chest 1984; 86:169.

Kinsey JH, Cortese DA, Sanderson DR. Detection of hematoporphyrin derivative during fiberoptic bronchoscopy to localize early bronchogenic cancer. Mayo Clin Proc 1978; 53:594.

Martini N, Melamed MR. Occult cancers of the lung. Ann Thorac Surg 1980; 30:215.

Melamed MR, Zaman MB, Flehingger BJ, Martini N. Radiologically occult in situ and incipient invasive epidermoid lung cancer: detection by sputum cytology in a survey of asymptomatic cigarette smokers. Am J Surg Pathol 1977; 1:5.

Tao LC, Chamberlain DW, Delarue NC, Pearson FG, Donat EE. Cytological diagnosis of radiologically occult squamous cell carcinoma of the lung. Cancer 1982; 50:1580.

Tyers GFO, McGavran MH. Diagnostic challenges following cytologic diagnosis of in situ cancer of the lung. Chest 1976; 69:33.

Woolner LB, Fantana RS, Cortese DA, et al. Roentgenographically occult lung cancer: pathologic finding and frequency of multicentric during a 10 year period. Mayo Clin Proc 1984; 59:453.

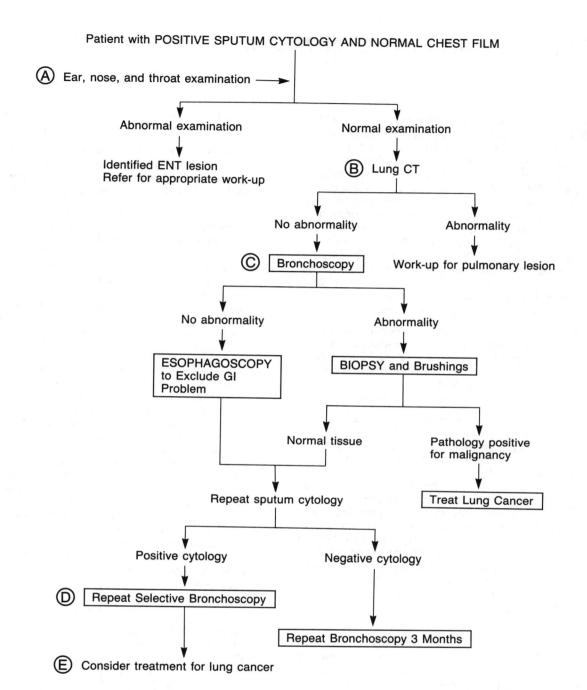

Patient with POSITIVE SPUTUM CYTOLOGY AND NORMAL CHEST FILM

(A) Ear, nose, and throat examination ⟶

Abnormal examination   Normal examination

Identified ENT lesion   (B) Lung CT
Refer for appropriate work-up

                          No abnormality   Abnormality

                    (C) Bronchoscopy   Work-up for pulmonary lesion

        No abnormality   Abnormality

ESOPHAGOSCOPY   BIOPSY and Brushings
to Exclude GI
Problem

                    Normal tissue   Pathology positive
                                           for malignancy

                    Repeat sputum cytology   Treat Lung Cancer

Positive cytology   Negative cytology

(D) Repeat Selective Bronchoscopy

                    Repeat Bronchoscopy 3 Months

(E) Consider treatment for lung cancer

SUPERIOR VENA CAVA SYNDROME

A. Patients usually present complaining of a feeling of head fullness that is sometimes accompanied by headache. Other common complaints include dyspnea, cough, syncope, dysphagia, hemoptysis, and swollen arms. Less common complaints, which occur in the setting of cerebral edema, include vertigo, visual disturbances, and depressed mentation and levels of consciousness. Physical examination reveals dilated neck veins, prominent thoracic venous pattern, and facial and arm edema. Cyanosis is common. The diagnosis can be made with a high degree of specificity at the bedside. In patients who have central venous catheters and who acutely develop the superior vena cava (SVC) syndrome, remove the catheters immediately to avoid progression of associated thrombosis, and reroute all pacemaker wires.

B. About two-thirds of all cases show mediastinal widening on the chest radiograph. Other findings include right hilar mass, pleural effusion, right upper lobe atelectasis, infiltrates, and anterior mediastinal mass. A normal chest film does not exclude the diagnosis if appropriate historical and physical findings are present.

C. If no abnormalities are seen on routine chest radiographs, other imaging procedures must be done to locate the pathology. These include CT of the thorax with or without contrast enhancement, superior vena caval venography, and MRI. When performed with contrast, the CT appearance of SVC obstruction is pathognomonic and is characterized by luminal compression of the SVC often accompanied by intraluminal thrombosis. SVC venography can be dangerous when venous pressure in the upper extremities and head is equal to or greater than 200 mm Hg and should therefore be employed with strict caution in such patients. The effectiveness of magnetic resonance scanning in this instance is still under investigation. If no pathologic abnormalities are seen with these imaging techniques, a nonmalignant etiology of SVC syndrome is likely.

D. Treatment of nonmalignant causes of the superior vena cava syndrome is mainly symptomatic, consisting of medical regimens. Aortic aneurysms may be surgically correctable and large goiters may be removed. Inflammatory disease may be treated with corticosteroids.

E. If a lesion is visualized, the diagnosis may be made by bronchoscopy (20 to 40 percent of all cases). This relatively noninvasive procedure is indicated in all cases where malignancy is suspected. It should be done to stage the patient even if the diagnosis has been made by sputum cytology.

F. If the results of the bronchoscopy are negative, other more invasive procedures must be done to make the diagnosis. These procedures include open-lung biopsy or mediastinoscopy with biopsy of lymph nodes.

G. Two-thirds of all cases of SVC syndrome are caused by neoplastic disease. Carcinoma of the lung is the leading cause of this syndrome; undifferentiated large cell, squamous cell, and small cell lung carcinoma are the most common cell types found. Breast carcinoma, lymphoma, and metastatic thymoma or testicular carcinoma metastatic to the mediastinum are other etiologies. Nonmalignant causes include fibrotic mediastinal disease, thrombosis of the SVC due to venous lines, large goiters, aortic aneurysms, and inflammatory disease of the mediastinal nodes.

H. The prognosis of SVC syndrome caused by malignant nonlymphomatous disease is poor, with an average survival of less than 1 year. However, symptoms may be ameliorated by surgical, radiotherapeutic, or chemotherapeutic means depending on the etiology. Surgical spinal vein bypass grafting is possible in some carefully selected cases, as is balloon angioplasty. These patients have almost complete or complete obstruction of the SVC with either antegrade flow in the azygous–right atrial path or reversal of azygous flow. Treat surgical bypass patients as well as all other cases of SVC syndrome caused by malignant disease on an emergent basis with radiotherapy alone or with a combination of radiation and chemotherapy. Treat obstruction caused by small cell carcinoma of the lung with emergency combined-agent chemotherapy, since this neoplasm is extremely chemosensitive.

References

Ali MK, Ewer MS, Balakrishnan PV, et al. Balloon angioplasty for superior vena cava syndrome. Ann Intern Med 1987; 107:856.

Lochridge SK, Knibbe P, Doty DB. Obstruction of the superior vena cava. Surgery 1979; 85:14.

Parish JM, Marschke RF Jr, Dines DE, Lee RE. Etiologic considerations in superior vena cava syndrome. Mayo Clin Proc 1981; 56:407.

Stanford W, Doty DB. The role of venography and surgery in the management of patients with superior vena cava obstruction. Ann Thorac Surg 1986; 41:158.

Patient with HEADACHE, FEELING OF HEAD FULLNESS, VERTIGO, SWOLLEN ARMS

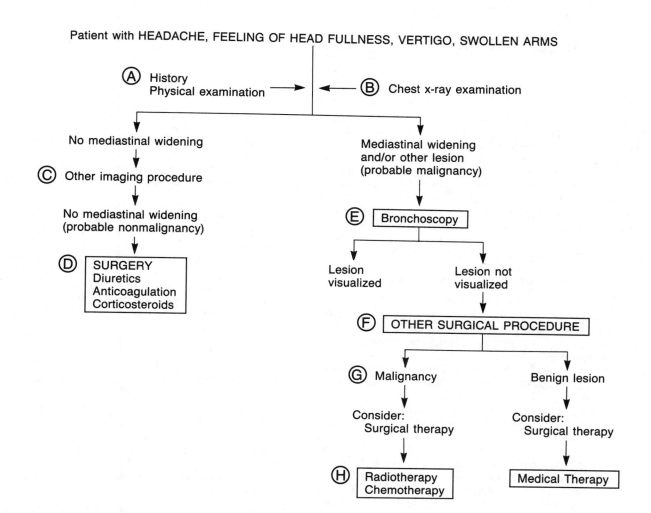

MULTIPLE PULMONARY NODULES

Most multiple lung nodules occur as hematogenous metastases in patients with known primary malignancies. Other conditions associated with multiple pulmonary nodules include infectious and *parasitic etiologies* such as tuberculosis, histoplasmosis, varicella pneumonia, septic pulmonary emboli, lung abscesses, echinococcosis (hydatid disease), dirofilariasis, and paragonimiasis; *immunologic and inflammatory etiologies* such as sarcoidosis, silicosis, rheumatoid arthritis, and Wegener's granulomatosis; *neoplastic diseases* such as non-Hodgkin's lymphoma, alveolar cell carcinoma, and atrial myxoma; and *other conditions* such as amyloidosis, arteriovenous fistula, hamartoma, intrapulmonary lymph nodes, and drug toxicity (bleomycin).

A. The history and physical examination are important to narrow the diagnostic possibilities. Since neoplastic metastases are the most common cause of multiple nodules, a thorough history and physical examination should be performed to exclude the presence of a primary neoplasm. Physical findings are highly variable and depend on the etiology of the nodules. Patients with granulomas caused by previous histoplasmosis are likely to be asymptomatic. Upper respiratory signs and symptoms are almost always present in patients with Wegener's granulomatosis. High fever, appearance of toxicity, and physical evidence of intravenous drug abuse may be found in patients with multiple septic emboli. Rheumatoid nodules over the extensor surfaces of extremities may be found in patients with rheumatoid arthritis; pulmonary nodules in these patients should not be assumed to be benign.

B. The radiographic appearance of pulmonary nodules often provides diagnostic clues as to the etiology. Nodules caused by metastases and non-Hodgkin's lymphoma are likely to be round, well circumscribed, and numerous (often more than 10); the size of these nodules may vary from 3 mm to 6 cm (many are larger than 2.5 cm), and they are more likely to be found in the lower lung fields. Small upper lung nodules are more likely to be seen in tuberculosis, sarcoidosis, silicosis, and eosinophilic granuloma. Sarcoidosis is often associated with hilar and mediastinal lymphadenopathy. Nodules caused by Wegener's granuloma range in size from 5 mm to 9 cm, tend to cavitate, and are distributed widely throughout the lung. Nodules caused by arteriovenous fistulas are more likely to be found in the lower lobes; they are variable in size and shape, are not calcified, and may cause hypoxemia and produce a bruit. Multiple pulmonary nodules may be seen in approximately 20 percent of patients with histoplasmosis; two-thirds of these nodules are calcified. Coccidiodomycosis and histoplas-

mosis nodules range in size between 0.5 and 3 cm; they appear round and well circumscribed and are sometimes calcified, and they have a predilection for upper lung fields. Comparisons with previous chest films will aid in determining the acuteness of the disease process. Rapidly growing nodules suggest metastases or infection.

C. The initial laboratory evaluation is guided by the history and findings on the physical examination. Septic pulmonary emboli due to endocarditis or other sources are frequently apparent and can readily be diagnosed by blood cultures; echocardiography can be used to detect valvular vegetation. Sputum evaluation should be performed to exclude active tuberculosis. Sputum cytology may reveal the presence of malignant cells. The urinalysis is frequently abnormal in patients with Wegener's granulomatosis.

D. Hematogenous metastases are the most common cause of multiple pulmonary nodules in patients with a history of extrapulmonary malignancy. Infections should be excluded in the initial evaluation. If the confirmation of metastases is important or alters management, fiberoptic bronchoscopy should be performed.

E. Patients without a definitive diagnosis should undergo further investigation. Chest CT often identifies nodules not apparent on plain chest films and provides a more accurate assessment of nodule size and other characteristics.

F. Fiberoptic bronchoscopy with transbronchial biopsy provides a diagnosis for most patients. The remaining patients should be considered for an open-lung biopsy. Work-up for a primary neoplasm should be initiated in patients found to have pulmonary metastases without a prior history of malignancy.

References

Connell JV, Muhm JR. Radiographic manifestations of pulmonary histoplasmosis: a 10-year review. Radiology 1976; 121:281.

Gross BH, Glazer GM, Bookstein FL. Multiple pulmonary nodules detected by computed tomography: diagnostic implications. J Comput Tomogr 1985; 9:880.

Jolles H, Moseley PL, Peterson MW. Nodular pulmonary opacities in patients with rheumatoid arthritis. A diagnostic dilemma. Chest 1989; 96:1022.

Kalifa LG, Schimmel DH, Gamsu G. Multiple chronic benign pulmonary nodules. Radiology 1976; 121:275.

Lillington GA. Pulmonary nodules: solitary and multiple. Clin Chest Med 1982; 3:361.

MULTIPLE PULMONARY NODULES Suspected

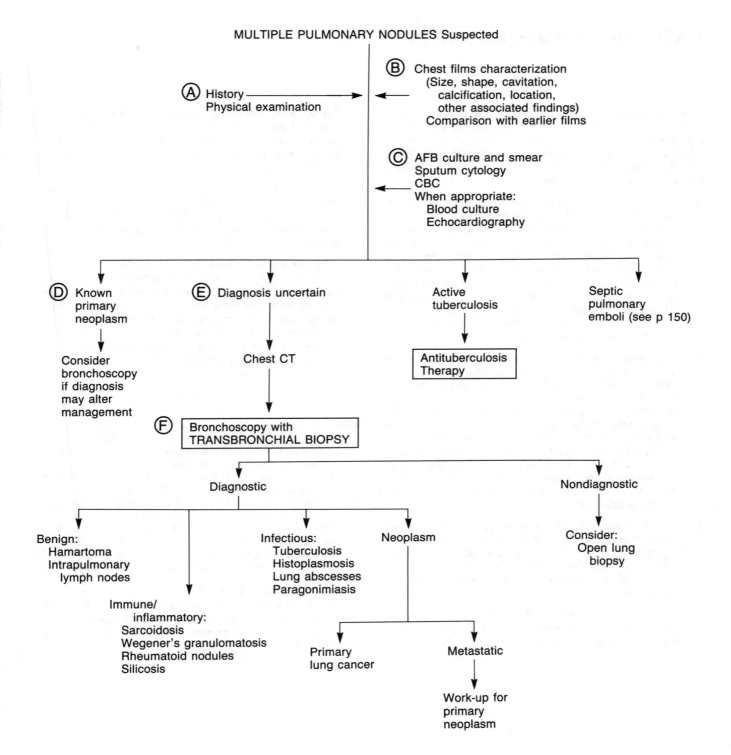

Ⓐ History
Physical examination

Ⓑ Chest films characterization
(Size, shape, cavitation,
calcification, location,
other associated findings)
Comparison with earlier films

Ⓒ AFB culture and smear
Sputum cytology
CBC
When appropriate:
Blood culture
Echocardiography

Ⓓ Known
primary
neoplasm

Consider
bronchoscopy
if diagnosis
may alter
management

Ⓔ Diagnosis uncertain

Chest CT

Active
tuberculosis

Antituberculosis
Therapy

Septic
pulmonary
emboli (see p 150)

Ⓕ Bronchoscopy with
TRANSBRONCHIAL BIOPSY

Diagnostic

Nondiagnostic

Benign:
Hamartoma
Intrapulmonary
lymph nodes

Infectious:
Tuberculosis
Histoplasmosis
Lung abscesses
Paragonimiasis

Neoplasm

Consider:
Open lung
biopsy

Immune/
inflammatory:
Sarcoidosis
Wegener's granulomatosis
Rheumatoid nodules
Silicosis

Primary
lung cancer

Metastatic

Work-up for
primary
neoplasm

RADIATION PNEUMONITIS

The acute effects of radiation generally begin 1 to 2 months after the initiation of radiation and may progress rapidly to a fatal outcome even if corticosteroids are used. The chronic effects of radiation begin 4 to 6 months after the completion of radiotherapy and are primarily vascular in nature. The injury may respond to corticosteroids.

A. The patient gives a history of intrathoracic neoplasm that was treated with radiation. Patients may present with dyspnea on exertion and cough, which may be due to an associated radiation pharyngitis, or dysphagia, which may be due to radiation esophagitis. Hemoptysis does not occur unless intrabronchial neoplasm is present. Patients may have fever, which is usually low-grade unless a bacterial infection has occurred distal to an obstructed airway. Physical examination of the chest reveals decreased breath sounds over the area of radiation. Fine expiratory rales may be heard.

B. Chest x-ray examination reveals the presence of an infiltrate, which may not be confined to the area of the radiation portal. A clear line of demarcation separating irradiated from nonirradiated lung may not be seen until fibrosis has occurred. It may be difficult to distinguish a mass within the infiltrate; thus, the diagnosis of recurrent neoplasm may not always be made from the chest x-ray examination. Analysis of arterial blood gas (ABG) may reveal hypoxemia, and pulmonary function reveals a restrictive defect. Examine sputum to rule out infection. Measure the diffusing capacity and use the results to follow effectiveness of treatment.

C. Bronchoscopy will rule out recurrence of neoplasm and ensure that the airway to the involved segment of lung is patent. If a mass is visualized, brushings and biopsies will confirm that the cytology of the lesion is the same as the original lung cancer, so that further therapy can be planned.

D. Depending on the dosage of radiation used to treat the initial neoplasm, recurrent obstructing bronchial lesions may be treated with additional radiation therapy once the radiation pneumonitis has cleared. However, when patients have received the full dose, laser therapy can be used to open the airway quickly and effectively. This therapy may be repeated over several days and can be used chronically.

E. Treat radiation pneumonitis with corticosteroids given either parenterally or orally and with antibiotics for possible infectious colonization or infection of the involved lung. Antibiotic coverage should include drugs effective against anaerobic organisms.

F. If no neoplastic lesion is present and the pneumonitis has not cleared, larger doses of parenteral corticosteroids may be used. In this situation it is unlikely that any significant improvement in pulmonary function or in the radiographic characteristics will occur. Improvement may be limited to pulmonary symptoms only. Persistent pulmonary infiltrates following radiation therapy indicate irreversible fibrotic changes in the pulmonary parenchyma.

References

Botterman J, Tasson J, Schelstraete K, et al. Scintigraphic, spirometric, and roentgenologic effects of radiotherapy on normal lung tissue. Short-term observations in 14 consecutive patients with breast cancer. Chest 1990; 97:97.

Duane P. Pulmonary insults due to transfusions, radiation, and hyperoxia. Sem Respir Infect 1988; 3:240.

Rubin P, McDonald S, Maasilta P, et al. Serum markers for prediction of pulmonary radiation syndromes. Part I: Surfactant apoprotein. Int J Radiat Oncol Biol Phys 1989; 17:553.

Tillman BF, Loyd JE, Malcolm AW, Holm BA, Brigham KL. Unilateral radiation pneumonitis in sheep: physiological changes and bronchoalveolar lavage. J Appl Physiol 1989; 66:1273.

Wechsler RJ, Ayyangar K, Steiner RM, Yelovich R, Moylan DM. The development of distant pulmonary infiltrates following thoracic irradiation: the role of computed tomography with dosimetric reconstruction in diagnosis. Comput Med Imag Graph 1990; 14:43.

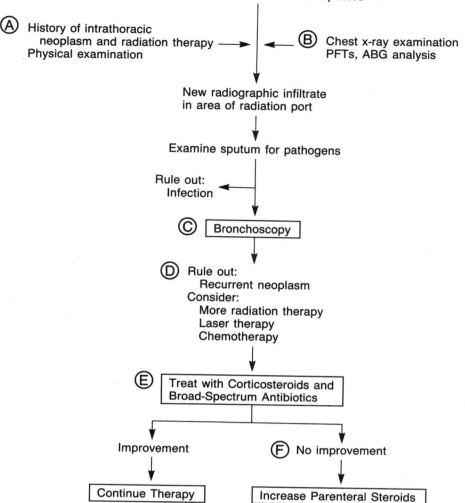

RADIATION PNEUMONITIS Suspected

Ⓐ History of intrathoracic
neoplasm and radiation therapy ——→ ←—— Ⓑ Chest x-ray examination
Physical examination   PFTs, ABG analysis

New radiographic infiltrate
in area of radiation port

Examine sputum for pathogens

Rule out: ←
Infection

Ⓒ Bronchoscopy

Ⓓ Rule out:
    Recurrent neoplasm
  Consider:
    More radiation therapy
    Laser therapy
    Chemotherapy

Ⓔ Treat with Corticosteroids and
   Broad-Spectrum Antibiotics

Improvement   Ⓕ No improvement

Continue Therapy   Increase Parenteral Steroids

INFECTIOUS DISEASES OF THE LUNG, PLEURA, AND AIRWAY

Calcified Pulmonary Lesions
Middle Lobe Syndrome
Acute Bronchitis
Community-Acquired Pneumonia
Pneumococcal Pneumonia
Recurrent Bacterial Pneumonia
Anaerobic Lung Infections
Pulmonary Involvement in Patients with
  Acquired Immunodeficiency Sydrome
Nosocomial Pneumonia

Legionnaires' Disease
Pneumocystis carinii Pneumonia
Lung Abscess
Air-Fluid Level in Bullae
Empyema
Pulmonary Infiltrates in the (Non-AIDS)
  Immunocompromised Host
Acute Epiglottitis
Mediastinitis

CALCIFIED PULMONARY LESIONS

The majority of calcified pulmonary lesions represent dystrophic or healing processes, although bronchogenic carcinomas are sometimes associated with calcifications (scar carcinoma). Metastatic calcifications may also occur in patients with longstanding hypercalcemia or chronic renal failure. Calcified pulmonary lesions can be categorized into four groups; solitary calcified nodules, diffuse or multiple parenchymal calcifications, calcified lymph nodes, and pleural calcifications.

A. The history may aid the diagnosis of calcified pulmonary lesions. Ask about a history of travel, past residence, and exposures to asbestos, silica, and other mineral dusts. A past medical history of empyema, hemothorax, histoplasmosis, tuberculosis, or varicella pneumonia may suggest the diagnosis. There are no specific physical findings that differentiate the various calcified pulmonary lesions, although physical examination may identify patients with mitral stenosis or evidence of chronic renal failure. Patients with diffuse interstitial lung diseases caused by silicosis and asbestosis may have symptoms of chronic nonproductive cough, dyspnea, and clubbing of fingers.

B. Solitary nodules in the lung parenchyma are the most common calcified pulmonary lesions and most likely represent a healed granulomatous process that was caused by histoplasmosis or tuberculosis. Histoplasmosis often produces calcified laminar layers; these are pathognomonic. Another cause of solitary calcified pulmonary lesions is hamartoma, which produces a characteristic "popcorn" type of calcification. Eccentrically calcified nodules should raise the suspicion of malignancy, because these are often associated with scar carcinoma.

C. In patients with severe mitral stenosis, recurrent hemoptysis may result in deposits of hemosiderin in the lungs, and calcifications may occur as a result. The lower lung fields are most likely to be involved. Histoplasmosis, disseminated pulmonary tuberculosis, and varicella pneumonia may produce diffuse nodular calcifications. Calcifications caused by previous histoplasmosis infection may also be found in spleen, liver, and adrenals.

D. Lymph node calcifications are generally amorphous and distributed irregularly within the node. Amorphous lymph node calcifications are most often healed granulomas caused by tuberculosis and histoplasmosis. Eggshell calcifications are less common and have been found to be associated with silicosis, pneumoconiosis, sarcoidosis, and postirradiation Hodgkin's disease; they have been rarely seen in patients with scleroderma, blastomycosis, or histoplasmosis. Eggshell calcification is defined as shell-like calcifications up to 2 mm thick present in the peripheral zone of at least two lymph nodes; the calcifications may be solid or broken, but in at least one of the lymph nodes, the ringlike shadow must be complete. The central part of the lymph node may show additional calcifications, and one of the affected lymph nodes must be at least 1 cm in its greatest diameter.

E. Pleural calcifications are often caused by a remote hemothorax, pyothorax, or tuberculous effusion. The pleura is often thickened over the entire surface of the involved lung. The calcifications typically occur over the visceral surface and may appear as a continuous sheet or multiple plaques. Silicatosis, talcosis, and asbestosis typically produce calcifications along the parietal pleura with plaques forming along the diaphragm.

References

Gross BH, Schneider HJ, Proto AV. Eggshell calcification of lymph nodes: an update. AJR 1980; 135:1265.

Rosenthal DI, Chandler HL, Azizi F, Schneider PB. Uptake of bone imaging agents by diffuse pulmonary metastatic calcification. Am J Roentgenol 1977; 129:871.

Patient with CALCIFIED PULMONARY LESIONS

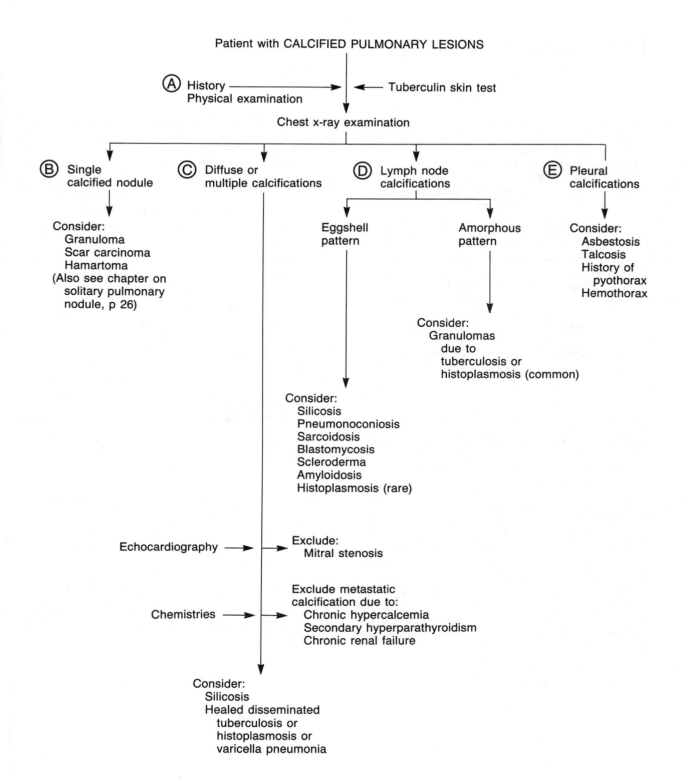

Ⓐ History ──────────→ ←── Tuberculin skin test
Physical examination

Chest x-ray examination

Ⓑ Single calcified nodule

Ⓒ Diffuse or multiple calcifications

Ⓓ Lymph node calcifications

Ⓔ Pleural calcifications

Consider:
  Granuloma
  Scar carcinoma
  Hamartoma
(Also see chapter on
  solitary pulmonary
  nodule, p 26)

Eggshell pattern

Amorphous pattern

Consider:
  Asbestosis
  Talcosis
  History of
    pyothorax
  Hemothorax

Consider:
  Granulomas
  due to
  tuberculosis or
  histoplasmosis (common)

Consider:
  Silicosis
  Pneumonoconiosis
  Sarcoidosis
  Blastomycosis
  Scleroderma
  Amyloidosis
  Histoplasmosis (rare)

Echocardiography ──────→ Exclude:
  Mitral stenosis

Chemistries ──────→ Exclude metastatic
  calcification due to:
    Chronic hypercalcemia
    Secondary hyperparathyroidism
    Chronic renal failure

Consider:
  Silicosis
  Healed disseminated
    tuberculosis or
    histoplasmosis or
    varicella pneumonia

MIDDLE LOBE SYNDROME

The definition of middle lobe syndrome has evolved since it was first described in 1948 and is now used to delineate various degrees of right middle lobe or lingular atelectasis or consolidation. It is due to various causes. In some patients, the right middle lobe is believed to be especially susceptible to atelectasis because of a lengthy right mainstem bronchus and the acute angle of takeoff of the middle lobe bronchus. Enlargement of peribronchial lymph nodes due to acute or chronic inflammation and fibrosis contributes to the development of this condition. In some cases, total separation of the middle lobe from the remainder of lung parenchyma by complete minor fissures results in a lack of collateral ventilation, predisposing these patients to right middle lobe atelectasis. Infectious processes are the most common pathologic etiology and are found in 40 to 60 percent of all patients; neoplastic lesions are found in 20 to 40 percent of cases. Actual obstruction is found in about half of all patients during bronchoscopy; the resulting recurrent infections and atelectasis may cause a nonfunctional lobe.

A. Recurrent pneumonia is the most common presentation of middle lobe syndrome. Hemoptysis and pleuritic chest pain may be present in about half of these patients. The underlying cause of the atelectasis dictates any additional signs and symptoms that may be observed. Other etiologies include sarcoidosis, tuberculosis (Brock's syndrome), bronchogenic carcinoma, bronchiectasis, and esophageal diverticula.

B. Routine laboratory evaluation of sputum is aimed at identifying the etiologic organism causing pneumonia and at excluding tuberculosis. Sputum cytologies should be performed to exclude bronchogenic carcinoma.

C. Standard posteroanterior and lateral chest films identify the atelectasis. The frontal view may show an ill-defined infiltrate obscuring the adjacent right (or left) heart border. The atelectatic right middle lobe characteristically appears as a wedge-shaped density overlying the heart on the lateral view. Chest films may reveal large neoplastic lesions that cause the atelectasis.

D. The atelectasis resolves in many patients after a course of broad-spectrum antibiotics coupled with chest physio-therapy. When this therapy fails, perform chest CT, which may identify obstructing intrabronchial lesions or mucus directly producing atelectasis or lesions that are externally compressing the affected mainstem bronchus.

E. All patients with middle lobe atelectasis that does not quickly resolve with antibiotics and bronchodilators or with atelectasis that is recurrent in the same lobe should undergo bronchoscopy to exclude obstructing endobronchial lesions.

F. If atelectasis persists and no lesions are present, continue treatment with antibiotics and chest physiotherapy. Recurrent atelectasis and pneumonia may occur.

G. Patients who do not respond to medical therapy, those without evidence of obstructive lesions on chest computed tomography, and those who require fiberoptic bronchoscopy should be periodically followed with repeated imaging studies (chest films, CT). Patients with complete bronchial obstruction, those with bronchiectasis due to chronic infection, with or without hemoptysis, and those who have significant parenchymal damage should be considered for surgical resection of the involved lobe.

References

Bertelsen S. Isolated middle lobe atelectasis: aetiology, pathogenesis, and treatment of the so-called middle lobe syndrome. Thorax 1980; 35:449.

Inners CR, Terry PB, Traystman RJ, Menkes HA. Collateral ventilation and the middle lobe syndrome. Am Rev Resp Dis 1978; 118:305.

Rosenbloom SA, Ravin CE, Putman CE, et al. Peripheral middle lobe syndrome. Radiology 1983; 149:17.

Saha SP, Mayo P, Long GA, McElvein RB. Middle lobe syndrome: diagnosis and management. Ann Thorac Surg 1982; 33:28.

Wagner RB, Johnston MR. Middle lobe syndrome. Ann Thorac Surg 1983; 35:679.

Patient with MIDDLE LOBE SYNDROME

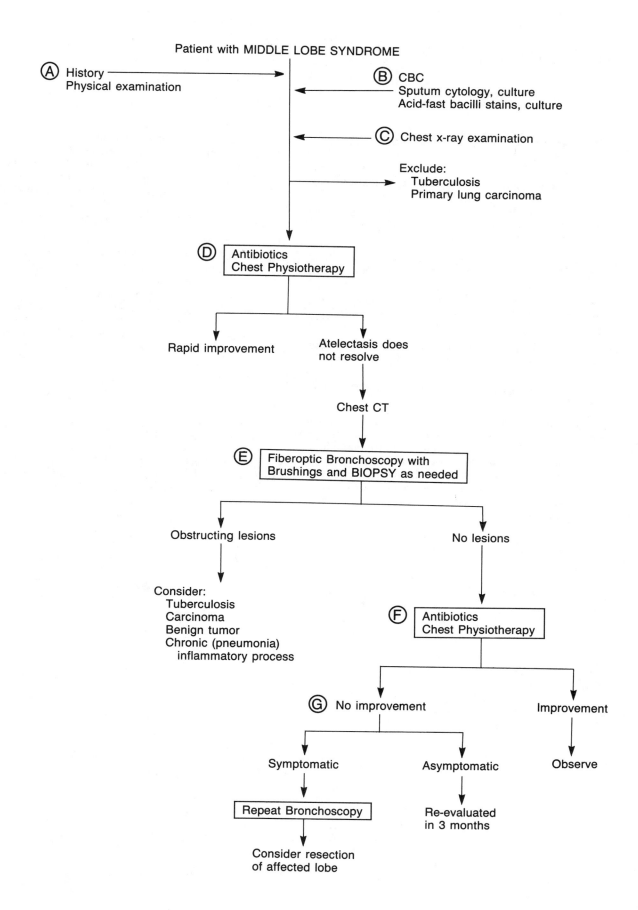

A History
   Physical examination

B CBC
   Sputum cytology, culture
   Acid-fast bacilli stains, culture

C Chest x-ray examination

Exclude:
   Tuberculosis
   Primary lung carcinoma

D Antibiotics
   Chest Physiotherapy

Rapid improvement   Atelectasis does
                           not resolve

Chest CT

E Fiberoptic Bronchoscopy with
   Brushings and BIOPSY as needed

Obstructing lesions   No lesions

Consider:
   Tuberculosis
   Carcinoma
   Benign tumor   F Antibiotics
   Chronic (pneumonia)   Chest Physiotherapy
      inflammatory process

                         G No improvement   Improvement

Symptomatic   Asymptomatic   Observe

Repeat Bronchoscopy   Re-evaluated
                      in 3 months

Consider resection
of affected lobe

ACUTE BRONCHITIS

Acute bronchitis in otherwise healthy patients is a self-limiting disease often with a viral etiology. It generally lasts for 1 to 2 weeks, although occasionally it may last longer than a month. Because acute bronchitis is primarily viral in origin, the diagnostic approach is aimed at excluding other conditions such as bacterial pneumonias and influenza A infections. The use of antibiotics in the treatment of acute bronchitis is controversial, and there have not been adequate clinical trials to demonstrate its efficacy.

A. Acute bronchitis presents with acute onset of cough, frequently productive of clear or purulent sputum. Low-grade fever and night sweats as well as other symptoms of upper respiratory tract infections such as sore throat are also common findings. Bronchospasm may be present in some patients.

B. There are no specific radiographic findings in patients with acute bronchitis. The primary purpose of the chest x-ray examination is to exclude pneumonia in patients with fever and pulmonary findings on physical examination.

C. Influenza A virus epidemic is generally confined to winter months. During the epidemic season for influenza A, amantadine therapy should be considered for patients with acute bronchitis, especially elderly patients who are at increased risk for morbidity. The timely use of amantadine could significantly reduce the morbidity of the symptoms and prevent the development of influenza A pneumonia.

D. Sputum analysis is of limited value in the diagnosis of acute bronchitis, although it may be useful to detect early pneumonias. A clinically significant sputum Gram stain on an uncontaminated specimen would contain more than five polymorphonuclear leukocytes and a single predominating organism. Sputum from most patients with acute bronchitis typically has five or less polymorphonuclear leukocytes per high-power field.

E. Elderly patients, those with comorbidity factors such as congestive heart failure or diabetes mellitus, and patients with significant sputum may be considered for antibiotic therapy. Antibiotics that have been used to treat acute bronchitis include ampicillin, erythromycin, tetracycline, and trimethoprim-sulfamethoxazole. Patients without comorbidities or those who have insignificant sputum could be treated symptomatically with cough suppressants and bronchodilators if needed.

References

Ellner JJ. Management of acute and chronic respiratory tract infections. Am J Med 1988; 85(Suppl 3A):2

Gleckman RA. Bronchial infections: acute bronchitis and acute exacerbation in chronic bronchitis. Compr Ther 1987; 13:44.

Rodnick JE, Gude JK. The use of antibiotics in acute bronchitis and acute exacerbations of chronic bronchitis. West J Med 1988; 149:347.

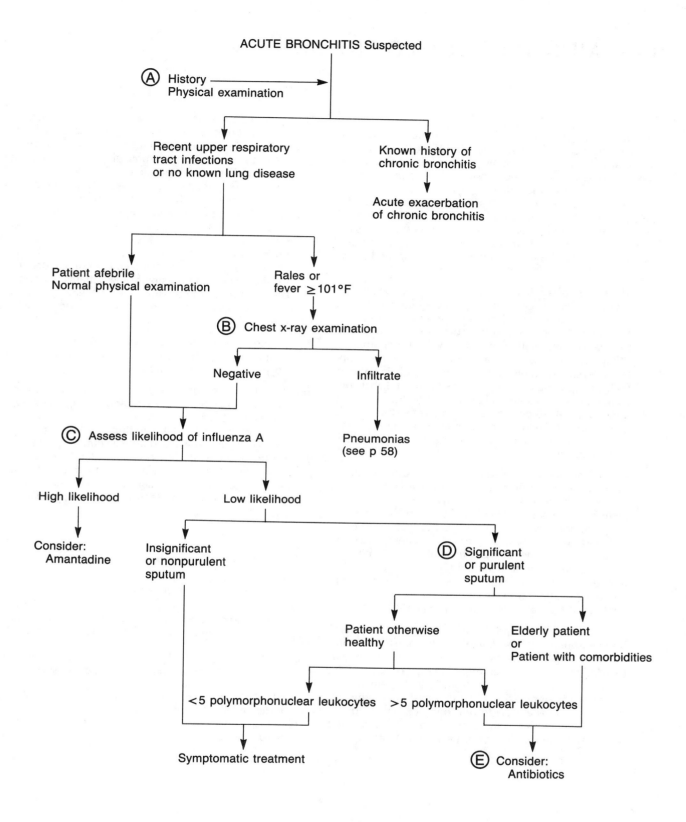

ACUTE BRONCHITIS Suspected

(A) History
Physical examination

Recent upper respiratory
tract infections
or no known lung disease

Known history of
chronic bronchitis

Acute exacerbation
of chronic bronchitis

Patient afebrile
Normal physical examination

Rales or
fever ≥101°F

(B) Chest x-ray examination

Negative

Infiltrate

(C) Assess likelihood of influenza A

Pneumonias
(see p 58)

High likelihood

Low likelihood

Consider:
Amantadine

Insignificant
or nonpurulent
sputum

(D) Significant
or purulent
sputum

Patient otherwise
healthy

Elderly patient
or
Patient with comorbidities

<5 polymorphonuclear leukocytes

>5 polymorphonuclear leukocytes

Symptomatic treatment

(E) Consider:
Antibiotics

COMMUNITY-ACQUIRED PNEUMONIA

Community-acquired pneumonia arises in a broad spectrum of patients, is caused by a wide variety of infectious agents, and is associated with a myriad of clinical presentations. Patients range from normal healthy young adults to debilitated nursing home residents. The prevalences of various etiologic microorganisms are difficult to estimate because most studies are performed on patients who are hospitalized. The predominant etiologic organism is *Pneumococcus*, followed by *Mycoplasma* and viruses. Other common organisms include *Haemophilus influenzae*, *Staphylococcus*, gram-negative bacteria, *Legionella*, anaerobic bacteria, and tuberculosis.

A. The history of sudden onset with rigor, high fever, cough productive of rust-colored sputum, pleuritic chest pain, and a preceding upper respiratory infection along with the physical findings of lobar consolidation constitute the classic presentation of pneumococcal pneumonia. Many patients, however, have variations of these symptoms. *Mycoplasma* pneumonia is more likely in patients with a nonproductive cough and a sore throat. Lobar consolidation is less likely, and bullous myringitis occurs in approximately 20 percent of patients with *Mycoplasma* pneumonia. Influenza virus pneumonia occurs during epidemic seasons and causes high fever, cough, headache, and diffuse myalgia.

B. Chest films are not particularly useful in differentiating the types of pneumonia, although they are essential for assessing the extent of parenchymal involvement and identifying the presence of pleural effusion. Pneumococcal pneumonia typically produces homogeneous consolidation with air-bronchogram; this pattern, however, is not universal. The radiographic features of *Mycoplasma* pneumonia are also variable, including patchy infiltrates and mixed interstitial and alveolar patterns. Radiographic findings may be absent in dehydrated patients until they are adequately hydrated.

C. Debilitated patients and those with significant comorbidities should be hospitalized. Intravenous fluids, antibiotics, oxygen, and other supportive measures should be administered. Reported mortality rates of patients requiring hospitalization range from 10 to 25 percent. Patients with significant pleural effusion require a diagnostic thoracentesis to rule out empyema. Obtain early blood cultures as these may be positive and diagnostic when sputum cultures are unrevealing.

D. Sputum Gram stain is important to guide the initial selection of antibiotics. An adequate sputum specimen should contain 25 or more white blood cells and few epithelial cells. A sputum specimen containing many gram-positive diplococci and polymorphic neutrophils is virtually diagnostic of pneumococcal pneumonia. Penicillin or erythromycin would be the appropriate antibiotics in this case. A sputum of predominant pleomorphic gram-negative rods suggests *Haemophilus influenzae*, especially if the patient has a history of chronic obstructive pulmonary disease. Gram-negative bacteria and mouth anaerobes should be considered as etiologic organisms for debilitated and nursing home patients. During epidemic seasons, the possibility of influenza pneumonia must be considered, since amantadine therapy could be effective.

E. Empiric therapy based on clinical presentation, patient characteristics, and sputum examination should be started prior to culture results.

F. The clinical response to antibiotics and supportive therapy must be closely followed and management adjusted as necessary. Sputum culture results should be interpreted in light of the findings on the sputum Gram stains. Organisms isolated from a sputum specimen that do not show white blood cells on the Gram stain are more likely to be upper airway or mouth contaminants. Monitor patients with influenza viral pneumonia for possible development of *Staphylococcus* superinfection.

References

Atmar RL, Greenberg SB. Pneumonia caused by *Mycoplasma* pneumoniae and the TWAR agent. Semin Respir Infect 1989; 4:19.

Marrie TJ, Durant H, Yates L. Community-acquired pneumonia requiring hospitalization: 5-year prospective study. Rev Infect Dis 1989; 11:586.

McKellar PP. Treatment of community-acquired pneumonias. Am J Med 1985; 79(Suppl 2A):25.

Sullivan CJ, Jordan MC. Diagnosis of viral pneumonia. Semin Respir Infect 1988; 3:148.

Patient with COMMUNITY-ACQUIRED PNEUMONIA

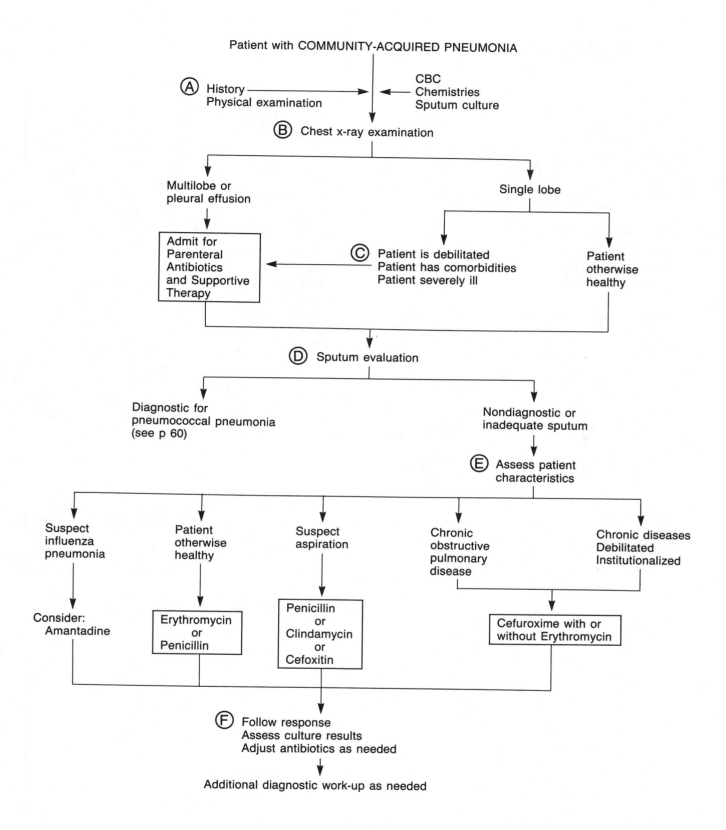

(A) History ——— CBC
Physical examination ←——— Chemistries
Sputum culture

(B) Chest x-ray examination

Multilobe or pleural effusion

Single lobe

Admit for Parenteral Antibiotics and Supportive Therapy

(C) Patient is debilitated
Patient has comorbidities
Patient severely ill

Patient otherwise healthy

(D) Sputum evaluation

Diagnostic for pneumococcal pneumonia (see p 60)

Nondiagnostic or inadequate sputum

(E) Assess patient characteristics

Suspect influenza pneumonia

Patient otherwise healthy

Suspect aspiration

Chronic obstructive pulmonary disease

Chronic diseases Debilitated Institutionalized

Consider: Amantadine

Erythromycin or Penicillin

Penicillin or Clindamycin or Cefoxitin

Cefuroxime with or without Erythromycin

(F) Follow response
Assess culture results
Adjust antibiotics as needed

Additional diagnostic work-up as needed

PNEUMOCOCCAL PNEUMONIA

Pneumococcal pneumonia remains the most common community-acquired bacterial pneumonia, making up more than 50 percent of the cases in many studies. It is caused by *Streptococcus pneumoniae*, a gram-positive organism. Up to 30 percent of blood cultures are positive. Despite advances in antibiotics and supportive therapy, the reported mortality rate among bacteremic patients remains high.

A. The classic clinical presentation of acute pneumococcal pneumonia is abrupt onset associated with fever and shaking chills, pleuritic chest pain, and cough, often with bloody or rust-colored sputum. The presentation is highly variable and is often less dramatic in elderly and debilitated patients.

B. Most past studies reported that lobar consolidation is the most common radiographic pattern in pneumococcal pneumonia. Recent studies suggest that the findings of bronchopneumonia or interstitial pattern are becoming more common, perhaps due to earlier presentation of the patient. Occasionally among elderly or dehydrated patients, radiographic evidence of infiltrate does not appear until after the patient is rehydrated. Up to 25 percent of the cases may involve two or more lobes. Multiple lobe involvement is associated with a higher mortality. Small amounts of pleural effusion are commonly seen, especially on lateral decubitus chest films, although clinically significant empyema is uncommon.

C. Patients with single-lobe infiltrate and insignificant pleural effusion, stable vital signs, and without significant risk factors generally can be treated effectively as outpatients with oral antibiotics. Unstable or debilitated patients and those with special risk factors such as pre-existing lung diseases, sickle cell disease, splenectomy, or immunocompromised host should be admitted for intravenous antibiotics and observation.

D. Admit patients with complicated pneumonia or those at risk for parenteral therapy and respiratory support. Patients with significant effusion or effusion that does not resolve with treatment require thoracentesis. When empyema is present, drainage with a chest tube is necessary.

E. Obtain a properly collected sputum specimen for Gram stain and culture. A good sputum Gram stain should show many polymorphonuclear leukocytes, predominant diplococci, and none or only a few squamous cells. Patients with a diagnostic sputum may be given oral penicillin; those with an inadequate sputum specimen and nondiagnostic sputum, or penicillin allergy may be given erythromycin.

F. Treat hospitalized patients, who have complications and a diagnostic sputum specimen with intravenous or intramuscular penicillin. Patients with nondiagnostic sputum should be treated with a third-generation cephalosporin or a combination of ampicillin and an aminoglycoside to provide a broader antimicrobial coverage.

G. Follow the culture results and clinical response and adjust antibiotics as needed. Culture of the sputum may or may not yield the causative organism.

References

Austrian R. Pneumococcal pneumonia: diagnostic, epidemiologic, therapeutic and prophylactic considerations. Chest 1986; 90:738.

Palmer DL, Jones CC. Diagnosis of pneumococcal pneumonia. Semin Respir Infect 1988; 3:131.

Segreti J, Bone RC. Overwhelming pneumonia. Dis Mon. January 1987:1.

Stratton CW. Bacterial pneumonias: An overview with emphasis on pathogenesis, diagnosis, and treatment. Heart Lung 1986; 15:226.

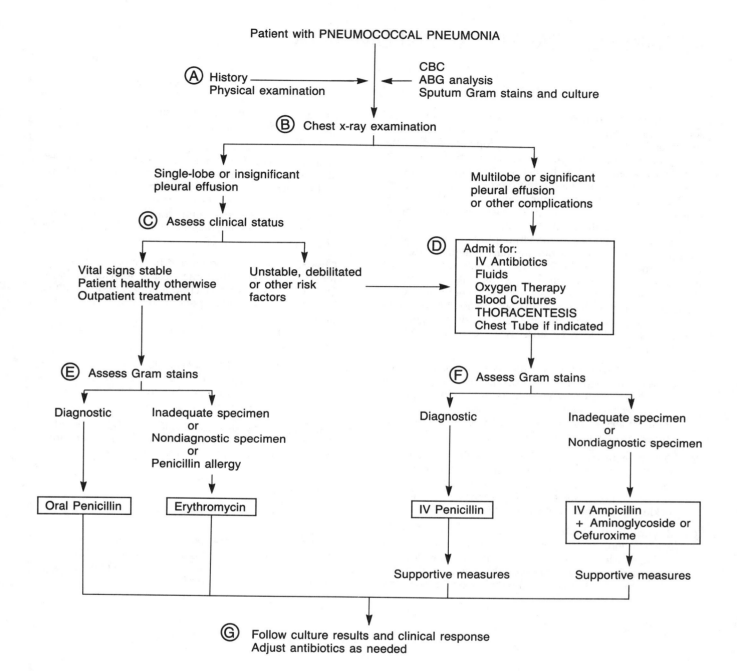

Patient with PNEUMOCOCCAL PNEUMONIA

(A) History ——————→ ←—— CBC
Physical examination   ABG analysis
                              Sputum Gram stains and culture

(B) Chest x-ray examination

Single-lobe or insignificant   Multilobe or significant
pleural effusion   pleural effusion
                                      or other complications

(C) Assess clinical status

Vital signs stable   Unstable, debilitated   (D) Admit for:
Patient healthy otherwise   or other risk   IV Antibiotics
Outpatient treatment   factors   Fluids
                                                               Oxygen Therapy
                                                               Blood Cultures
                                                               THORACENTESIS
                                                               Chest Tube if indicated

(E) Assess Gram stains   (F) Assess Gram stains

Diagnostic   Inadequate specimen   Diagnostic   Inadequate specimen
                    or   or
                    Nondiagnostic specimen   Nondiagnostic specimen
                    or
                    Penicillin allergy

Oral Penicillin   Erythromycin   IV Penicillin   IV Ampicillin
                                                                      + Aminoglycoside or
                                                                      Cefuroxime

                                                 Supportive measures Supportive measures

(G) Follow culture results and clinical response
Adjust antibiotics as needed

RECURRENT BACTERIAL PNEUMONIA

Recurrent bacterial pneumonia is defined as two or more episodes of nontuberculous pneumonias separated by an interval of at least 1 month, or by a documented complete radiographic resolution of the previous infection. Although recurrent pneumonia may be caused by many conditions, most patients have an underlying predisposing factor. The most common associated conditions include alcoholism, chronic obstructive pulmonary disease, congestive heart failure, diabetes mellitus, asthma, and bronchiectasis. Other less common conditions include multiple myeloma, chronic sinusitis, cystic fibrosis, extrapulmonary malignancies, and hypogammaglobulinemia. Recurrent pneumonias are common in human immunodeficiency virus (HIV)–positive individuals. In young adults recurrent pneumonias may be associated with chronic granulomatous disease, IgG deficiency, pulmonary sequestration, and Job's syndrome (generalized eczema, staphylococcal abscesses, recurrent bronchitis, and pneumonia).

A. The history usually reveals the presence of one of the above-mentioned associated risk factors. Alcoholic patients have a history of excessive drinking in the period preceding the pneumonia. The physical examination demonstrates signs consistent with acute pneumonia: cough, fever, sputum production, rales, and rhonchi.

B. Obtain Gram stains and culture to identify the infectious agent. Laboratory studies confirm the infection and assess the severity of any known associated conditions such as cystic fibrosis, diabetes, otitis, sinusitis, heart failure, sickle cell anemia, or chronic lymphocytic leukemia.

C. Regardless of whether *Pneumocystis* is the infectious agent found, an HIV test should be performed in individuals who have no other risk factors for the development of recurrent pneumonias. Abnormally high or low serum globulin levels should be followed up by protein and quantitative immunoelectrophoresis to make the diagnoses of hypogammaglobulinemia or multiple myeloma.

D. In approximately two-thirds of the cases, review of chest films reveals infiltrates located in the right lung. Most of these are in the lower or middle lobe. Comparisons with previous films may indicate that the pneumonia is recurrent in the same location; this is found in about 40 percent of all cases and does not depend on the presence of previous lung disease.

E. Chest CT should be performed in patients with recurrent pneumonias in the same location to visualize bronchial obstruction or bronchopulmonary sequestration. Bronchoscopy should be performed if bronchial obstruction is detected.

F. For individuals with nondiagnostic bronchoscopies, rule out associated conditions.

G. Individuals with a history of sinusitis, recurrent bronchitis, and infertility should first undergo sinus evaluation and, if negative, be evaluated for the immotile cilia syndrome and cystic fibrosis.

H. Esophagography detects occult esophageal disorders leading to aspiration in patients without apparent predisposing factors for recurrent pneumonia.

References

Roth RM, Gleckman RA. Recurrent bacterial pneumonia: a contemporary perspective. South Med J 1985; 78:573.

Winterbauer RH, Bedon GA, Ball WC Jr. Recurrent pneumonia. Ann Intern Med 1969; 70:689.

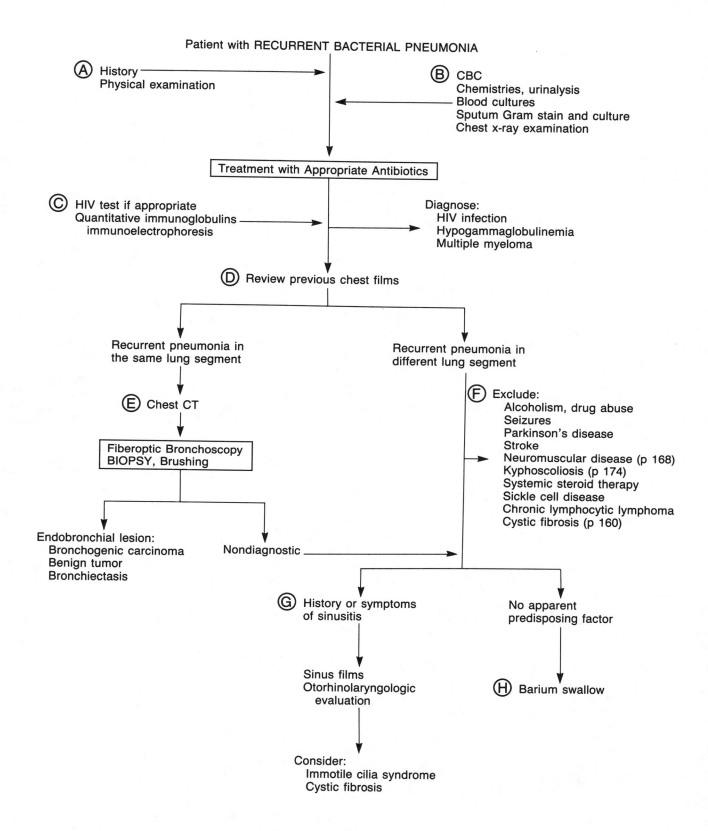

Patient with RECURRENT BACTERIAL PNEUMONIA

(A) History
Physical examination

(B) CBC
Chemistries, urinalysis
Blood cultures
Sputum Gram stain and culture
Chest x-ray examination

Treatment with Appropriate Antibiotics

(C) HIV test if appropriate
Quantitative immunoglobulins
immunoelectrophoresis

Diagnose:
HIV infection
Hypogammaglobulinemia
Multiple myeloma

(D) Review previous chest films

Recurrent pneumonia in
the same lung segment

Recurrent pneumonia in
different lung segment

(E) Chest CT

(F) Exclude:
Alcoholism, drug abuse
Seizures
Parkinson's disease
Stroke
Neuromuscular disease (p 168)
Kyphoscoliosis (p 174)
Systemic steroid therapy
Sickle cell disease
Chronic lymphocytic lymphoma
Cystic fibrosis (p 160)

Fiberoptic Bronchoscopy
BIOPSY, Brushing

Endobronchial lesion:
Bronchogenic carcinoma
Benign tumor
Bronchiectasis

Nondiagnostic

(G) History or symptoms
of sinusitis

No apparent
predisposing factor

Sinus films
Otorhinolaryngologic
evaluation

(H) Barium swallow

Consider:
Immotile cilia syndrome
Cystic fibrosis

ANAEROBIC LUNG INFECTIONS

Clinical manifestations of anaerobic lung infections include acute and chronic pneumonitis, lung abscess, necrotizing pneumonia, septic pulmonary infarction, and empyema. The incidence of anaerobic lung infections in the community setting has been estimated to be between 20 and 35 percent. Most anaerobic pleuropulmonary infections are mixed infections and are caused by aerobic or facultative bacteria as well as by anaerobic species. The most common anaerobic bacterial isolates include *Fusobacterium nucleatum*, *Peptostreptococcus*, and *Bacteroides* species.

Predisposing factors associated with anaerobic lung infections include aspiration in patients with altered consciousness due to ingestion of alcohol, general anesthesia, or seizures, and in patients with preceding extrapulmonary anaerobic infection caused by periodontal disease, pharyngitis, otitis, mastoiditis, infections of the female genital tract, infections of the gastrointestinal tract, and endocarditis. Anaerobic infections are also found post-thoracotomy or after penetrating chest trauma, and less commonly are associated with other conditions such as bronchogenic carcinoma, bronchiectasis, aspiration of foreign body, and diabetes mellitus; they are also seen in the setting of corticosteroid or immunosuppressive therapy.

Recovery from anaerobic infections of the lung and pleura, which are treated by appropriate antibiotics, surgical drainage of pus, and debridement of necrotic tissue, may be quite slow, averaging 9 weeks for a solitary lung abscess and longer for necrotizing pneumonia and empyema. Prolonged antibiotic therapy is often necessary to prevent relapse or residual damage.

A. Based on clinical features alone, most cases of anaerobic lung infection are difficult to differentiate from other bacterial pneumonias. Fever, productive cough, and chest pain are commonly present. Anaerobic lung infection may sometimes be confused with malignancy due to their similar presentations, with weight loss and an indolent course. Physical findings are not specific. Poor gingival conditions may be the only clue to the etiology of the infection.

B. The sputum is considered to be diagnostic for anaerobic lung infection if the characteristic putrid odor is present. This odor may be found in about 50 percent of patients with the late suppurative manifestations of anaerobic infection such as lung abscesses, necrotizing pneumonitis, or empyema, but only in about 5 percent of patients with simple pneumonitis. Expectorated sputum is generally not suitable for anaerobic culture because of mouth flora contamination. For cultures, use sputum obtained from transtracheal aspiration, percutaneous transthoracic aspiration, or bronchoscopy using the protected brush technique. Maintain strict anaerobic culture techniques to ensure the recovery of anaerobic organisms. Blood cultures are seldom positive in confirmed cases of anaerobic pulmonary infections. Gram stain and acid-fast bacilli (AFB) stains of the sputum will exclude the presence of specific bacterial infections, including tuberculosis.

C. Suspect anaerobic lung infection on the basis of the proper clinical setting, a history of, or predisposition to, aspiration, and radiographic evidence of pulmonary infiltrates in the dependent portions of the lung. The radiographic appearance of uncomplicated anaerobic pneumonitis is nonspecific. Necrotizing pneumonia may be diagnosed when the radiographic appearance of the pneumonia is consistent with spread of the infection beyond the initially involved lobe to adjacent parenchyma combined with evidence of multiple small cavitations formed within the necrotizing tissue. Extension of the process to the pleural surfaces may lead to the formation of anaerobic empyema.

D. Most cases of uncomplicated community-acquired pneumonia are treated with penicillins; these cases include many cases of unrecognized anaerobic pneumonitis. Aqueous penicillin G has been the traditional treatment of choice for aspiration pneumonia. High-dose penicillin (10 million units or more per day) may be required for the treatment of necrotizing pneumonitis or lung abscess. Use clindamycin if penicillin-resistant *Bacteroides fragilis* is suspected. Add an aminoglycoside or a broad-spectrum second-generation cephalosporin to increase antibiotic coverage if concurrent gram-negative bacteria infection is suspected.

E. Thoracentesis must be performed in patients found to have pleural effusion. Empyemas require chest tube drainage in addition to the proper antibiotics.

F. Although most anaerobic pneumonias are not specifically diagnosed, they will respond to empiric antibiotic therapies. Fiberoptic bronchoscopy with protected brush and transbronchial biopsies may be performed to facilitate diagnosis when patients do not respond to therapy.

References

Bartlett JG. Anaerobic bacterial infections of the lung. Chest 1987; 91:901.

Bartlett JG. Treatment of anaerobic pulmonary infections. J Antimicrob Chemother 1989; 24:836.

Finegold SM, George WL, Mulligan ME. Anaerobic infections. Dis Mon 1985; 31:8.

Pennza PT. Aspiration pneumonia, necrotizing pneumonia, and lung abscess. Emerg Clin North Am 1989; 7:279.

Patient with ANAEROBIC LUNG INFECTION

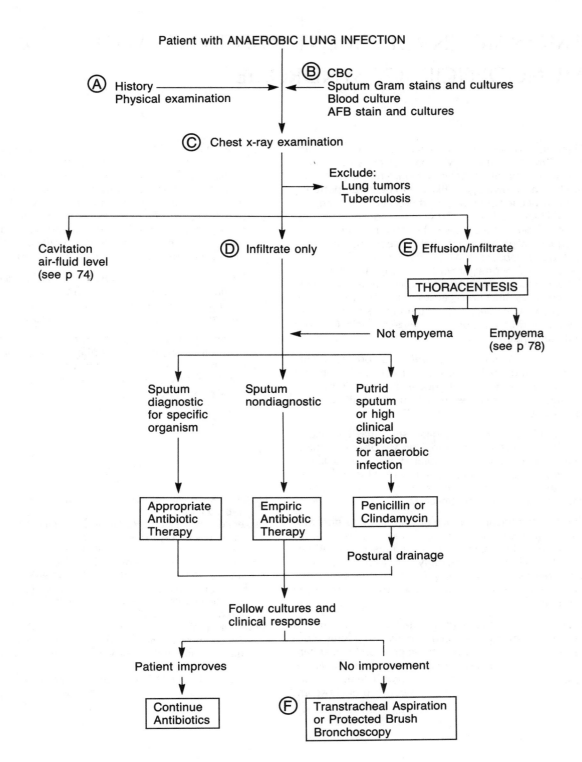

PULMONARY INVOLVEMENT IN PATIENTS WITH ACQUIRED IMMUNODEFICIENCY SYNDROME

The diagnostic and therapeutic approach to pulmonary symptoms or infiltrate in patients who have or are suspected of having acquired immunodeficiency syndrome (AIDS) should be guided by the knowledge of likely etiologies. Opportunistic infections occur commonly in these patients. Many series reported that in AIDS patients with pulmonary infections, more than 60 percent are caused by *Pneumocystis carinii*. Other frequent infectious agents that cause pulmonary infections include *Mycobacteria* (*M. avium-intracellulare* and *M. tuberculosis*), and cytomegalovirus. Although less common, bacterial pneumonia caused by *Pneumococcus* and *Legionella* also occurs. Noninfectious causes of pulmonary infiltrate include lymphocytic interstitial pneumonitis, Kaposi's sarcoma, lymphoma, drug reactions, and oxygen toxicity for those on ventilator support.

A. Symptoms of *Pneumocystis carinii* pneumonia are highly variable, although increasing shortness of breath and dyspnea on exertion are frequent findings. Pulmonary findings on physical examination generally are unremarkable.

B. Sputum Gram stain and acid-fast stain may be used to identify patients with bacterial or *Mycobacteria* infections. Special stains of expectorated or sputum obtained through suction for pneumocystis are seldom diagnostic; if the results were positive, however, this would obviate the need for bronchoscopy.

C. The radiographic appearance of *Pneumocystis pneumonia* is nonspecific. It often appears as a diffuse interstitial process, although normal chest films are sometimes seen. Pleural effusion generally is not seen in patients with *Pneumocystis pneumonia*; its presence suggests other diagnoses or concurrent diseases that need to be investigated.

D. Because of the high rate of simultaneous occurrence of multiple pulmonary problems in these patients, continued close monitoring of their progress under treatment must be made even after a diagnosis has been made. Patients who do not improve after appropriate therapy has been initiated should undergo fiberoptic bronchoscopy.

E. A normal chest film along with a normal alveolar-arterial oxygen (A-a O_2) gradient will exclude most pulmonary diseases. Pulmonary diseases such as asthma, bronchitis, and pulmonary embolism should be excluded at this time. Abnormal oxygen gradients are likely to be found in patients with *Pneumocystis pneumonia* with normal chest films. Some authorities have advocated the use of gallium scan or carbon monoxide diffusion capacity to detect the presence of interstitial diseases.

F. For many patients, fiberoptic bronchoscopy is necessary to make the diagnosis. Depending on the biopsy risks, brushings, bronchoalveolar lavage, or transbronchial biopsy may be used to make the diagnosis.

G. Patients with abnormal chest films and a nondiagnostic fiberoptic bronchoscopy require open lung biopsy to establish the diagnosis. Patients with normal chest films may be observed or may undergo repeat fiberoptic bronchoscopy.

References

Donath J, Khan FA. Pulmonary infections in AIDS. Compr Ther 1987; 13:49.

Fitzgerald W, Bevelaqua FA, Garay SM, Aranda CP. The role of open lung biopsy in patients with the acquired immunodeficiency syndrome. Chest 1987; 91:659.

Hopewell PC, Luce JM. Pulmonary involvement in the acquired immunodeficiency syndrome. Chest 1985; 87:104.

Polsky B, Gold JWM, Whimbey E, et al. Bacterial pneumonia in patients with acquired immunodeficiency syndrome. Ann Intern Med 1986; 104:38.

Stover DE, White DA, Romano PA, Gellene RA, Robeson WA. Spectrum of pulmonary diseases associated with the acquired immunodeficiency syndrome. Am J Med 1985; 78:429.

Talavera W, Mildvan D. Pulmonary infections in the acquired immunodeficiency syndrome. Semin Respir Infect 1986; 1:202.

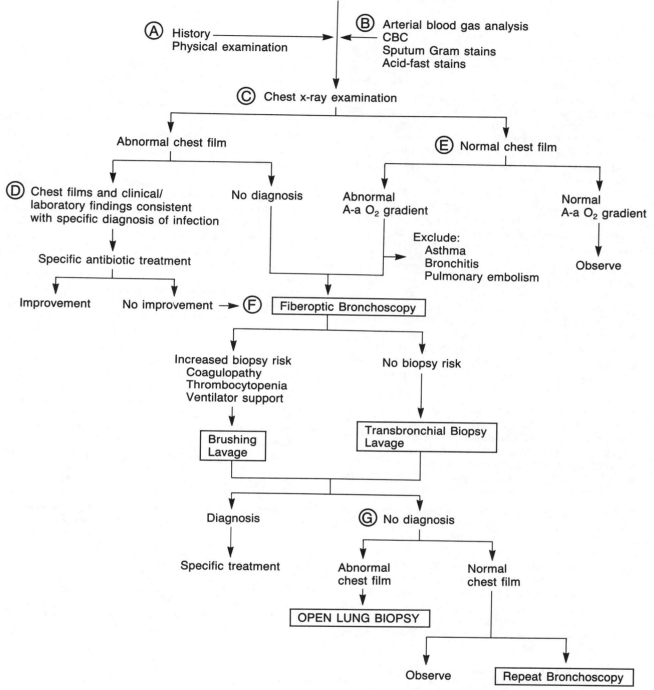

PULMONARY SYMPTOMS IN PATIENTS
WITH, OR SUSPECTED OF HAVING, AIDS

Ⓐ History
Physical examination

Ⓑ Arterial blood gas analysis
CBC
Sputum Gram stains
Acid-fast stains

Ⓒ Chest x-ray examination

Abnormal chest film

Ⓔ Normal chest film

Ⓓ Chest films and clinical/
laboratory findings consistent
with specific diagnosis of infection

No diagnosis

Abnormal
A-a O₂ gradient

Normal
A-a O₂ gradient

Specific antibiotic treatment

Exclude:
Asthma
Bronchitis
Pulmonary embolism

Observe

Improvement

No improvement → Ⓕ Fiberoptic Bronchoscopy

Increased biopsy risk
Coagulopathy
Thrombocytopenia
Ventilator support

No biopsy risk

Brushing
Lavage

Transbronchial Biopsy
Lavage

Diagnosis

Ⓖ No diagnosis

Specific treatment

Abnormal
chest film

Normal
chest film

OPEN LUNG BIOPSY

Observe

Repeat Bronchoscopy

NOSOCOMIAL PNEUMONIA

Nosocomial pneumonia occurs 48 to 72 hours after hospitalization in patients who had no signs of symptoms upon admission. It is the second most common hospital-acquired infection and often occurs in critically ill patients. The diagnosis of nosocomial pneumonia is often difficult to make, and it is sometimes only recognized at autopsy. Gram-negative bacteria account for approximately half of these infections; *Pseudomonas* is the most common type. *Staphylococcus aureus* commonly causes gram-positive bacterial nosocomial pneumonia. Other bacteria causing nosocomial pneumonias include *Enterobacteriaceae* species and a number of anaerobic organisms. *Legionella*, fungi, and viruses have also been associated with nosocomial pneumonia. Despite advances in diagnostic techniques and antibiotics, reported mortality rates range from 15 to 50 percent.

A. The diagnostic process must take into account the patient's underlying problems and clinical status. Patients with stroke are predisposed to aspiration. Patients with recent thoracoabdominal surgery are at an increased risk of acquiring nosocomial pneumonia. The clinical findings usually associated with pneumonia, such as fever, cough, and sputum, may be absent in patients with nosocomial pneumonia. Pneumonia in elderly patients may present as decreased responsiveness or increased mental confusion.

B. There are no specific laboratory findings associated with nosocomial pneumonia. Elevated white blood cell counts may not be present because of depressed immune response in some patients. Hospitalized patients often are critically ill with comorbidities such as congestive heart failure or pre-existing pulmonary disease, making the interpretation of the chest film difficult.

C. Examination of the sputum provides the most important clue to the nature of the infection. However, one of the difficulties of making an accurate diagnosis is that patients often are colonized with potential pathogenic organisms soon after hospitalization. Sputum often becomes contaminated by organisms from the upper airway. In addition, many patients often are unable to produce sputum. Invasive procedures such as transtracheal aspiration or percutaneous aspiration have been advocated as an accurate method of obtaining adequate specimens for analysis.

D. Several lines of clinical reasoning should be considered in assessing the likely etiologic organism. *Haemophilus influenzae* should be considered in patients with history of chronic lung disease. *Klebsiella pneumoniae* should be considered in patients with history of alcoholism. Patients with strokes, decreased gag reflex, seizures, and poor dentition are at special risk of aspirating mouth flora and developing anaerobic pneumonia. Nosocomial pneumonia is often caused by mixed organisms; in these cases, the pneumonia is more likely located in the lower lobes of the lung, especially in the right lower lobe. In addition to patient characteristics, the local hospital bacterial epidemiology should be taken into consideration when one is evaluating a patient with nosocomial pneumonia.

E. Empiric treatment of nosocomial pneumonia with antibiotics should be started before culture results become available and should include coverage for aerobic gram-negative bacilli such as *Pseudomonas aeruginosa*, *Klebsiella*, *Enterobacter*, *Escherichia coli*, *Serratia*, *Proteus*, and gram-positive cocci such as *S. aureus*. Effective regimens generally include an aminoglycoside plus a second- or third-generation cephalosporin. Erythromycin is added if the patient is severely ill or if *Legionella* is suspected. Patients suspected of aspiration require coverage for mouth anaerobes; cefoxitin as simple coverage or clindamycin plus an aminoglycoside may be used.

F. The patient's clinical condition must be evaluated at 24 to 48 hours to assess the response to therapy. Results of cultures should be used to modify antibiotic regimens. Invasive diagnostic procedures are seldom needed in the management of patients with nosocomial pneumonia, but severely ill patients who do not respond to empiric antibiotics and those without a definitive bacterial diagnosis should have fiberoptic bronchoscopy with bronchoalveolar lavage, transtracheal aspiration, or percutaneous aspiration performed to acquire a specimen and determine whether a change of management is needed. Thoracentesis to exclude empyema is recommended for patients with pleural effusion.

References

Bamberger DM. Diagnosis of nosocomial pneumonia. Semin Respir Infect 1988; 3:140.

Bartlett JG, O'Keefe P, Thomas FP, Louie TJ, Gorbach SL. Bacteriology of hospital-acquired pneumonia. Arch Intern Med 1986; 146:868.

Hessen MT, Kaye D. Nosocomial pneumonia. Crit Care Clin 1988; 4:245.

Pennington JE. New therapeutic approaches to hospital-acquired pneumonia. Semin Respir Infect 1987; 2:67.

Winterbauer RH, Dries DF. New diagnostic approaches to the hospitalized patient with pneumonia. Semin Respir Infect 1987; 2:57.

NOSOCOMIAL PNEUMONIA Suspected

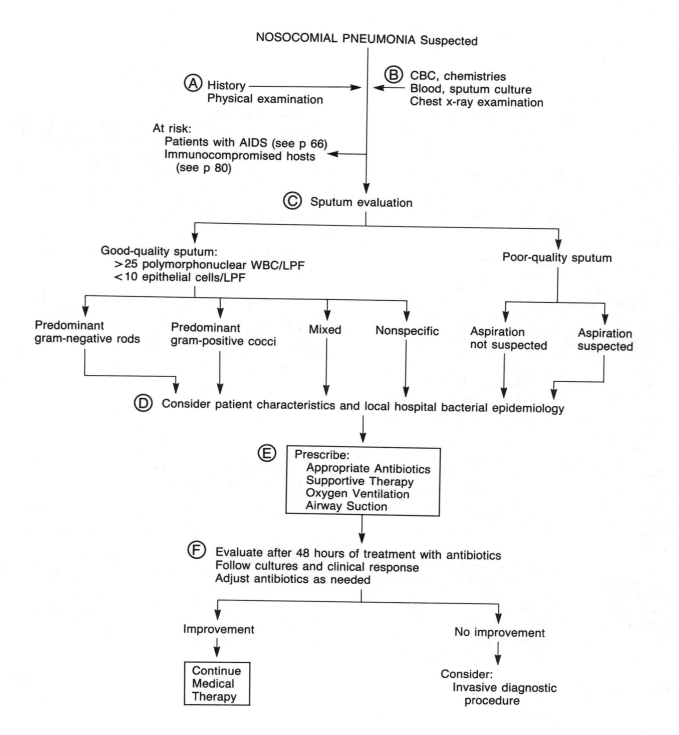

LEGIONNAIRES' DISEASE

Legionella pneumophilia is a ubiquitous aerobic gram-negative bacillus which grows best in warm water. Airborne spread is the usual mode of transmission. The organism is a common cause of community-acquired pneumonia (1 to 15 percent). There is no person-to-person transmission. Approximately 65 percent of cases occur in smokers or patients with other medical problems, including neoplasms, renal transplantation, and rheumatologic or inflammatory diseases. Patients with hairy cell leukemia appear to have a predisposition to develop Legionnaires' disease.

A. The illness is characterized by a high fever and a nonproductive cough. Patients may have abdominal pain, diarrhea, abnormal liver function tests (LFTs) and hematuria and hypophosphatemia. However, these findings do not differentiate Legionnaires' disease from other pneumonias. Neurologic abnormalities are common and include headache, encephalopathy with confusion and disorientation, myopathies, and neuropathies. Hyponatremia occurring early in the course of the disease is more common in Legionnaires' disease than in other pneumonias. Bradycardia occurs in about 50 percent of patients.

B. Chest x-ray examination shows consolidation, which often begins as a patchy or round infiltrate and then rapidly progresses to involve other areas of lung. Abscess formation is common (25 percent). Effusions may occur in more than 50 percent of cases, but empyema is rare.

C. Direct immunofluorescence of sputum samples or of transtracheal aspirates is a rapid test with moderate to high sensitivity for *Legionella*. Because of laboratory variation, the usefulness of this test varies from one institution to another.

D. Moderate to severe disease requires intravenous erythromycin therapy for at least 3 weeks as a first measure. Tetracycline has also been used, but the results are inconsistent. The combination of erythromycin and rifampin should be reserved for seriously ill patients.

E. A negative sputum smear does not exclude the diagnosis. Patients with a clinical picture consistent with *Legionella* and negative smears should undergo serologic testing and specific sputum cultures. Serologic conversion may take as long as 8 weeks and may not occur in approximately 10 to 25 percent of cases, so negative serology results also do not exclude the diagnosis.

F. Patients with clinical evidence of Legionnaires' disease but in whom a firm diagnosis has not been established should begin receiving erythromycin.

G. Some studies recommend combined therapy of erythromycin and rifampin for immunocompromised patients or those with a poor response to erythromycin alone.

H. If the disease progresses despite antibiotic therapy, a tissue diagnosis is required. Progression may be caused by the unresponsiveness of *Legionella* to therapy or to other associated medical conditions. An open-lung biopsy or a transbronchoscopic biopsy will confirm the diagnosis. The exact procedure performed depends on the status of the patient.

References

Chiodini PL, Williams AJ, Barker J, Innes JA. Bronchial lavage and transbronchial lung biopsy in the diagnosis of Legionnaires' disease. Thorax 1985; 40:154.

Davis GS, Winn WC. Legionnaires' disease: respiratory infections caused by *Legionella* bacteria. Clin Chest Med 1987; 8:419.

Edelstein PH, Meyers RD. Legionnaires' disease. Chest 1984; 85:114.

Edelstein PH, Meyers RD, Finegold SM. Laboratory diagnosis of Legionnaires' disease. Am Rev Respir Dis 1980; 121:317.

Fairbank JT, Mamourian AC, Dietrich FA, Girod JC. The chest radiograph in Legionnaires' disease. Radiology 1983; 147:33.

Yu VL, Kroboth JF, Shannard J, Brown A, McDearman S, Magnussen M. Legionnaires' disease: new clinical perspective from a prospective pneumonia study. Am J Med 1982; 73:357.

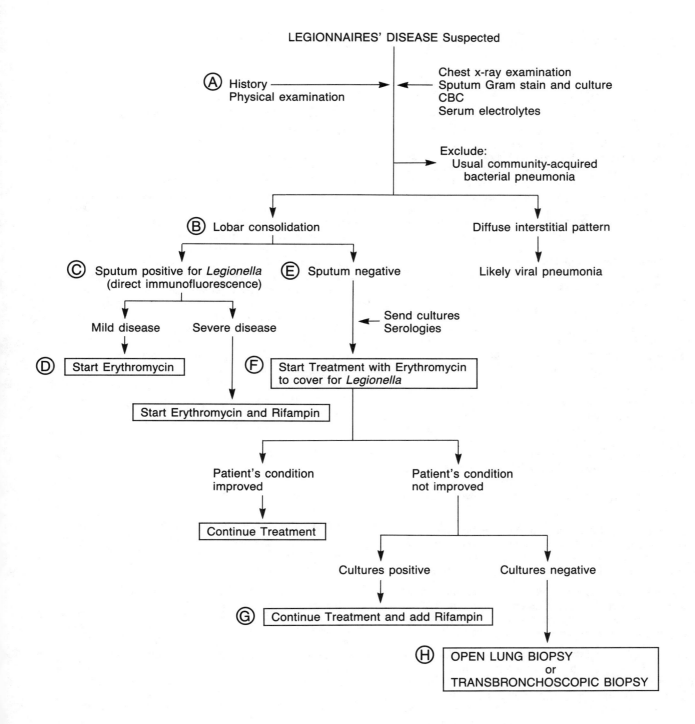

LEGIONNAIRES' DISEASE Suspected

Ⓐ History —————→ Chest x-ray examination
Physical examination ←——— Sputum Gram stain and culture
CBC
Serum electrolytes

Exclude:
————→ Usual community-acquired
bacterial pneumonia

Ⓑ Lobar consolidation   Diffuse interstitial pattern

Ⓒ Sputum positive for *Legionella*   Ⓔ Sputum negative   Likely viral pneumonia
(direct immunofluorescence)

←——— Send cultures
Serologies

Mild disease   Severe disease

Ⓓ │ Start Erythromycin │   Ⓕ │ Start Treatment with Erythromycin │
to cover for *Legionella*

│ Start Erythromycin and Rifampin │

Patient's condition   Patient's condition
improved   not improved

│ Continue Treatment │

Cultures positive   Cultures negative

Ⓖ │ Continue Treatment and add Rifampin │

Ⓗ │ OPEN LUNG BIOPSY
or
TRANSBRONCHOSCOPIC BIOPSY │

PNEUMOCYSTIS CARINII PNEUMONIA

Pneumocystis carinii is a protozoon. Prior to 1981, *Pneumocystis carinii* pneumonia (PCP) was a relatively uncommon opportunistic infection usually seen in patients with primary immunodeficiency disorders and underlying hematologic malignancies such as lymphoma, in patients receiving immunosuppressive therapy, in neonates, and rarely, in normal individuals with no apparent immunologic defects. Acquired immunodeficiency syndrome (AIDS) has now become the most common etiologic factor predisposing patients to PCP.

A. The clinical presentation of patients with PCP is variable. The symptoms are often initially mild, and the onset is insidious. Fever, dyspnea, and nonproductive cough are the most common presenting symptoms. Some patients may be asymptomatic. Physical findings are not reliable when one is diagnosing PCP, because up to half of patients have normal pulmonary findings on auscultation. Fever is present in up to 75 percent of patients, and tachypnea is present in approximately two-thirds.

B. There are no characteristic radiographic findings in patients with PCP. Although some patients have normal chest films on presentation, ground-glass–like perihilar infiltrates are often seen in the early stage of the disease; these progress to diffuse interstitial or alveolar infiltrations which may be asymmetric. Pneumothorax and pleural effusion associated with PCP have been reported in a number of patients. Arterial blood gas findings often demonstrate hypoxemia and an increased arterial-alveolar oxygen gradient.

C. Sputum examined with methenamine-silver, Giemsa, or toluidine blue-O will be positive in only approximately 15 percent of patients. Most patients required bronchoscopy to obtain specimens adequate for diagnosis.

D. Fiberoptic bronchoscopy with bronchoalveolar lavage and transbronchial biopsy is an effective method of obtaining specimens for the diagnosis of PCP. The sensitivity of this procedure exceeds 90 percent.

E. In seriously ill patients or in those in whom PCP is suspected, an open lung biopsy or a repeat bronchoscopy should be performed. Some authors, however, believe that the sensitivity of the combination of bronchoalveolar lavage and transbronchial biopsy is sufficiently high that there is little to be gained from additional procedures.

F. Pentamidine and trimethoprim-sulfamethoxazole (TMP-SMX) are the two major therapeutic options available. They are similarly effective with a treatment survival rate of approximately 70 percent. The choice of the initial drug must be made in view of the patient's allergy history, clinical status, and concurrent problems. TMP-SMX is usually the first drug used. However, adverse reactions to TMP-SMX, including leukopenia, skin rash, fever, elevated liver enzymes, azotemia, and thrombocytopenia, are common when one is using doses necessary to treat PCP; reported adverse reaction rates have varied from 50 to 100 percent. More than half of patients have adverse reactions severe enough to require that therapy be discontinued. These patients and those who fail to respond to TMP-SMX are switched to pentamidine. Because pentamidine has a toxicity rate similar to that of TMP-SMX, discontinuation of this therapy also occurs in over half of the patients treated. Common toxicities include nephrotoxicity, liver dysfunction, neutropenia, hypoglycemia, hypotension, anemia, and thrombocytopenia. Patients successfully treated for PCP should be considered for prophylaxis with aerosolized pentamidine to reduce the risk of reinfection.

References

Bigby TD, Margolskee D, Curtis JL, et al. The usefulness of induced sputum in the diagnosis of *Pneumocystis carinii* pneumonia in patients with the acquired immunodeficiency syndrome. Am Rev Respir Dis 1986; 133:515.

DeLorenzo LJ, Huang CT, Maguire GP, Stone DJ. Roentgenographic patterns of *Pneumocystis carinii* pneumonia in 104 patients with AIDS. Chest 1987; 91:323.

Goldin JA, Hollander H, Stulbarg MS, Gamsu G. Bronchoalveolar lavage as the exclusive diagnostic modality for *Pneumocystis carinii* pneumonia. Chest 1986; 90:18.

Kovacs JA, Hiemenz JW, Macher AM, et al. *Pneumocystis carinii* pneumonia: a comparison between patients with the acquired immunodeficiency syndrome and patients with other immunodeficiencies. Ann Intern Med 1984; 100:663.

Levine SJ, White DA. Pulmonary effects of AIDS: *Pneumocystis carinii*. Clin Chest Med 1988; 9:395.

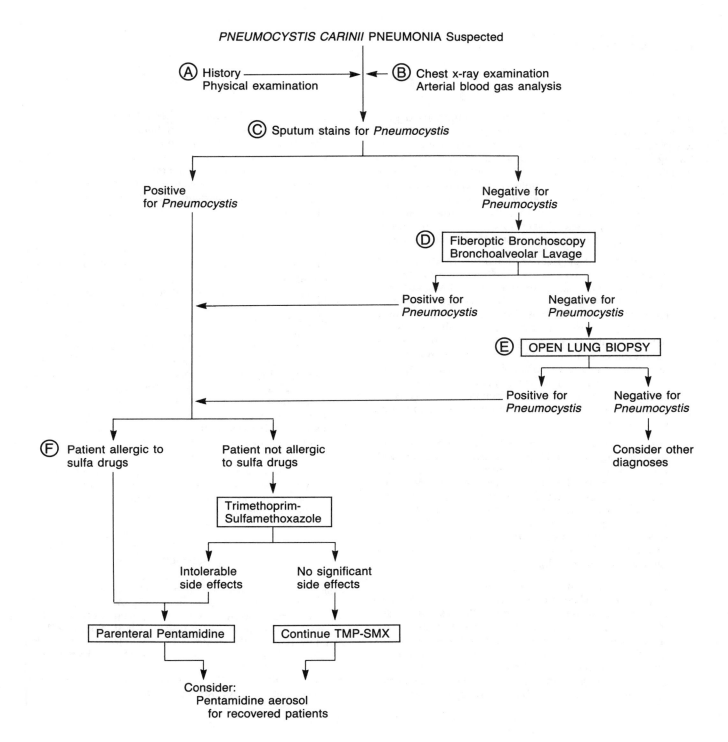

PNEUMOCYSTIS CARINII PNEUMONIA Suspected

(A) History
Physical examination

(B) Chest x-ray examination
Arterial blood gas analysis

(C) Sputum stains for Pneumocystis

Positive
for Pneumocystis

Negative for
Pneumocystis

(D) Fiberoptic Bronchoscopy
Bronchoalveolar Lavage

Positive for
Pneumocystis

Negative for
Pneumocystis

(E) OPEN LUNG BIOPSY

Positive for
Pneumocystis

Negative for
Pneumocystis

Consider other
diagnoses

(F) Patient allergic to
sulfa drugs

Patient not allergic
to sulfa drugs

Trimethoprim-
Sulfamethoxazole

Intolerable
side effects

No significant
side effects

Parenteral Pentamidine

Continue TMP-SMX

Consider:
Pentamidine aerosol
for recovered patients

LUNG ABSCESS

A lung abscess develops from a pneumonia caused by a necrotizing organism such as *Staphylococcus* or from a mixture of aerobic and anaerobic organisms that might occur following an aspiration. Mixed aerobic and anaerobic infection resulting from aspiration of mouth contents is the most common cause of lung abscess. Simple aspiration pneumonia may progress to lung abscess, depending on the quantity and nature of the aspirated material. Usually a mixture of aerobic and anaerobic organisms is necessary to provide the correct microenvironment for the development of lung abscess.

A. The history and physical examination are useful in the evaluation of lung abscess. The presence of signs of chronic infection such as weight loss and low-grade fever supports the diagnosis of lung abscess secondary to aspiration of aerobic and anaerobic organisms. In addition, any history of loss of consciousness, swallowing disorders, upper airway or pharyngeal pathology increases the likelihood of aspiration pneumonia. Sputum examination should provide an indication as to whether a specific organism such as *Staphylococcus* or *Klebsiella* is responsible for the infection. Usually when the abscess is secondary to aspiration, a mixture of organisms is found on Gram stain.

B. Infection in a pre-existing bulla is suggested by the presence of an air-fluid level in a cavity with a thin wall. Cavities with thick walls are commonly caused by lung abscess or cavitary lung malignancies. A lung malignancy usually causes a discrete mass lesion with well-circumscribed borders. Cytologic examination of sputum may yield malignant cells; however, in other cases, differentiation is difficult, and malignancy is considered when the patient fails to respond to appropriate antibiotics as described below.

C. Lung abscesses that are community-acquired usually respond to high-dose penicillin therapy. This improvement occurs whether or not penicillin-resistant organisms are present, because penicillin disrupts the microenvironment necessary for abscess formation. Some physicians prefer to use clindamycin because *B. fragilis*, a common penicillin-resistant organism, is sensitive to this drug. Hospital-acquired infections are treated with broad-spectrum antibiotic coverage.

D. When the air-fluid level is located adjacent to the pleural space, it becomes necessary to differentiate lung abscess from empyema. Both of these processes occur in similar settings and may present a similar clinical picture, but require somewhat different treatment. CT of the chest will demonstrate the presence of pleural fluid and air in the pleural space and indicate the need for chest tube drainage.

E. Most lung abscesses respond to antibiotic treatment. A persistently high fever, an elevated white blood cell count, and an increase in the amount of involved lung parenchyma suggest the need for more aggressive treatment. In patients who are surgical candidates, the lung abscess can be resected. A double-lumen endotracheal tube is placed to prevent spillage of the abscess contents into the bronchus and the development of multilobar infections, a serious complication that could lead to refractory infection and respiratory failure. In patients who are not surgical candidates, the abscess can be drained percutaneously with a chest tube or a pig-tailed catheter, placed under CT guidance. This procedure must be used cautiously because of the possibility of creating a bronchopleural fistula or an empyema.

F. Failure to respond to treatment suggests the possibility of a malignancy causing bronchial obstruction. Sputum cytology and bronchoscopic examination of the airway should be performed.

References

Schachter EN, Kreisman H, Putman C. Diagnostic problems in suppurative lung disease. Arch Intern Med 1976; 136:167.

Snow N, Lucas A, Horrigan TP. Utility of pneumonectomy in the treatment of cavitary lung disease. Chest 1985; 87:731.

Stark DD, Federle MP, Goodman PC, Podrasky AE, Webb WR. Differentiating lung abscess and empyema. Am J Roentgenol 1983; 141:163.

Vainrub B, Musher DM, Guinn GA, et al. Percutaneous drainage of lung abscess. Am Rev Respir Dis 1978; 117:153.

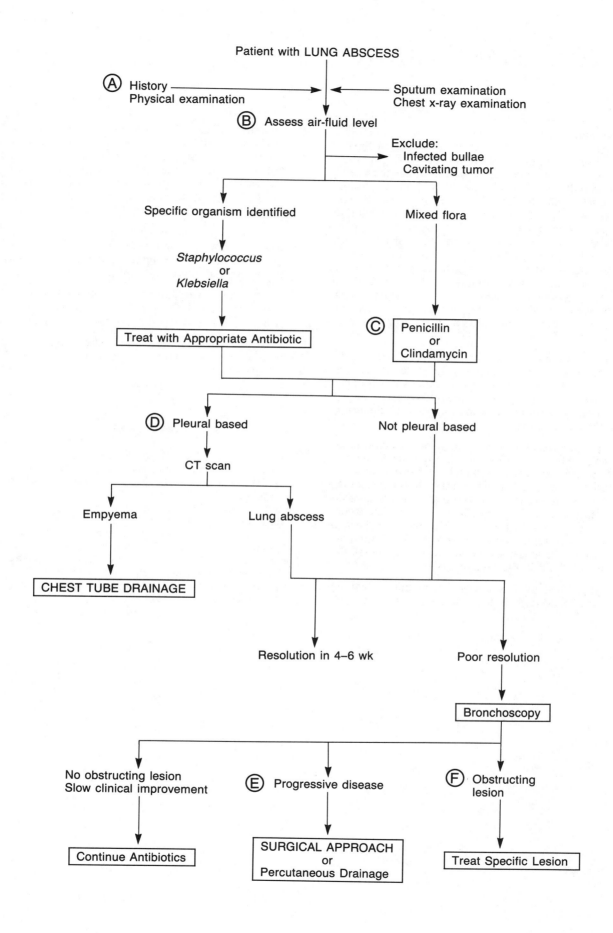

Patient with LUNG ABSCESS

Ⓐ History ——→ ←—— Sputum examination
Physical examination   Chest x-ray examination

Ⓑ Assess air-fluid level

Exclude:
Infected bullae
Cavitating tumor

Specific organism identified   Mixed flora

Staphylococcus
or
Klebsiella

Treat with Appropriate Antibiotic

Ⓒ Penicillin
or
Clindamycin

Ⓓ Pleural based   Not pleural based

CT scan

Empyema   Lung abscess

CHEST TUBE DRAINAGE

Resolution in 4–6 wk   Poor resolution

Bronchoscopy

No obstructing lesion   Ⓔ Progressive disease   Ⓕ Obstructing
Slow clinical improvement   lesion

Continue Antibiotics   SURGICAL APPROACH   Treat Specific Lesion
                              or
                              Percutaneous Drainage

AIR-FLUID LEVEL IN BULLAE

Bullae are thin-walled cavities within the lung parenchyma. These bullae may contain fluid as demonstrated by the development of an air-fluid level on the chest film. The most common cause of fluid collecting within bullae is an adjacent pneumonitis with transudation of fluid, the equivalent of a parapneumonic effusion. The bullae may have originated as a developmental abnormality or may be the result of an infectious or traumatic process. The diagnosis is suggested by a previous chest film that demonstrates the presence of a thin-walled cavity. In the absence of a previous film, a bulla with an air-fluid level can be distinguished from acute lung abscess or cavitating carcinoma on clinical grounds. In general, the presence of an air-fluid level in a bulla usually is a relatively benign finding. However, under certain circumstances it is important to exclude an obstructing airway lesion as an etiology.

A. Patients with lung abscess are usually symptomatic for several weeks and show signs of an acute or a chronic illness. Associated predisposing features of aspiration pneumonia and lung abscess are often present, including an episode of loss of consciousness, or gingival or esophageal disease.

B. Lung cavities resulting from malignancy or active tuberculosis are usually thick-walled. It is unusual for a tuberculous cavity to have an air-fluid level. Nevertheless, skin test all patients for tuberculosis and send sputum for cytologic examination and bacterial culture. Finally, consider and exclude an air-fluid level loculated within the pleural space as a diagnostic possibility. The presence of a large effusion, bullae located in lower lobes, or air-fluid levels crossing fissure lines should suggest the possibility of air and fluid in the pleural space.

C. If signs of infection are present, treat patients with antibiotics for 10 days. In the absence of these signs, observation suffices. The usual course is resolution of the air-fluid level. It has been noted that bullae may disappear following the resolution of an infection within the bullae. Presumably this is the result of inflammation in the walls of the bleb, causing adhesions and the collapse of the bleb. These patients may have a small residual scar or a normal-appearing lung on the chest film.

D. If the air-fluid level fails to resolve after several weeks, bronchoscopy is recommended to exclude an obstructing lesion such as a malignancy. Persistent hemoptysis or recurrent air-fluid levels are particularly worrisome.

E. If the index of suspicion for malignancy is high, a CT scan should also be performed. The risk of malignancy is high in a middle-aged patient who is a smoker.

F. Repeat the chest x-ray examination in 3 months to document complete resolution of the bullae or the need for a re-evaluation.

References

Gross DC, Lerner SD, Rohatgi PK. Intrabullous carcinoma: a diagnostic dilemma. Eur J Respir Dis 1984; 65:229.

Mahler DA. Air-fluid levels with lung bullae associated with pneumonitis. Lung 1981; 159:163.

Sanford HS, Green RA. Air-fluid levels in emphysematous bullae. Dis Chest 1963; 43:193.

Stark P, Gadziala N, Green R. Fluid accumulation in pre-existing pulmonary air spaces. Am J Roentgenol 1980; 134:701.

Zinn WL, Naidich DP, Whelan CA, et al. Fluid within pre-existing pulmonary air spaces: a potential pitfall in the CT differentiation of pleural from parenchymal disease. J Comput Assist Tomogr 1987; 11:441.

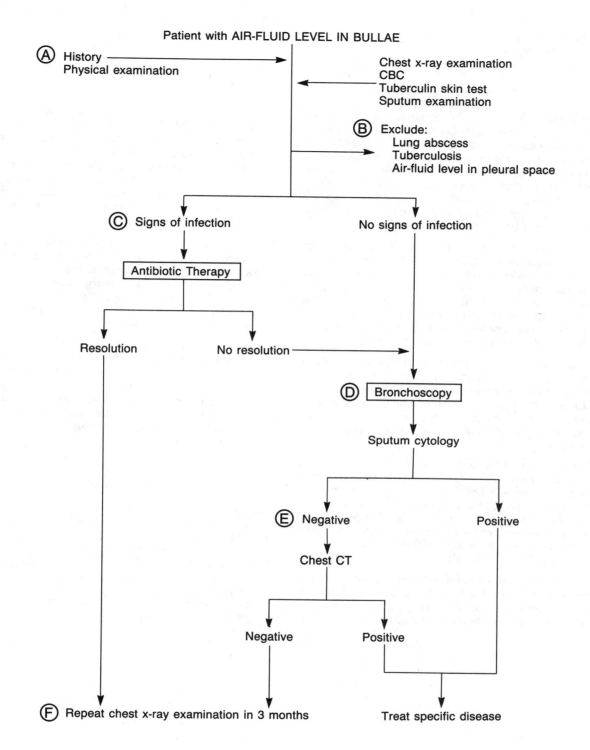

Patient with AIR-FLUID LEVEL IN BULLAE

A History ——————————→ Chest x-ray examination
Physical examination   CBC
                             Tuberculin skin test
                             Sputum examination

B Exclude:
   Lung abscess
   Tuberculosis
   Air-fluid level in pleural space

C Signs of infection   No signs of infection

Antibiotic Therapy

Resolution   No resolution ——————————→

                                    D Bronchoscopy

                                    Sputum cytology

                              E Negative   Positive

                                Chest CT

                          Negative   Positive

F Repeat chest x-ray examination in 3 months   Treat specific disease

EMPYEMA

An empyema is defined as the accumulation of purulent material in the pleural space. Controversy surrounds much of the literature regarding the diagnosis and treatment of empyemas. In recent years, the use of the term "empyema" has been broadened to include parapneumonic effusions that have relatively low white blood cell counts but contain organisms on Gram stain. In addition, exudative effusions of low pH associated with mixed aerobic-anaerobic infections are considered to be impending empyemas.

A. Patients with empyema present with the signs and symptoms of an acute infection. The most common cause of empyema is extension of a subpleural bacterial pneumonia into the pleural space. In some cases, the pneumonia dominates the clinical picture, whereas in other cases the pleural effusion dominates the clinical findings. A history of persistent fevers for weeks or months suggests the possibility of a tuberculous empyema.

B. A pleural effusion in a patient with clinical signs of infection should be rapidly investigated by performing thoracentesis, whether or not a pulmonary infiltrate is also present. A Gram stain should be obtained and the fluid sent for culture, cell counts, cytologies, and chemistries. Pleural fluid caused by empyema is exudative in character.

C. The presence of bacteria in pleural fluid indicates the need for a chest tube unless the amount of fluid is small and can be removed by thoracentesis. The rationale for the use of a chest tube is to drain infected material in an area where antibiotic penetration is suboptimal. In addition, removal of the fluid prevents potential loculation and walled-off areas of infection. These measures usually prevent the development of a fibrothorax.

D. Acidic pleural effusions caused by infections are known to loculate rapidly. The finding of a low pleural fluid pH in a patient suspected of having a pulmonary infection indicates the need for a chest tube. Markedly elevated white blood cell counts in pleural fluid in patients with pulmonary infections also suggest empyema and the need for a chest tube. These fluids may be highly viscous and difficult to withdraw from the pleural space using a needle. Effusions with low white blood cell counts and normal pH should be removed by thoracentesis if possible and the patient observed for recurrence. Exudative effusions of unknown etiology require further evaluation.

E. Empyemas usually respond to antibiotics and chest tube drainage. Failure to respond suggests the possibility of a necrotizing pneumonia or multiple loculations in the pleural space, with poor drainage through only one chest tube. A CT scan will distinguish these possibilities. If multiple loculations are found, early decortication can result in a more rapid recovery.

F. In some patients, the infection in the pleural space becomes walled off and persistently drains purulent material through the chest tube. A surgical procedure is necessary (Eloesser flap) to establish open drainage to the outside and enable lavage of the space with antibiotics. In these cases, the space may eventually close by the ingrowth of granulation tissue when the infection is adequately treated.

References

Mandal AK, Thadepalli H. Treatment of spontaneous bacterial empyema thoracis. J Thorac Cardiovasc Surg 1987; 94:414.

Potts DE, Taryle DA, Sahn SA. The glucose-pH relationship in parapneumonic effusions. Arch Intern Med 1978; 138:1378.

Silverman SG, Mueller PR, Saini S, et al. Thoracic empyema: management with image-guided catheter drainage. Radiology 1988; 169:5.

Snider GL, Saleh SS. Empyema of the thorax in adults: review of 105 cases. Dis Chest 1968; 54:410.

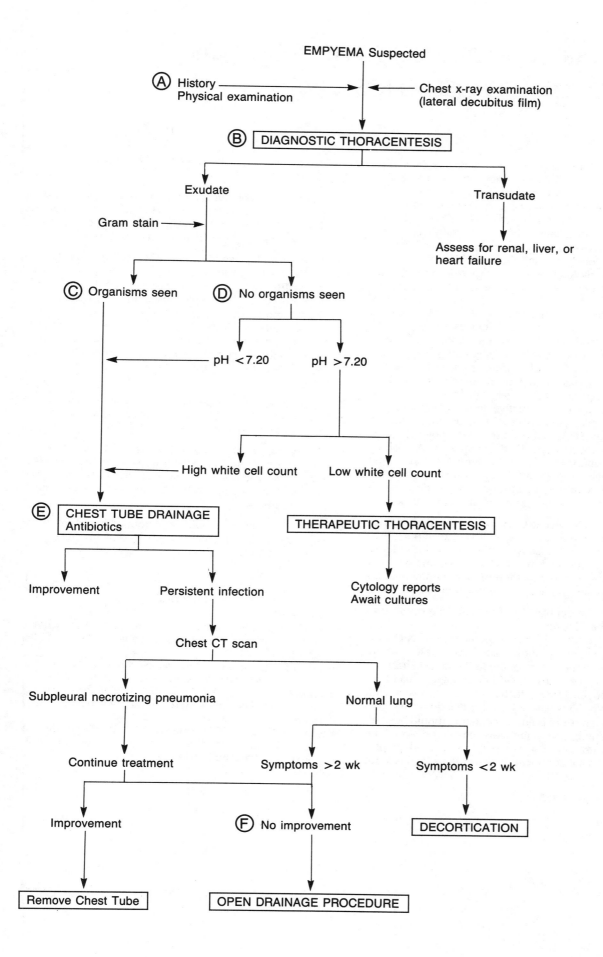

EMPYEMA Suspected

(A) History ——————————→ ←—————— Chest x-ray examination
Physical examination   (lateral decubitus film)

(B) | DIAGNOSTIC THORACENTESIS |

Exudate   Transudate

Gram stain ——————→   Assess for renal, liver, or
                                            heart failure

(C) Organisms seen   (D) No organisms seen

                    pH <7.20   pH >7.20

            High white cell count   Low white cell count

(E) | CHEST TUBE DRAINAGE
      Antibiotics | | THERAPEUTIC THORACENTESIS |

Improvement   Persistent infection   Cytology reports
                                         Await cultures

                Chest CT scan

Subpleural necrotizing pneumonia   Normal lung

Continue treatment   Symptoms >2 wk   Symptoms <2 wk

Improvement   (F) No improvement | DECORTICATION |

| Remove Chest Tube | | OPEN DRAINAGE PROCEDURE |

PULMONARY INFILTRATES IN THE (NON-AIDS) IMMUNOCOMPROMISED HOST

Defects in the host immunologic system may be caused by a number of diseases and therapies, including (1) autoimmune diseases; (2) malignant disorders such as lymphoma, leukemia, and widespread metastatic cancers; (3) immunosuppressive therapy such as corticosteroids, alkylating and antimetabolites; (4) renal failure; (5) chronic malnutrition; and (6) general debilitated states. Immunocompromised hosts are at increased risk for developing the usual bacterial and opportunistic infections. Knowledge of the specific immunologic defect is useful to determine the causative organism. Impairment of the B-lymphocyte antibody formation predisposes patients to infections caused by the usual bacteria as well as by *Pneumocystis* and cytomegalovirus. Impaired T-lymphocyte cell-mediated immunity predisposes patients to infections caused by mycobacteria; fungi such as *Cryptococcus, Aspergillus,* and *Candida*; viruses such as herpes and cytomegalovirus; parasites such as *Pneumocystis* and *Toxoplasma*; and opportunistic bacteria such as *Listeria* and *Nocardia*. Quantitative or qualitative defects of granulocytes predispose patients to infections caused by gram-negative bacteria and fungi. Two or all of these immunologic dysfunctions can be present concurrently in the same patient. While the majority of pulmonary infiltrates in immunocompromised hosts are infectious, sometimes they may be caused by the progression of the underlying disease process, drug toxicities, pulmonary edema, hemorrhage, and embolism.

A. In addition to knowledge of the patient's underlying disease and immunologic defects, it is also important to review the patient's history of past medical problems, travels, and medications. Perform a complete and thorough physical examination to identify potential infectious foci and other areas of involvement.

B. Gram stain and acid-fast bacilli (AFB) stain of the sputum may be diagnostic of the pulmonary infiltrate. However, a negative sputum examination does not exclude the presence of these infections. Chest films are used to define the nature of the infiltrate. Localized infiltrates may be caused by hemorrhage, infarction, tumors, and bacterial infections. A comparison with previous chest films may be useful to determine the etiology. The diagnosis of pulmonary edema should be readily established, and pulmonary embolism could be excluded with lung scan and pulmonary arteriography. Fungal and viral serologies confirm the diagnosis but

generally do not contribute to the immediate care of the patient.

C. Neutropenic patients with fever or a high index of suspicion for bacterial infections are at high risk for fatality. They must be promptly covered with broad-spectrum antibiotics after cultures have been obtained.

D. In severely ill patients, empiric antibiotic coverage should include a third-generation cephalosporin, an aminoglycoside, an anti-*Pseudomonas* penicillin, and erythromycin. Observe patients on this regimen for 1 to 3 days and modify antibiotics when culture results become available. When patients do not improve on this regimen, perform fiberoptic bronchoscopy. Do not initiate antifungal therapy until a firm diagnosis has been established or until other therapies have proven ineffective.

E. Patients without fever or evidence of infections need not be covered with empiric broad-spectrum antibiotics. Fiberoptic bronchoscopy establishes the diagnosis.

F. Fiberoptic bronchoscopy is also reserved for patients who do not respond to broad-spectrum antibiotic coverage and those without a definite diagnosis. Bronchoalveolar lavage and transbronchial biopsy often yield diagnostic specimens.

G. Open-lung biopsy should be performed in patients with nondiagnostic bronchoscopy. The risks of this procedure, even in gravely ill patients, are acceptably low.

References

Masur H, Shelhamer J, Parrillo JE. The management of pneumonias in immunocompromised patients. JAMA 1985; 253:1769.

McCabe RE. Diagnosis of pulmonary infections in immunocompromised patients. Med Clin North Am 1988; 72:1067.

Rosenow EC III, Wilson WR, Cockerill FR III. Pulmonary disease in the immunocompromised host (first of two parts). Mayo Clin Proc 1985; 60:473.

Wilson WR, Cockerill FR III, Rosenow EC III. Pulmonary disease in the immunocompromised host (second of two parts). Mayo Clin Proc 1985; 60:610.

PULMONARY SYMPTOMS AND ABNORMAL CHEST FILMS
IN NON-AIDS IMMUNOCOMPROMISED HOST

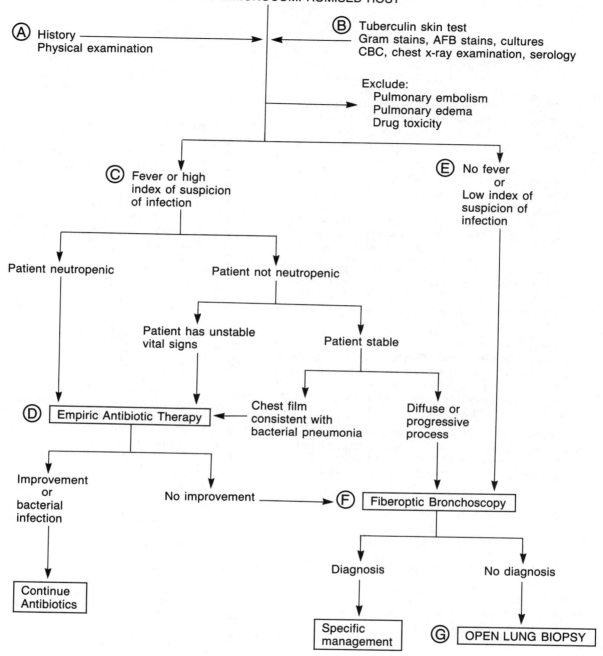

Ⓐ History
Physical examination

Ⓑ Tuberculin skin test
Gram stains, AFB stains, cultures
CBC, chest x-ray examination, serology

Exclude:
Pulmonary embolism
Pulmonary edema
Drug toxicity

Ⓒ Fever or high
index of suspicion
of infection

Ⓔ No fever
or
Low index of
suspicion of
infection

Patient neutropenic

Patient not neutropenic

Patient has unstable
vital signs

Patient stable

Ⓓ Empiric Antibiotic Therapy

Chest film
consistent with
bacterial pneumonia

Diffuse or
progressive
process

Improvement
or
bacterial
infection

No improvement

Ⓕ Fiberoptic Bronchoscopy

Continue
Antibiotics

Diagnosis

No diagnosis

Specific
management

Ⓖ OPEN LUNG BIOPSY

ACUTE EPIGLOTTITIS

Acute epiglottitis is an infectious process involving the epiglottis with or without the involvement of the supraglottic structures. This condition is potentially fatal by obstruction of the airway. The more common organisms that have been isolated in this infection include *Haemophilus influenzae*, *Streptococcus pneumoniae*, Group A *Streptococcus*, Group F *Streptococcus*, *Staphylococcus aureus*, *Staphylococcus pyogenes*, and *Streptococcus viridans*.

A. Although this condition is rare among adults, if not diagnosed in time, its serious nature mandates that the disease be considered in all patients with complaints of new onset of sore throat and dysphagia. Unfortunately the degree of respiratory symptoms has not been found to be a reliable predictor of impending airway obstruction.

B. Patients with cyanosis, stridor, or other signs of respiratory compromise must have the airway protected as a first priority. Endotracheal intubation or cricothyrotomy should be performed followed by indirect laryngoscopy to confirm the diagnosis.

C. Characteristic radiographic changes of epiglottitis can be seen in 90 percent of cases. Because of instances of sudden airway obstruction without warning, patients should be accompanied by someone skilled in intubation or cricothyrotomy while soft tissue neck films are being obtained.

D. A normal soft tissue neck film does not completely exclude the presence of epiglottitis. Patients with indeterminate or normal neck films should undergo indirect laryngoscopy or fiberoptic rhinolaryngoscopy.

E. There are no reliable clinical predictors for respiratory arrest caused by total airway obstruction, and the management of the airway is somewhat controversial. Some authors believe that selected patients could be observed closely without intubation. However, cases of sudden death have been reported even in hospitalized patients. All patients with epiglottitis should have endotracheal or nasotracheal intubation to protect the airway. Tracheostomy should be performed if intubation is not possible.

F. Treat patients with epiglottitis with intravenous antibiotics to cover the spectrum of likely organisms, and provide airway and general supports. Generally patients may be extubated after 2 to 3 days of appropriate antibiotic therapy if they can breathe around the closed endotracheal tube. The use of corticosteroids is controversial.

References

Baxter FJ, Dunn GL. Acute epiglottitis in adults. Can J Anaesth 1988; 35:428.

MayoSmith MF, Hirsch PJ, Wodzinski SF, Schiffman FJ. Acute epiglottitis in adults. An eight-year experience in the state of Rhode Island. N Engl J Med 1986; 314:1133.

Tveteras K, Kristensen S. Acute epiglottis in adults: bacteriology and therapeutic principles. Clin Otolaryngol 1987; 12:337.

Warshawski J, Havas TE, McShane DP, Gullane PJ. Adult epiglottitis. J Otolaryngol 1986; 15:362.

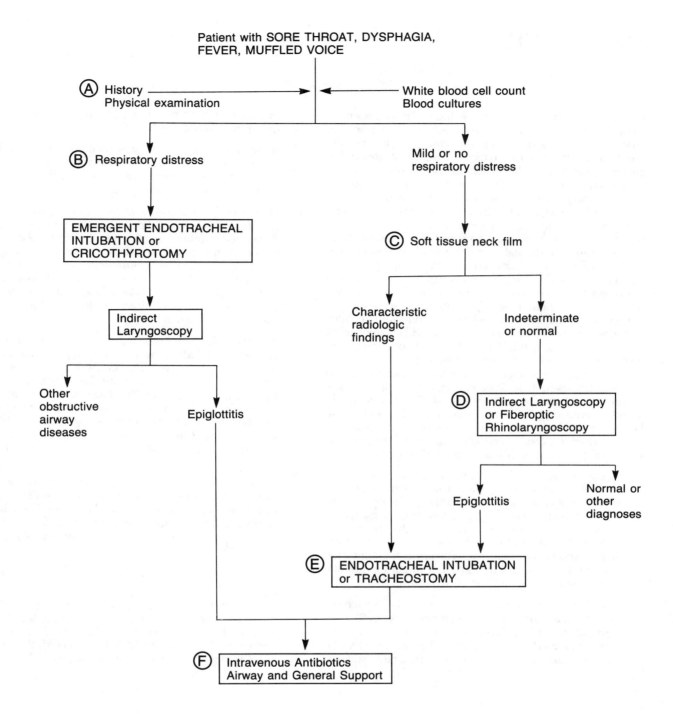

Patient with SORE THROAT, DYSPHAGIA, FEVER, MUFFLED VOICE

Ⓐ History — Physical examination → ← White blood cell count / Blood cultures

Ⓑ Respiratory distress

Mild or no respiratory distress

EMERGENT ENDOTRACHEAL INTUBATION or CRICOTHYROTOMY

Ⓒ Soft tissue neck film

Indirect Laryngoscopy

Characteristic radiologic findings

Indeterminate or normal

Other obstructive airway diseases

Epiglottitis

Ⓓ Indirect Laryngoscopy or Fiberoptic Rhinolaryngoscopy

Epiglottitis

Normal or other diagnoses

Ⓔ ENDOTRACHEAL INTUBATION or TRACHEOSTOMY

Ⓕ Intravenous Antibiotics Airway and General Support

MEDIASTINITIS

The incidence of mediastinitis has increased as a result of the increasing number of head and neck and cardiothoracic procedures and esophageal and bronchial instrumentations. Esophageal perforation due to cancer, instrumentation, or foreign body ingestion is the most common cause of nonsurgically related mediastinitis, with odontogenic, peritonsillar, and retropharyngeal abscesses, cervical lymphadenitis, Ludwig's angina, subphrenic abscesses, sternal or vertebral osteomyelitis, trauma-related and endotracheal intubation–related infections as other less common etiologies. Infection extends along and through one or more of the three potential mediastinal spaces (pretracheal, retrovisceral, perivascular) and can also disseminate hematogenously. Infections in the pretracheal space are most often caused by extensions of tracheal and lateral pharyngeal infections, with those in the retrovisceral space caused by oropharyngeal infections and those in the perivascular space caused by extension of infections from the cervical area. The most common pathogens that are found after surgically related mediastinitis include *Staphylococcus aureus* or *S. epidermidis*, gram-negative aerobes, beta-hemolytic *Streptococcus*, and mixed gram-negative and gram-positive infections. Those commonly found in nonsurgically related mediastinitis include beta-hemolytic *Streptococcus*, *S. aureus*, *Streptococcus pneumoniae*, *Bacteroides fragilis* and other anaerobic bacilli, and gram-negative aerobes. Mortality exceeds 40 percent.

A. Acute mediastinitis that occurs secondary to a surgically related procedure or aspiration usually presents with fever, dysphagia, increasing dyspnea, and chest pain. Chronic mediastinitis may be asymptomatic except for chest pain, which may be pleuritic. The chest pain usually leads to a cardiopulmonary evaluation and the eventual diagnosis of mediastinitis. The physical examination may be within normal limits or may reveal signs of one of the associated conditions listed above.

B. The chest radiograph may reveal mediastinal widening, defined as a width greater than 8 cm at the level of the aortic knob on a supine anteroposterior film. Air-fluid levels may also be seen. However, the chest film may be normal. Examination of the sputum by Gram stain and culture should be performed but may not identify the organism causing the infection.

C. If the clinical features suggest mediastinitis, CT of the chest should be performed as soon as possible to delineate the process and to help determine whether early surgical intervention is necessary.

D. In patients with postsurgical mediastinitis, start broad-spectrum antibiotics and perform a drainage procedure. If the mediastinitis is confined to the region above the carina (fourth thoracic vertebra), transcervical drainage may be adequate. If the mediastinitis is more extensive, subxiphoid or chest incisions may be necessary to effect adequate drainage. Endotracheal intubation may be necessary for complete airway control. Nutritional support will be necessary.

E. If mediastinitis is not postsurgical, start broad-spectrum antibiotics, including anaerobic coverage, as soon as the diagnosis is made; in addition, perform cine-esophagography to diagnose perforation. This may be followed by endoscopy to confirm the diagnosis and to remove any foreign body that is visualized. Surgical treatment may be necessary to remove the foreign body and to effect drainage. Closure of the esophageal perforation should not be attempted in the presence of active mediastinitis.

F. In patients without perforation, medical management is warranted. Nutritional support should be instituted, and airway management by tube may be required. Antibiotic coverage should not be specific unless definitive organisms are recovered. Treatment may take several weeks to months.

References

Friedman BC, Pickul DC. Acute mediastinitis. What to do when the cause is nonsurgical. Postgrad Med 1990; 87:273.

Wheatley MJ, Stirling MC, Kirsh MM, Gago O, Orringer MB. Descending necrotizing mediastinitis: transcervical drainage is not enough. Ann Thorac Surg 1990; 49:780.

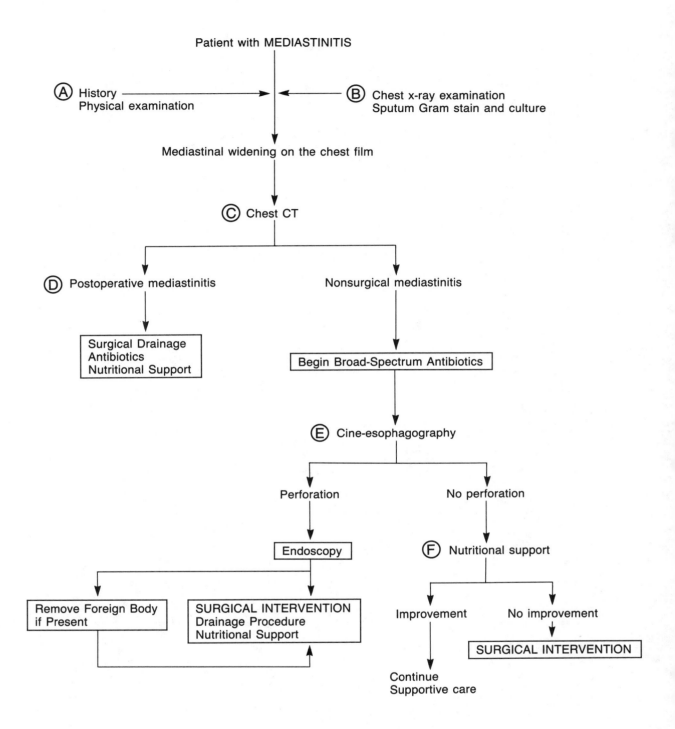

Patient with MEDIASTINITIS

(A) History — Physical examination

(B) Chest x-ray examination
Sputum Gram stain and culture

Mediastinal widening on the chest film

(C) Chest CT

(D) Postoperative mediastinitis

Nonsurgical mediastinitis

Surgical Drainage
Antibiotics
Nutritional Support

Begin Broad-Spectrum Antibiotics

(E) Cine-esophagography

Perforation

No perforation

Endoscopy

(F) Nutritional support

Remove Foreign Body
if Present

SURGICAL INTERVENTION
Drainage Procedure
Nutritional Support

Improvement

No improvement

SURGICAL INTERVENTION

Continue
Supportive care

MYCOBACTERIAL AND FUNGAL DISEASE OF THE LUNG

Isoniazid Chemoprophylaxis for Tuberculosis
Primary Tuberculous Infection
Nontuberculous Mycobacterial Infection
Histoplasmosis

Coccidioidomycosis
Mycetoma (Aspergilloma)
Allergic Bronchopulmonary Aspergillosis
Invasive Aspergillosis

ISONIAZID CHEMOPROPHYLAXIS FOR TUBERCULOSIS

The efficacy of isoniazid (INH) in preventing tuberculosis in patients with tuberculous infection has clearly been established. Treatment with a 6- to 12-month course of INH reduces the risk of future tuberculosis by as much as 90 percent among compliant patients. Patients at risk for developing tuberculosis include contacts of newly discovered cases of tuberculosis, tuberculin-negative contacts (especially children), newly infected persons, tuberculin reactors with radiographic abnormalities, tuberculin reactors of special-risk categories, and tuberculin reactors without special risks. Among these patients, the risk of developing clinical tuberculosis varies with the risk status. The major risk of INH therapy is the potentially fatal complication of hepatic necrosis. Prophylactic therapy should be recommended after the risk of developing clinical tuberculosis has been weighed against the risks and benefits of the treatment.

A. When patients at risk have been identified, efforts should be made to identify those with active tuberculosis. Chest x-ray examination and sputum acid-fast bacilli (AFB) stains and cultures should be done. Active tuberculosis must be treated with multiple antituberculosis agents in a regimen sufficient to prevent the emergence of resistant organisms (see p 90).

B. Recent tuberculin converters, tuberculin-negative household members, and close contacts should be treated with INH prophylaxis. There is a 10 percent lifetime risk of developing tuberculosis among close contacts (Table 1). The drug resistance of the organism infecting the individual with active tuberculosis should be determined. Contacts of patients with nonresistant organisms could be treated with INH alone. The treatment of contacts of patients with resistant organisms is more controversial; in addition to rifampin, INH has also been recommended by some authorities.

C. Among patients with positive tuberculin infection of unknown duration, increased risks of developing clinical tuberculosis are seen in patients with silicosis, diabetes mellitus, prolonged corticosteroid therapy, immunosuppressive therapy, chronic dialysis, chronic malnutrition, rapid weight loss, abnormal chest films consistent with old tuberculosis, and in those with HIV infection. Patients without special risks have a 1-percent lifetime risk of developing tuberculosis.

TABLE 1 Lifetime Risk of Developing Tuberculosis

Category	Risk
Close contact	10%
Recent converter	10%
Special risk group	Unknown

TABLE 2 Risk of Isoniazid-Induced Hepatitis

Age (yr)	Risk
≤20	0.05%
21–34	0.3%
35–49	1.2%
≥50	2.3%

D. The current controversy with regard to recommending INH to patients without special risk surrounds the cutoff age. The major INH toxicity is drug-induced hepatitis. If the condition is undetected and the drug is not stopped in time, it could progress to fatal hepatic necrosis. Fatal complications occur in approximately 8 percent of patients with INH hepatitis. The risk of isoniazid hepatitis is age-dependent. The risk of INH-induced hepatitis is summarized in Table 2. The lowest risk occurs in patients younger than 21 years of age. The American Thoracic Society recommends prophylactic INH for persons under the age of 35 years without special risk factors. Several recent studies challenged this age threshold; these analyses concluded that in patients older than 20 years of age, there is little to be gained with INH prophylaxis. Another side effect of isoniazid therapy is peripheral neuropathy, which can be treated with pyridoxine supplement.

E. Patients should be warned about the signs and symptoms of hepatitis and cautioned against excessive consumption of alcohol, which is a risk cofactor. At the earliest sign of hepatic damage, the drug should be discontinued. Routine liver enzyme testing for patients under 35 years of age to monitor the liver condition generally is not recommended, because 10 to 20 percent of patients taking INH develop transient elevation of liver enzymes. It is recommended, however, that in patients over 35 years of age, a baseline value should be obtained and periodic enzyme evaluations should be performed.

References

American Thoracic Society. Treatment of tuberculosis and tuberculosis infection in adults and children. Am Rev Respir Dis 1986; 134:355.

Johnson JR. Chemoprophylaxis of pulmonary tuberculosis: current recommendations and controversies. Postgrad Med 1983; 74:64.

National consensus conference on tuberculosis. Preventive treatment of tuberculosis. Chest 1985; 87(Suppl):128S.

Tsevat J, Taylor WC, Wong JB, Pauker SG. Isoniazid for tuberculin reactor: take it or leave it. Am Rev Respir Dis 1988; 137:215.

ISONIAZID PROPHYLAXIS

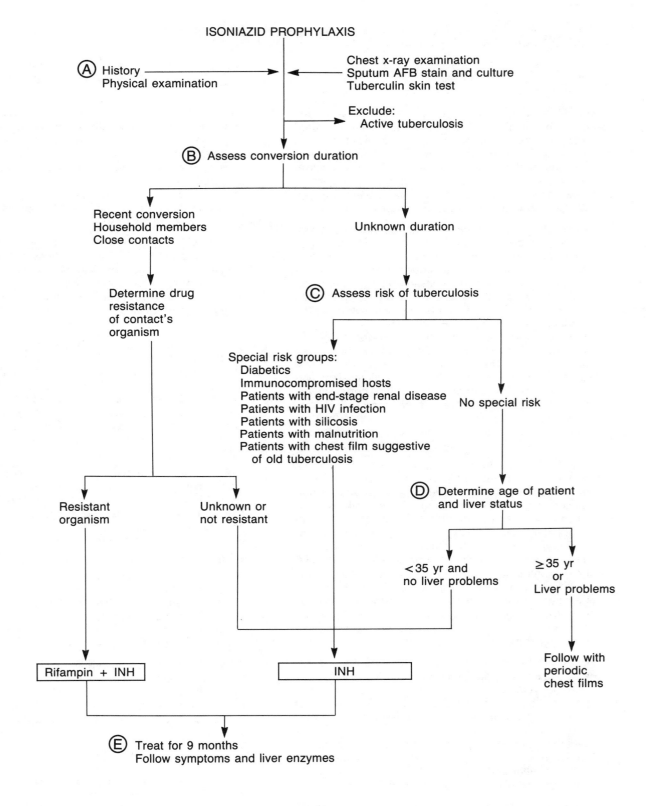

A History ——————→   ←—————— Chest x-ray examination
Physical examination   Sputum AFB stain and culture
                                    Tuberculin skin test

                                    Exclude:
                                        Active tuberculosis

B Assess conversion duration

Recent conversion   Unknown duration
Household members
Close contacts

Determine drug   C Assess risk of tuberculosis
resistance
of contact's
organism

                    Special risk groups:
                        Diabetics
                        Immunocompromised hosts
                        Patients with end-stage renal disease   No special risk
                        Patients with HIV infection
                        Patients with silicosis
                        Patients with malnutrition
                        Patients with chest film suggestive
                            of old tuberculosis

                                                        D Determine age of patient
                                                           and liver status

Resistant   Unknown or
organism   not resistant
                                            <35 yr and   ≥35 yr
                                            no liver problems   or
                                                                    Liver problems

                                                                    Follow with
                                                                    periodic
                                                                    chest films

Rifampin + INH   INH

            E Treat for 9 months
               Follow symptoms and liver enzymes

PRIMARY TUBERCULOUS INFECTION

The incidence of tuberculosis in the United States was steadily declining until the mid 1980s. The increased rate since then has been attributed to the increasing number of patients with human immunodeficiency virus (HIV) infection. Most cases of active pulmonary tuberculosis are still caused by reactivation of infectious foci, although in an increasing percentage of cases, primary infections and atypical presentations associated with HIV infections are the cause.

A. Up to one-fifth of patients with active pulmonary tuberculosis are asymptomatic. Small apical infiltrates sometimes may be present for months before detection. Progression of the infection frequently results in the development of nonspecific constitutional symptoms including night sweats, fever, chills, anorexia, and weight loss. Pleuritic chest pain and nonproductive or mildly productive cough may be present. Hemoptysis may be present in advanced disease and, when present, is generally mild, although occasional exsanguinations have been reported. Often a history of tuberculosis contacts can be elicited. Patients with diabetes, alcoholism, and chronic disability, immunocompromised hosts, and patients with HIV infection are at increased risk. Pulmonary findings may be absent; in many cases they are similar to those seen in other air-space pneumonias and are not specific to the diagnosis of tuberculosis.

B. Sputum Gram stain may be used to exclude bacterial pneumonia. The total white blood cell count is usually normal, although monocytosis may be present. A normochromic, normocytic anemia is frequently present. Chemistries are not helpful in the diagnosis of pulmonary tuberculosis, although they may identify patients with complications such as the syndrome of inappropriate secretion of antidiuretic hormone, Addison's disease, or extrapulmonary tuberculosis; they also evaluate the liver function prior to the initiation of antituberculous therapy. A positive tuberculin skin test is useful in the diagnosis of tuberculosis, but high false-negative test rates have been found in older age groups and in patients with HIV infections (up to 50 percent).

C. Chest films identify the location and extent of the disease and enable evaluation of the response to treatment. The most common roentgenographic finding of postprimary tuberculosis is an apical infiltrate with or without cavitation. Sometimes the superior segment of the lower lobe may be first involved. Primary tuberculosis has variable roentgenographic presentations, including airspace consolidation (50 percent), pleural effusion (24 percent), hilar and mediastinal lymphadenopathy (35 percent), and disseminated miliary disease (6 percent).

D. Mycobacteria smears and cultures of the sputum are diagnostic in many patients. An adequate number of specimens must be collected to ensure the successful recovery of organisms. Patients unable to produce sputum should be induced with aerosolized hypertonic saline solution. Three sputum specimens should be sent for cultures if acid-fast bacilli (AFB) are seen on smears, and additional sputum specimens should be sent if smears are negative for AFB. Cultures of mycobacteria require 3 to 8 weeks, but they are necessary in order to identify the drug sensitivity of the organism.

E. Patients with negative smears on repeated sputum specimens and patients with HIV infections with uncertain diagnosis should undergo fiberoptic bronchoscopy with bronchoalveolar lavage and transbronchial lung biopsy to obtain specimens. Specimens should be smeared and cultured for mycobacteria and other opportunistic organisms.

F. Treat pulmonary tuberculosis with isoniazid and rifampin for 9 months or isoniazid and rifampin for 6 months along with pyrazinamide for the first 2 months. Adjust the regimen according to the resistant pattern of the organism, and instruct patients about the symptoms of drug-induced hepatitis. Obtain a baseline measurement of hepatic and renal functions and monitor these at regular intervals in order to identify patients who may develop this complication.

G. Patients with a nondiagnostic bronchoscopy and for whom there is a high index of suspicion for tuberculosis may be considered for a short-term trial of antituberculous therapy with isoniazid and rifampin while awaiting culture results. Nonresponders should have additional diagnostic procedures.

H. While awaiting culture results, patients with a nondiagnostic bronchoscopy and for whom there is a low index of suspicion for tuberculosis may be started on isoniazid therapy alone if they have a positive tuberculin skin test or if they are younger than 60 years old. Additional diagnostic procedures should be considered for patients who do not fit this category.

I. Additional diagnostic procedures such as repeat bronchoscopy or open-lung biopsy should be considered for those who do not respond to a trial of antituberculous therapy or those patients for whom an empiric trial of antituberculous therapy is contraindicated.

References

Fertel D, Pitchenik AE. Tuberculosis in acquired immune deficiency syndrome. Semin Respir Infect 1989; 4:198.

Glassroth J, Robin AG, Snider DE. Tuberculosis in the 1980s. N Engl J Med 1980; 302:1441.

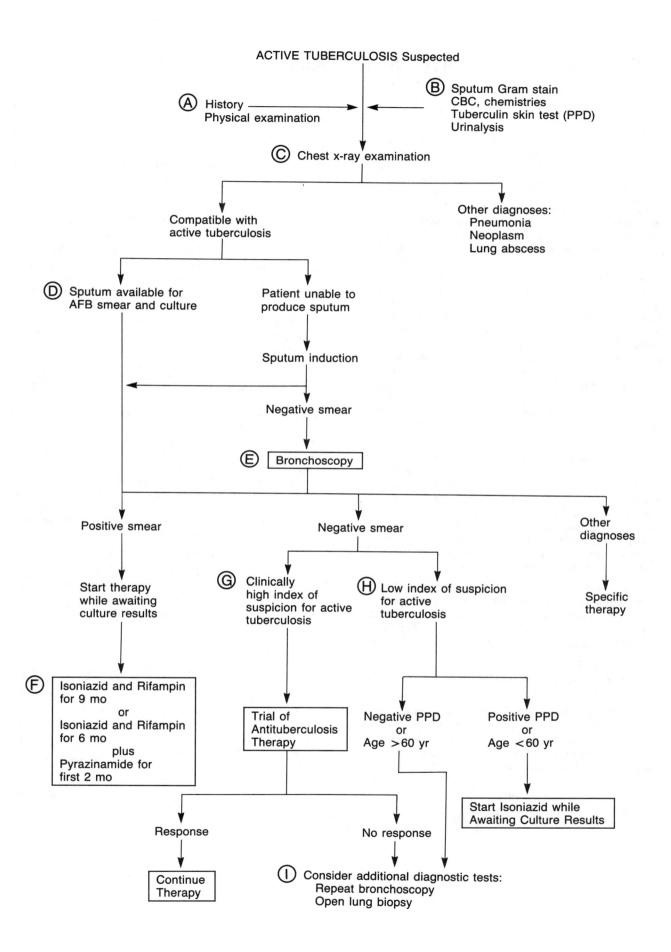

ACTIVE TUBERCULOSIS Suspected

(A) History
Physical examination

(B) Sputum Gram stain
CBC, chemistries
Tuberculin skin test (PPD)
Urinalysis

(C) Chest x-ray examination

Compatible with
active tuberculosis

Other diagnoses:
Pneumonia
Neoplasm
Lung abscess

(D) Sputum available for
AFB smear and culture

Patient unable to
produce sputum

Sputum induction

Negative smear

(E) Bronchoscopy

Positive smear

Negative smear

Other
diagnoses

Start therapy
while awaiting
culture results

(G) Clinically
high index of
suspicion for active
tuberculosis

(H) Low index of suspicion
for active
tuberculosis

Specific
therapy

(F) Isoniazid and Rifampin
for 9 mo
  or
Isoniazid and Rifampin
for 6 mo
  plus
Pyrazinamide for
first 2 mo

Trial of
Antituberculosis
Therapy

Negative PPD
or
Age >60 yr

Positive PPD
or
Age <60 yr

Start Isoniazid while
Awaiting Culture Results

Response

No response

Continue
Therapy

(I) Consider additional diagnostic tests:
Repeat bronchoscopy
Open lung biopsy

NONTUBERCULOUS MYCOBACTERIAL INFECTION

Mycobacterium avium complex and *M. kansasii* usually cause slowly progressive pulmonary disease in individuals with underlying parenchymal lung disease (chronic obstructive pulmonary disease, bronchiectasis, idiopathic pulmonary fibrosis, bullous lung disease). Organisms of the *M. avium* complex are found in water and enter the body through the respiratory or gastrointestinal tract. These organisms may be transmitted among humans through aerosolization; they commonly cause opportunistic infection in human immunodeficiency virus (HIV)–positive individuals and may disseminate and cause multiple organ failure. Dissemination is rare in immunocompetent hosts. Since colonization of the lung with nontuberculous mycobacteria (NTM) is common, assurance that progression of lung disease is due to NTM infection rather than worsening of the underlying condition may be difficult to ascertain (see below). Isolated extrapulmonary sites of infection include the cervical and submandibular lymph glands and (rarely) dermis, bone, and kidneys. Individuals may react weakly to purified protein derivative (PPD) but more strongly to specific mycobacterial antigens. Many other NTMs exist in the environment but rarely cause human disease (e.g., *M. bovis, M. leprae, M. ulcerans, M. fortuitum, M. scrofulaceum*).

A. Symptoms generally are similar to those found in patients with *M. tuberculosis*, but they may be attenuated and more chronic, except in patients with acquired immunodeficiency syndrome (AIDS) who have fulminant courses. Severe rapid weight loss, high fevers, and soaking sweats are not common in NTM. Patients present with symptoms caused by underlying lung disease including dyspnea, cough, and sputum production. The physical examination does not reveal any specific findings.

B. Perform routine laboratory studies to rule out anemia and to determine whether bone marrow involvement has occurred. The chest radiograph may demonstrate cavitation, but the patterns in NTM are no different from those seen with *M. tuberculosis*. Disease is usually multilobar.

C. Treatment for *M. tuberculosis* should be started when positive acid-fast smears are obtained and culture reports are pending (see p 90).

D. NTM is the probable diagnosis when the specific organism is identified on culture in large numbers of colonies, particularly when it is recovered from multiple sputum cultures. In addition, isolation of organisms from blood, cerebrospinal fluid, bone marrow, or lymph tissue is di-

agnostic. Other circumstances in which a diagnosis of NTM is likely include positive *M. avium* stool cultures in a patient with AIDS, repeated positive NTM cultures grown from a nonsterile source in an individual with the appropriate clinical findings, and in a patient with a positive acid-fast bacilli (AFB) stain and few NTM on culture, clinical worsening while he or she is receiving antituberculous (*M. tuberculosis*) therapy.

E. Appropriate combination chemotherapy must be individually tailored. Individuals with *M. avium* complex and moderate to severe disease should begin a three- to four-drug therapy including isoniazid (600 mg per day) in high doses, rifampin, ethambutol, and streptomycin. If cultures are negative after these drugs are used, this therapy may be continued. If cultures remain positive or the clinical course worsens, other drugs such as ethionamide and cycloserine may be added, either alone or in combination. If the initial disease is severe or disseminated, the above-mentioned drugs should be used as initial therapy supplemented by rifabutin, ciprofloxacillin, and clofazimine. Toxicities will be high, and the disease may progress despite therapy. Treatment should be continued for as long as possible. *M. kansasii* may be successfully treated with regimens containing rifampin. Initial therapeutic regimens include isoniazid (600 mg per day) and ethambutol. Rifampin resistance may develop quickly; additional drugs may then need to be added. Other mycobacterium species should be treated as well when progressive pulmonary disease is documented.

F. If NTM is confined to a single anatomic location in the lung and if remaining pulmonary function is sufficient, resection can be performed. It is unclear whether durable cures can be obtained after resection.

References

Collins FM. Mycobacterial disease, immunosuppression, and acquired immunodeficiency syndrome. Clin Microbiol Rev 1989; 10:360.

Davidson PT. The diagnosis and management of disease caused by *M. avium* complex, *M. kansasii*, and other mycobacteria. Clin Chest Med 1989; 10(3):431.

Woodring JH, Vandiviere HM. Pulmonary disease caused by nontuberculous mycobacteria. J Thorac Imaging 1990; 5:64.

NONTUBERCULOUS MYCOBACTERIA (NTM) Suspected

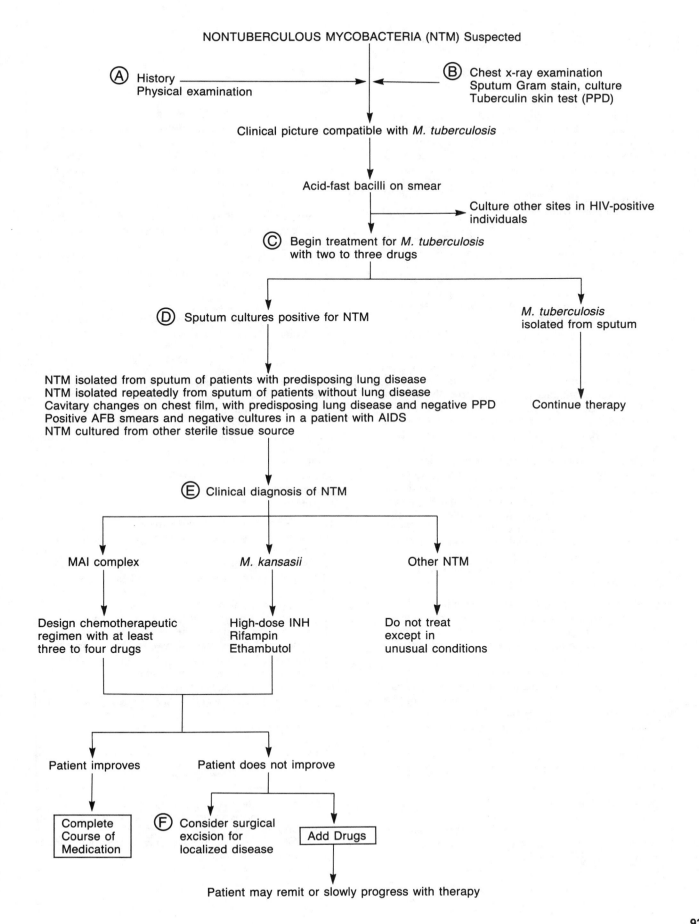

(A) History
Physical examination

(B) Chest x-ray examination
Sputum Gram stain, culture
Tuberculin skin test (PPD)

Clinical picture compatible with *M. tuberculosis*

Acid-fast bacilli on smear

Culture other sites in HIV-positive individuals

(C) Begin treatment for *M. tuberculosis* with two to three drugs

(D) Sputum cultures positive for NTM

M. tuberculosis isolated from sputum

NTM isolated from sputum of patients with predisposing lung disease
NTM isolated repeatedly from sputum of patients without lung disease
Cavitary changes on chest film, with predisposing lung disease and negative PPD
Positive AFB smears and negative cultures in a patient with AIDS
NTM cultured from other sterile tissue source

Continue therapy

(E) Clinical diagnosis of NTM

MAI complex

M. kansasii

Other NTM

Design chemotherapeutic regimen with at least three to four drugs

High-dose INH
Rifampin
Ethambutol

Do not treat except in unusual conditions

Patient improves

Patient does not improve

Complete Course of Medication

(F) Consider surgical excision for localized disease

Add Drugs

Patient may remit or slowly progress with therapy

HISTOPLASMOSIS

Histoplasmosis is caused by a small (2 to 4 μ) dimorphic fungus (mold in soil, yeast at body temperature), *Histoplasma capsulatum*. It is the most common systemic fungal infection in the United States and is an important opportunistic infection in immunocompromised hosts, including those with acquired immunodeficiency syndrome (AIDS). Histoplasmosis is endemic along the Ohio, Mississippi, and St. Lawrence River valleys. Histoplasmosis organisms have also been found in soil contaminated with bat and bird droppings. A low level of inoculum exposure results in only 1 percent of persons developing symptomatic illness, whereas 50 to 100 percent develop symptoms after heavy exposure. The majority of these cases are acute self-limiting illnesses. Only one of 2,000 infected individuals develops progressive disseminated or cavitary infection; these infections usually occur in patients with impaired cellular immune responses.

A. The majority of symptomatic patients present with a flu-like syndrome including fever, chills, headache, myalgia, and nonproductive cough. Enlarged mediastinal lymph nodes may be seen in approximately 10 percent of patients. A small percentage of patients, mostly women, may also develop rheumatologic symptoms of arthritis and arthralgias. Physical examination in most patients is nonspecific, but cervical or supraclavicular lymphadenopathy, pulmonary rales, and skin rashes may be found. Patients with disseminated disease have variable clinical manifestations depending on the severity of the condition, the immunocompetence of the patient, and the involved sites. Hepatosplenomegaly may be seen in the majority of patients with disseminated disease. Adult respiratory distress syndrome (ARDS) may develop in patients with acquired immunodeficiency syndrome (AIDS) who have diffuse pulmonary infiltrates due to histoplasmosis or in normal individuals who have had a heavy inoculum exposure.

B. Routine laboratory blood tests are nonspecific for the diagnosis of histoplasmosis. Owing to their small size, organisms are not generally seen on sputum examinations. Routine sputum examination excludes bacterial and acid-fast bacillary (AFB) infections. Serology is useful in identifying nonimmunocompromised patients with histoplasmosis infection, since the majority of these patients have a positive test result. The titer of the complement fixation test, however, does not predict the severity of the infection, nor does it identify those patients requiring therapy. Histoplasmosis skin testing is not generally performed for individual diagnosis, as it may boost the antibody titers and confuse the interpretation of future serologic results.

C. Nodules and infiltrates are commonly seen on chest films in symptomatic patients. Nodules are mostly solitary and less than 3 cm in diameter, and they may be calcified. Noncalcified nodules may be diagnostic dilemmas, and some patients may require thoracotomy to exclude malig-

nancy. Infiltrates due to histoplasmosis are characterized by nonsegmental homogeneous parenchymal consolidations that tend to clear and reappear in other areas of the parenchyma. Mediastinal or hilar adenopathy and cavitating lesions may also be seen. Pleural effusion is an uncommon finding.

D. Disseminated disease occurs primarily in immunocompromised hosts. Patients may be receiving immunosuppressive therapy or have diseases that suppress the cellular immune response, such as AIDS, lymphoma, and lymphocytic leukemia. Other factors that may predispose to disseminated disease include old age, diabetes, and renal or hepatic failure.

E. In patients with pulmonary involvement only, fiberoptic bronchoscopy with transbronchial biopsy is performed to obtain adequate tissue specimens for culture and histology. Wright Giemsa or methenamine silver staining may reveal histiocytes containing *H. capsulatum*.

F. Bone marrow, liver, or lymph node biopsy should be considered in those patients with extrapulmonary involvement and in patients with nondiagnostic pulmonary work-ups. Positive cultures may be found in as many as 75 percent of bone marrow specimens. Using centrifugation-lysis techniques, blood cultures may be positive in 50 to 70 percent of these patients. Urine and sputum cultures have also been found to be positive in approximately 60 percent of patients with disseminated disease.

G. Use intravenous amphotericin B to treat patients with disseminated disease, patients with AIDS and localized histoplasmosis infections, patients with complicated acute pulmonary histoplasmosis infections who develop ARDS, patients with progressive pulmonary histoplasmosis, and those with mediastinal granulomas with symptomatic bronchial obstruction. A total of 1 to 2 g of amphotericin B may be needed. Even with amphotericin B treatment, more than 90 percent of patients with AIDS have clinically significant relapses; suppressive therapy with oral ketoconazole is indicated in these cases. Patients not known to be immunocompromised who relapse after therapy should be investigated for the presence of adrenal insufficiency, endocarditis, meningitis, intravascular infection, and unrecognized immunosuppression.

References

Connell JV Jr, Muhm JR. Radiographic manifestations of pulmonary histoplasmosis: a 10-year review. Radiology 1976; 121:281.

Davies SF. Diagnosis of pulmonary fungal infections. Semin Respir Infect 1988; 3:162.

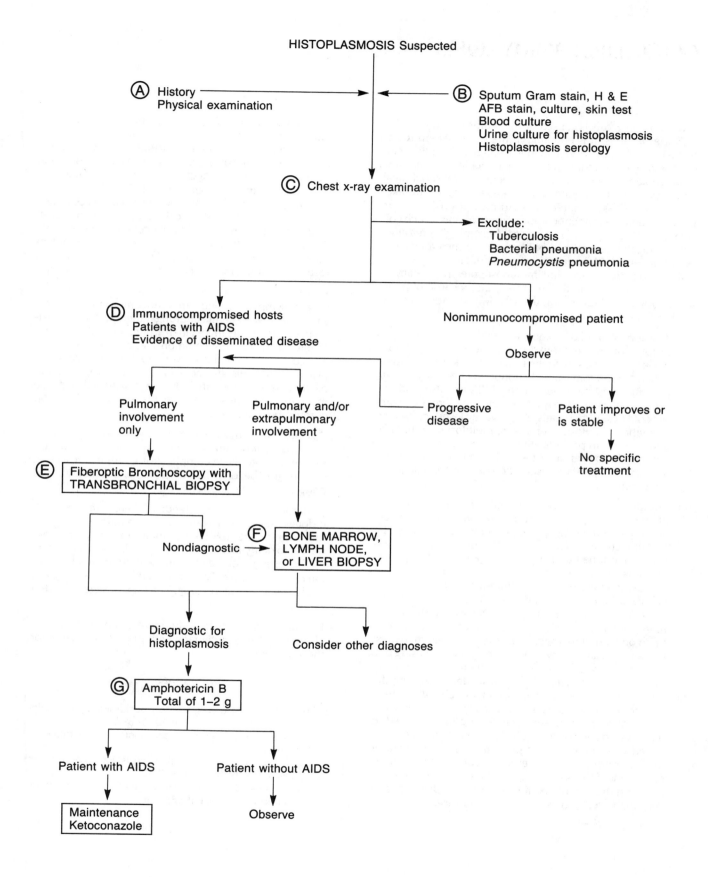

HISTOPLASMOSIS Suspected

Ⓐ History
Physical examination

Ⓑ Sputum Gram stain, H & E
AFB stain, culture, skin test
Blood culture
Urine culture for histoplasmosis
Histoplasmosis serology

Ⓒ Chest x-ray examination

Exclude:
Tuberculosis
Bacterial pneumonia
Pneumocystis pneumonia

Ⓓ Immunocompromised hosts
Patients with AIDS
Evidence of disseminated disease

Nonimmunocompromised patient

Observe

Pulmonary
involvement
only

Pulmonary and/or
extrapulmonary
involvement

Progressive
disease

Patient improves or
is stable

No specific
treatment

Ⓔ Fiberoptic Bronchoscopy with
TRANSBRONCHIAL BIOPSY

Nondiagnostic →

Ⓕ BONE MARROW,
LYMPH NODE,
or LIVER BIOPSY

Diagnostic for
histoplasmosis

Consider other diagnoses

Ⓖ Amphotericin B
Total of 1–2 g

Patient with AIDS

Patient without AIDS

Maintenance
Ketoconazole

Observe

COCCIDIOIDOMYCOSIS

Coccidioidomycosis is caused by the dimorphic fungus *Coccidioides immitis*. It is endemic in the southwestern region of the United States, Mexico, and in Central and South America. The disease is acquired through inhalation of organisms from contaminated soil. Most infections are subclinical, although patients frequently may experience a "flu-like" syndrome. Disseminated coccidioidomycosis occurs predominantly in immunocompromised patients. Once considered to be a regional disease, it is becoming increasingly geographically generalized because of the increased number of patients with acquired immunodeficiency syndrome (AIDS) and patients receiving immunosuppressive therapy for organ transplants and other diseases, and because of population growth and tourism in the southwestern region of the United States.

A. A history of travel or residence in endemic areas is usually forthcoming. A flu-like syndrome occurring 1 to 3 weeks after exposure to the fungus may develop in some patients. Symptoms include nonproductive cough, fever, pleuritic chest pain, headache, chills, malaise, and myalgia. Some patients may also develop the symptom complex of "desert rheumatism" or "valley fever" consisting of erythema nodosum, erythema multiforme, arthralgia, and arthritis. In patients with AIDS, the disease may occur months to years after the patient has left the endemic area; this represents reactivation of previously acquired infections.

B. Routine blood tests are nonspecific, although peripheral blood eosinophilia is a common finding. Exclude bacterial pneumonia and active pulmonary tuberculosis by sputum cultures, Gram stains, acid-fast bacilli (AFB) stains, and tuberculin skin testing. Perform the sputum examination for coccidioidomycosis with potassium hydroxide–digested sputum followed by periodic acid-Schiff, or hematoxylin and eosin (H & E) staining. The presence of characteristic spherules is diagnostic. *C. immitis* from lung secretions and tissues can be readily cultured on laboratory media; however, the specimen must be handled carefully by experienced personnel using biosafety equipment because of the extremely infectious nature of cultured material. Skin tests demonstrating the presence of delayed hypersensitivity to *C. immitis* have limited usefulness unless a recent skin test is known to be negative. Specific serologic testing may be used to diagnose coccidioidomycosis. Early infection may be detected with the tube precipitin, latex agglutination, or immunodiffusion test. Later in the course of the illness, complement fixation testing can be used. A fourfold increase in the complement fixation titer is diagnostic. A very high titer suggests disseminated disease.

C. The radiographic appearance of pulmonary coccidioidomycosis is variable. "Fleeting" patchy infiltrates with either segmental or lobar distribution may be seen. Hilar lymphadenopathy occurs in 20 percent of the cases. Pulmonary nodules, singular or multiple, ranging from 0.5 to 3 cm in diameter, are indistinguishable from other nodular pulmonary lesions. Cavitations caused by necrosis of these nodules are typically thin-walled and located in the upper lung fields; these occur in approximately 0.1 percent of all infections or in 2 to 8 percent of hospitalized patients. Pleural effusion may occur as a result of parapneumonic reactions or rupture of cavities.

D. Patients with evidence of disseminated infections, persistent symptoms, and immunocompromised status should receive systemic antifungal therapy. Disseminated infection occurs in less than 1 percent of all *C. immitis* infections; the most common sites are the skin, bones and joints, and central nervous system. Immunocompromised patients are more likely to develop disseminated disease; these include those with AIDS, those receiving immunosuppressive therapy, and those on chronic hemodialysis.

E. Cavitary lesions may cause hemoptysis and may rupture, resulting in pyopneumothorax. Surgery may be necessary to manage these complications. Surgical resection should also be considered for large, subpleural, and peripheral cavitary lesions.

F. Amphotericin B is the standard therapy for coccidioidomycoses. This drug must be given intravenously and has significant toxicities, including hypotension, nephrotoxicity, and electrolyte imbalance. Depending on the response of the patient, the required total dosage ranges from 1 to 3 g. Patients with relapses may be given additional doses of the drug. The total dosage is limited by nephrotoxicity.

G. Patients with AIDS have frequent relapses. Consider chronic suppressive therapy with oral ketoconazole for these patients.

References

Ampel NM, Wieden MA, Galgiani JN. Coccidioidomycosis: clinical update. Rev Infect Dis 1989; 11:897.

Davies SF. Diagnosis of pulmonary fungal infections. Semin Resp Infect 1988; 3:162.

Drutz DJ, Catanzaro A. Coccidioidomycosis. Parts I and II. Am Rev Respir Dis 1978; 117:559, 727.

Johnson PC, Sarosi GA. Community-acquired fungal pneumonias. Semin Resp Infect 1988; 4:56.

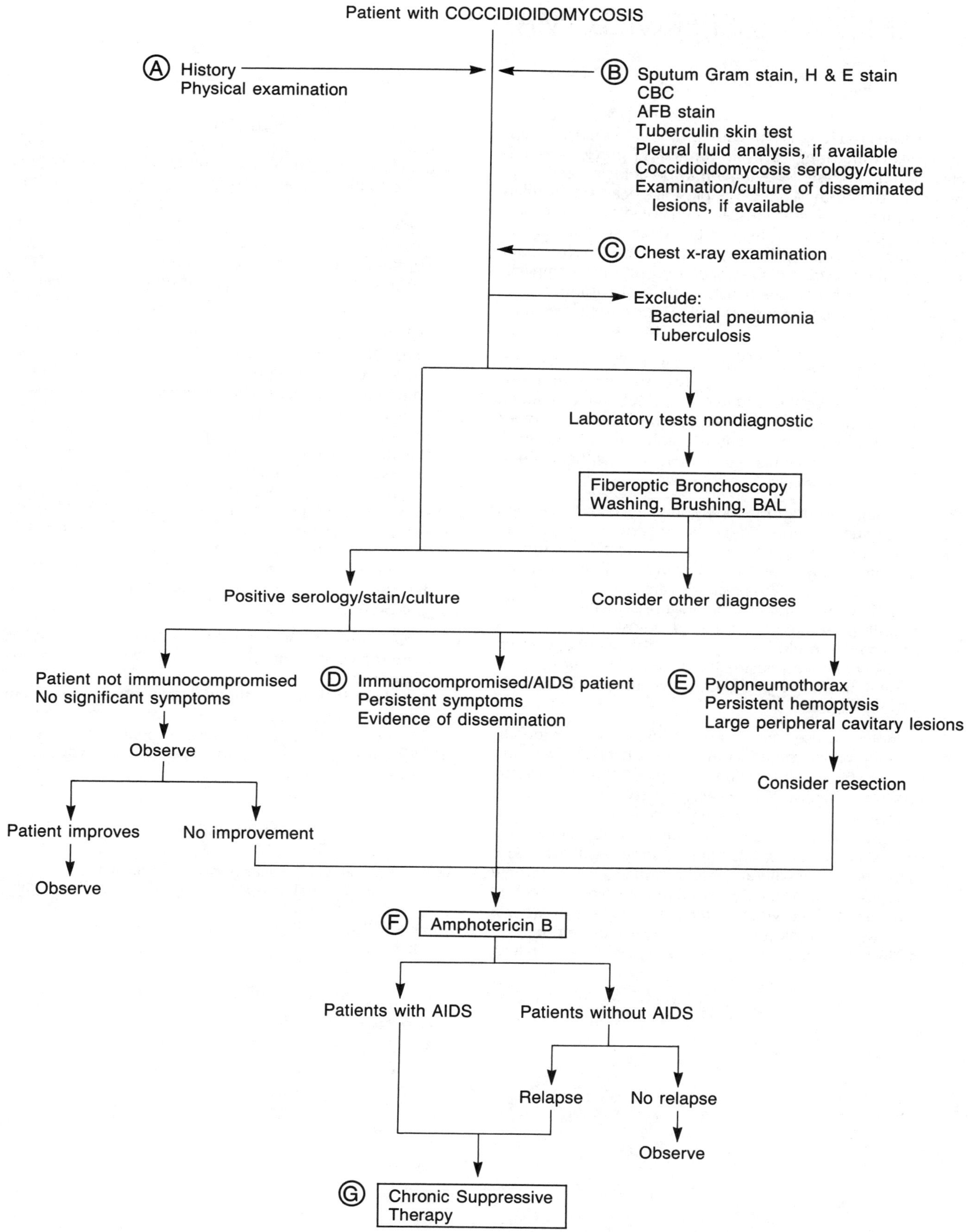

Patient with COCCIDIOIDOMYCOSIS

Ⓐ History
Physical examination

Ⓑ Sputum Gram stain, H & E stain
CBC
AFB stain
Tuberculin skin test
Pleural fluid analysis, if available
Coccidioidomycosis serology/culture
Examination/culture of disseminated
    lesions, if available

Ⓒ Chest x-ray examination

Exclude:
    Bacterial pneumonia
    Tuberculosis

Laboratory tests nondiagnostic

Fiberoptic Bronchoscopy
Washing, Brushing, BAL

Positive serology/stain/culture

Consider other diagnoses

Patient not immunocompromised
No significant symptoms

Ⓓ Immunocompromised/AIDS patient
Persistent symptoms
Evidence of dissemination

Ⓔ Pyopneumothorax
Persistent hemoptysis
Large peripheral cavitary lesions

Observe

Consider resection

Patient improves   No improvement

Observe

Ⓕ Amphotericin B

Patients with AIDS   Patients without AIDS

Relapse   No relapse

Observe

Ⓖ Chronic Suppressive
Therapy

MYCETOMA (ASPERGILLOMA)

A mycetoma is a fungus ball caused by *Aspergillus* infection of a pre-existing lung cavity in an area of previous parenchymal lung disease. Mycetoma may be detected and diagnosed on routine chest films. The presence of a partially filled cavity with an associated crescent sign noted on a chest radiograph or chest CT scan suggests the diagnosis. Local tissue invasion by the *Aspergillus* organism may be the dominant feature of the disease and the mycetoma only an accompanying feature. Such patients may complain of chronic cough or recurrent hemoptysis and are said to have chronic necrotizing aspergillosis.

A. Most cases of aspergillosis are caused by colonization of a pre-existing pulmonary cavity by the organism. These cavities may be the result of an old tuberculosis infection, an end-stage sarcoidosis, or any of a variety of other processes. Once the cavity is colonized with *Aspergillus*, its appearance may change over time, either becoming larger or smaller.

B. The diagnosis of a mycetoma can be made when a solid mass appears within a pre-existing cavity and is separated from the cavity wall by a crescent of air. The fungus ball may liquify, creating an air-fluid level, or it may calcify. Serum *Aspergillus* precipitins are usually present and are helpful in confirming the diagnosis. In atypical radiographic presentations, further diagnostic evaluation is warranted to exclude malignancy. Bronchoscopy determines whether an obstructing lesion of the bronchus is present. In all cases, rule out active tuberculosis or bacterial infection.

C. A more invasive form of aspergillosis occurs in debilitated or mildly immunocompromised patients. This form involves the upper lobes and is termed "chronic necrotizing aspergillosis." These cases are characterized by local tissue invasion by the organism. The diagnosis can be suspected from the roentgenographic appearance and the demonstration of *Aspergillus* in the sputum. These patients present with upper lobe cavities with or without mycetoma, accompanied by an intense pleural reaction adjacent to the cavities. The lesions may slowly worsen over weeks to months. The diagnosis can be firmly established by the demonstration of septate hyphae in lung tissue obtained by biopsy, but can also be made on clinical grounds. Most patients are symptomatic, with fever, cough, sputum production, and weight loss. Symptoms relate to the chronic, progressively necrotizing pulmonary process. Bronchoscopy is often performed to exclude malignancy and active tuberculosis. A course of broad-spectrum antibiotics is given to treat possible concurrent bacterial processes. Chronic necrotizing aspergillosis should be differentiated from invasive aspergillosis, which is a rapidly progressive disease.

D. Mild hemoptysis is very common in patients with mycetoma. The etiology is likely multifactorial and may involve physical abrasion of the cavity wall by the fungus ball, release of proteolytic enzymes from inflammatory cells present in the cavity wall, and granulation tissue formation. Occasionally, mycetomas may cause life-threatening hemoptysis. In these cases, cavitary resection is indicated in patients with localized lesions who are in relatively good health with good pulmonary function. However, postoperative complications including fistulae, empyema, and recurrent hemoptysis are common. In patients who are poor surgical candidates, intracavitary amphotericin B has been shown to be beneficial. Intravenous amphotericin B for mycetoma has not proved useful.

E. Treat patients with progressive necrotizing aspergillosis with intravenous amphotericin B. In addition, vigorous supportive treatment of their underlying medical problems including nutritional supplementation is indicated. Intracavitary amphotericin B may be initiated in unresponsive individuals. Surgical treatment may be indicated in patients with localized disease who cannot tolerate chemotherapy.

References

Binder RE, Faling LJ, Pugatch RD, Mahasaen C, Snider GL. Chronic necrotizing aspergillosis: a discrete clinical entity. Medicine 1982; 61:109.

Glimp RA, Bayer AS. Pulmonary aspergilloma. Arch Intern Med 1983; 143:303.

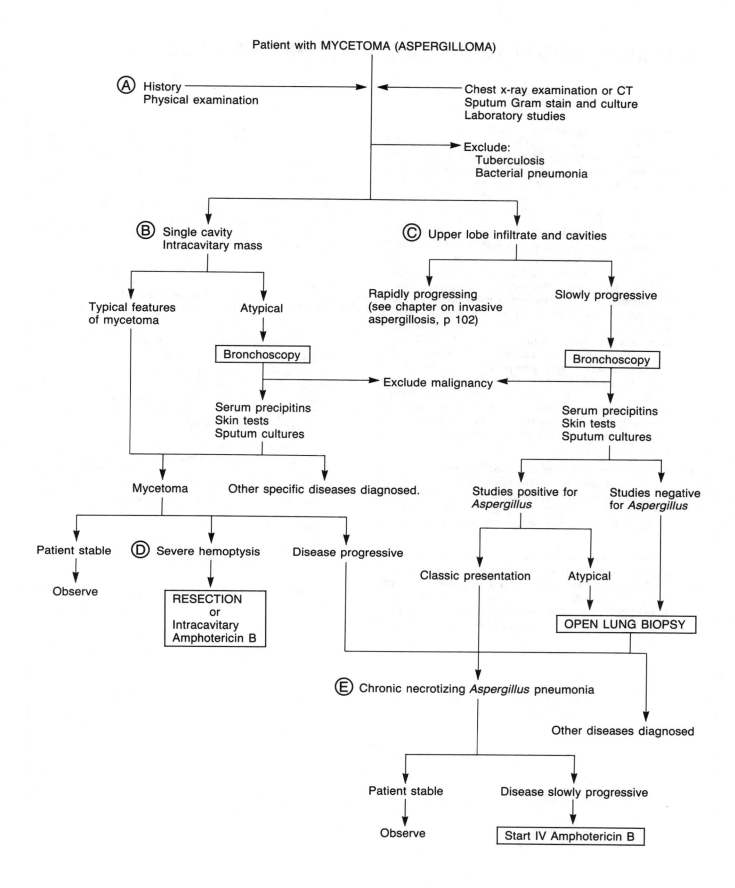

Patient with MYCETOMA (ASPERGILLOMA)

Ⓐ History —————————————— ← Chest x-ray examination or CT
Physical examination   Sputum Gram stain and culture
                                     Laboratory studies

→ Exclude:
    Tuberculosis
    Bacterial pneumonia

Ⓑ Single cavity   Ⓒ Upper lobe infiltrate and cavities
Intracavitary mass

Typical features   Atypical   Rapidly progressing   Slowly progressive
of mycetoma   (see chapter on invasive
                                              aspergillosis, p 102)

                        Bronchoscopy   Bronchoscopy

                        → Exclude malignancy ←

                        Serum precipitins   Serum precipitins
                        Skin tests   Skin tests
                        Sputum cultures   Sputum cultures

Mycetoma   Other specific diseases diagnosed.   Studies positive for   Studies negative
                                                          Aspergillus   for Aspergillus

Patient stable   Ⓓ Severe hemoptysis   Disease progressive   Classic presentation   Atypical

Observe   OPEN LUNG BIOPSY

          RESECTION
          or
          Intracavitary
          Amphotericin B

                        Ⓔ Chronic necrotizing Aspergillus pneumonia

                                                          Other diseases diagnosed

                        Patient stable   Disease slowly progressive

                        Observe   Start IV Amphotericin B

99

ALLERGIC BRONCHOPULMONARY ASPERGILLOSIS

Allergic bronchopulmonary aspergillosis (ABPA) is part of the spectrum of aspergillosis-related pulmonary diseases. Most patients with ABPA have a history suggestive of asthma. However, several unusual additional features suggest the diagnosis of ABPA. It is important to realize that because aspergillosis is a ubiquitous organism, the presence of the organism in the sputum does not definitively establish the diagnosis.

A. A history of episodic bronchial obstruction with peripheral eosinophilia is a characteristic feature of ABPA. Cough frequently presents with production of mucus plugs containing leukocytes, eosinophils, and *Aspergillus* organisms. Unlike typical asthma, recurrent febrile episodes are common, and the chest film is often abnormal. Fleeting infiltrates are often found and are usually confined to the upper lobes. It is essential to exclude bacterial pneumonia as the cause of these infiltrates. In patients with ABPA, the clinical response to inhaled beta-agonists and oral theophylline is often poor. Gram stain and culture of sputum should be performed in all patients. The combination of negative bacterial cultures, normal white blood cell count, and the lack of response to antibiotics effectively rules out bacterial infection. If recurrent bacterial pneumonia is noted, other diagnoses (such as cystic fibrosis) are likely.

B. Ill-defined infiltrates, often located in the upper lung zones, are a frequent finding. This pattern may suggest tuberculosis, which must be excluded with skin tests and sputum cultures. Other radiographic findings in ABPA include focal atelectasis, emphysematous changes, and cavitation.

C. A positive skin test for *Aspergillus* is suggestive of the diagnosis, but unfortunately is nonspecific. Patients with ABPA usually show both type I (immediate wheal and flare) and type III (Arthus reaction, occurring 4 to 10 hours after inoculation) reactions. Many false-negative and false-positive reactions occur because of differences in the antigenic purity of the preparations used in skin testing, the concurrent use of corticosteroid medications, and incidental environmental exposures. Serum precipitins for *Aspergillus* are usually elevated but are also relatively nonspecific. Elevated IgE levels, particularly elevated levels of *Aspergillus*-specific IgE, offer greater diagnostic specificity and also correlate with disease activity. Specific IgE levels should be obtained in any precipitin-negative patient when the diagnosis is strongly suspected.

D. The classic appearance of mucoid impaction (gloved finger pattern) on chest radiographs establishes the diagnosis. Additional studies are required when the radiographic presentation is atypical.

E. Negative *Aspergillus* skin tests and serology in a patient with sputum or tissue cultures that are positive for *Aspergillus* necessitate further diagnostic work-up. CT of the chest should be performed to look for saccular proximal bronchiectasis. The finding of saccular bronchiectasis is helpful in establishing the diagnosis of ABPA. Bronchography is potentially hazardous in asthmatic patients and should be avoided.

F. The treatment of choice in patients with ABPA is oral steroids. The duration of treatment necessary to control symptoms is not well defined, and some patients require intermittent courses of therapy. The activity of the disease can be monitored with total IgE levels. Treatment with cromolyn sodium or steroids by inhalation has not proven useful.

References

Fink JN. Allergic bronchopulmonary aspergillosis. Chest 1985; 87:81S.

Glimp RA, Bayer AS. Fungal pneumonias. Chest 1981; 80:85.

ALLERGIC BRONCHOPULMONARY ASPERGILLOSIS Suspected

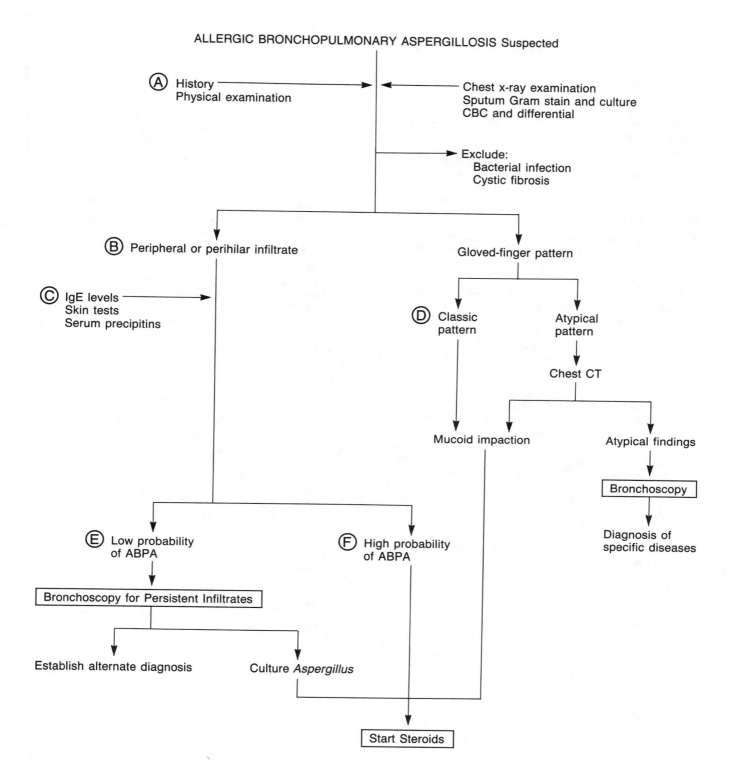

A History
Physical examination

Chest x-ray examination
Sputum Gram stain and culture
CBC and differential

Exclude:
    Bacterial infection
    Cystic fibrosis

B Peripheral or perihilar infiltrate

Gloved-finger pattern

C IgE levels
Skin tests
Serum precipitins

D Classic
pattern

Atypical
pattern

Chest CT

Mucoid impaction

Atypical findings

Bronchoscopy

Diagnosis of
specific diseases

E Low probability
of ABPA

F High probability
of ABPA

Bronchoscopy for Persistent Infiltrates

Establish alternate diagnosis

Culture *Aspergillus*

Start Steroids

INVASIVE ASPERGILLOSIS

Invasive aspergillosis is a common opportunistic infection that occurs in severely immunocompromised hosts. It rarely occurs in normal patients and in those with certain underlying chronic conditions such as cirrhosis. The *Aspergillus* species are soil saprophytes, which are widespread in nature. Air sampling within hospitals can frequently detect *Aspergillus*. Patients with chronic obstructive lung disease may be colonized with the organism.

A. Invasive aspergillosis should be suspected in immunocompromised patients with progressive pulmonary infiltrates that are resistant to antibiotic therapy. In particular, neutropenic patients receiving broad-spectrum antibiotics are at high risk for invasive aspergillosis. *Aspergillus* is less common in patients with acquired immunodeficiency disease. Physical findings are nonspecific and include fever, chills, cough, and dyspnea. Extrapulmonary involvement may be found in any organ system, including the brain, cranial sinuses, middle ear, gastrointestinal tract, liver, and spleen.

B. There is no specific chest film pattern in patients with invasive aspergillosis. The chest film may show progressive infiltrates that may be patchy, nodular, or diffuse. Cavitation may occur. *Aspergillus* often invades vessels, resulting in pulmonary infarcts and wedge-shaped densities. The presence of *Aspergillus* in sputum cultures is not generally helpful in making the diagnosis. However, in neutropenic patients who do not smoke, positive cultures may be of predictive value. Serologic tests for *Aspergillus* are of limited diagnostic value. Analysis of arterial blood gases (ABG) may reveal only mild hypoxemia.

C. Extrapulmonary involvement occurs in less than 25 percent of cases. However, involvement of the skin or gastrointestinal tract may provide an accessible biopsy site to demonstrate tissue invasion by the organism.

D. The diagnosis is established by finding septate hyphae with repeated branching at 45 degrees in tissues. The particular diagnostic procedure selected to obtain tissue depends on the status of the patient and the resources of the institution. Bronchial, transbronchial, and open lung biopsy have been used with success.

E. Successful treatment depends in part on the immune status of the patient. If possible, discontinue steroids and cytotoxic drugs. In experimental studies, corticosteroids have been found to exacerbate pulmonary aspergillosis. In neutropenic patients, an increase in the neutrophil count is a favorable sign.

F. Amphotericin B alone or in combination with rifampin is used to treat the infection. Serial determination of anti-*Aspergillus* precipitin antibody titers may provide a useful guide to the adequacy of therapy.

G. Refractory or recurrent infection localized to a single lobe may be resected.

References

Armstrong D. Problems in management of opportunistic fungal diseases. Rev Infect Dis 1989; 2:S1591.

Herbert PA, Bayer AS. Fungal pneumonia: invasive pulmonary aspergillosis. Chest 1981; 80:220.

Karam GH, Griffin FM. Invasive pulmonary aspergillosis in nonimmunocompromised non-neutropenic hosts. Rev Infect Dis 1986; 8:357.

Sidransky H, Friedman L. The effect of cortisone and antibiotic agents on experimental pulmonary aspergillosis. Am J Pathol 1959; 35:169.

Verea-Hernando H, Martin-Egana MT, Montero-Martinez C, Fontan-Bueso J. Bronchoscopic findings in invasive pulmonary aspergillosis. Thorax 1989; 44:822.

Yu VL, Muder RR, Poorsattar A. Significance of isolation of aspergillus from the respiration tract in the diagnosis of invasive pulmonary aspergillosis. Am J Med 1986; 81:249.

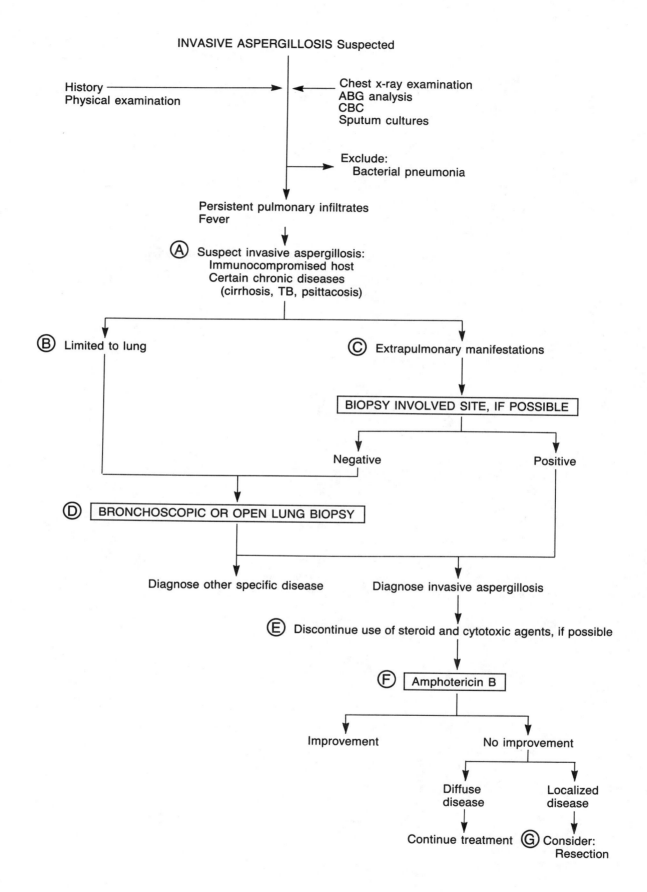

INVASIVE ASPERGILLOSIS Suspected

History —————
Physical examination

Chest x-ray examination
ABG analysis
CBC
Sputum cultures

Exclude:
    Bacterial pneumonia

Persistent pulmonary infiltrates
Fever

Ⓐ Suspect invasive aspergillosis:
    Immunocompromised host
    Certain chronic diseases
    (cirrhosis, TB, psittacosis)

Ⓑ Limited to lung

Ⓒ Extrapulmonary manifestations

BIOPSY INVOLVED SITE, IF POSSIBLE

Negative

Positive

Ⓓ BRONCHOSCOPIC OR OPEN LUNG BIOPSY

Diagnose other specific disease

Diagnose invasive aspergillosis

Ⓔ Discontinue use of steroid and cytotoxic agents, if possible

Ⓕ Amphotericin B

Improvement

No improvement

Diffuse
disease

Localized
disease

Continue treatment

Ⓖ Consider:
    Resection

OBSTRUCTIVE PULMONARY DISEASE

Upper Airway Obstruction
Asthma
Severe Asthma
Chronic Bronchitis
Bronchiectasis
Theophylline Toxicity

Emphysema
Respiratory Failure
Adult Respiratory Distress Syndrome
Weaning from Mechanical Ventilation
High-Frequency Ventilation
Pulmonary Rehabilitation

UPPER AIRWAY OBSTRUCTION

The causes of upper airway obstruction include aspiration of foreign body, inflammatory or neoplastic disorders of the pharynx, larynx, or trachea, lesions of the esophagus or middle mediastinum pushing into the posterior portion of the trachea, and post-traumatic obstruction resulting from acute bleeding or fracture. Diagnostic efforts should focus on determining the exact level of airway obstruction so that airway control can be established distally. Patients who develop airway obstruction after trauma must also be evaluated for cervical spine abnormalities and vascular injury. Rapid pulmonary decompensation can occur in patients with airway obstruction secondary to epiglottitis or large exophytic neoplasms of the trachea or major bronchi.

A. The most common symptoms of acute airway obstruction are all nonspecific; these include voice changes, dyspnea, dysphagia, local pain, and cough. Progressive dyspnea and stridor are the most common symptoms associated with nearly complete airway obstruction.

B. Hoarseness (aphonia) may be found in patients with laryngeal nerve paralysis, mucosal tear of the larynx, or laryngeal edema. Inspiratory stridor occurs with swelling at or proximal to the level of the vocal cords, whereas expiratory stridor occurs with lesions at or below the level of the cords, as in croup. The degree of severity of stridor cannot be used as a predictor of the degree of airway obstruction. Other findings include suprasternal retraction, restlessness due to hypoxia, drooling, bleeding from neoplastic lesions or inflamed mucosa, and subcutaneous emphysema secondary to injuries of the sinuses, hypopharynx, laryngotracheal complex, esophagus, or lung. In the setting of trauma, fractures of the facial skeleton, larynx, or trachea may be found.

C. Arterial blood gas should be analyzed to assess the adequacy of gas exchange, although decisions to intubate are not made solely upon findings from this test.

D. Patients deemed clinically unstable by vital signs or blood gas findings (hypoxemia, hypercapnemia) should be placed under close supervision in an intensive care unit and immediate otolaryngologic consultation should be sought. Patients should be placed on oxygen therapy. The otolaryngologist may be able to make a diagnosis by either indirect laryngoscopy (mirror) or by fiberoptic laryngoscopy and/or aid in immediate endotracheal intubation if it is required.

E. If the diagnosis is not known, imaging of the soft tissues of the neck as well as of the trachea and larynx, lung, and esophagus should be done. Possible studies include lateral films of the neck and cervical spine, radiography of the chest, and computed tomography of the neck and chest. These studies help establish the presence or absence of supraglottic edema and the integrity of the laryngeal ventricle, and demonstrate foreign bodies. Neoplastic lesions may be seen and the exact level of the obstruction clarified.

F. The condition of patients not requiring immediate intubation may worsen, and they may eventually require intubation. General medical and surgical support including antibiotic use, fluid management, and surgical reconstruction of the mandible or other structure may be necessary. Subcutaneous emphysema severe enough to cause airway obstruction occurs in intubated patients as a result of an improper intubation or as a result of barotrauma.

G. Patients who have significant airway obstruction due to exophytic obstruction of the trachea or larynx should be evaluated for laser excision or reduction of tumor mass. Lasers can be used when the obstruction is not total so that the lumen behind the mass can be visualized, and when the patient can tolerate the procedure. This procedure is generally palliative only, but symptomatic improvement occurs rapidly, and repeated excisions may be done. Radiation can also be used to reduce tumor size, but not all tumors respond, and days to weeks may be needed to effect improvement.

H. In patients who are stable at presentation, the same studies are required as in those who were initially unstable, but these can be done electively under the direction of the pulmonologist, otolaryngologist, and gastroenterologist.

I. Fiberoptic bronchoscopy can be emergently or electively performed to determine the level of obstruction and to make a diagnosis. Further work-up and treatment are the same as for patients requiring acute intubation.

References

Weymuller EA. Airway management. In: Fredrickson JM, ed. Otolaryngology–head and neck surgery. Vol. 3. St. Louis: CV Mosby, 1986: 2417.

UPPER AIRWAY OBSTRUCTION Suspected

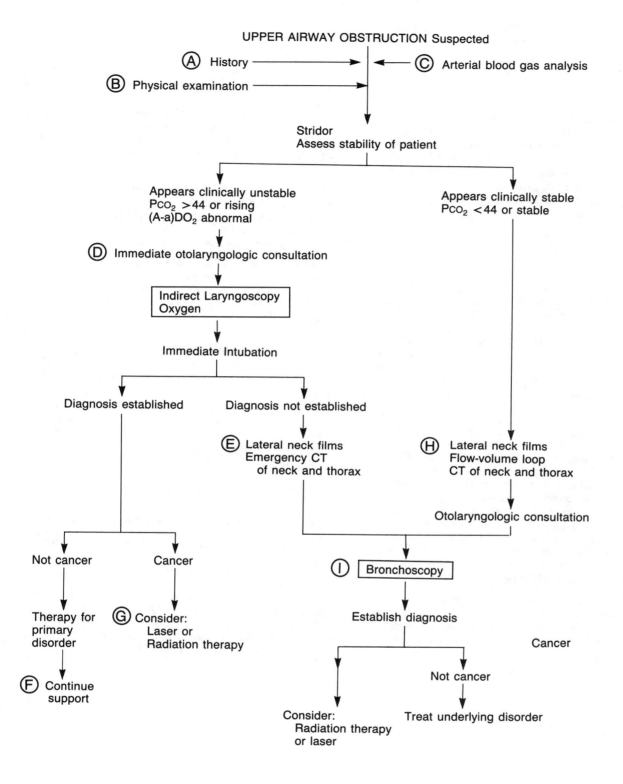

Ⓐ History

Ⓑ Physical examination

Ⓒ Arterial blood gas analysis

Stridor
Assess stability of patient

Appears clinically unstable
Pco₂ >44 or rising
(A-a)DO₂ abnormal

Appears clinically stable
Pco₂ <44 or stable

Ⓓ Immediate otolaryngologic consultation

Indirect Laryngoscopy
Oxygen

Immediate Intubation

Diagnosis established

Diagnosis not established

Ⓔ Lateral neck films
Emergency CT
of neck and thorax

Ⓗ Lateral neck films
Flow-volume loop
CT of neck and thorax

Otolaryngologic consultation

Not cancer

Cancer

Ⓘ Bronchoscopy

Therapy for
primary
disorder

Ⓖ Consider:
Laser or
Radiation therapy

Establish diagnosis

Cancer

Ⓕ Continue
support

Not cancer

Consider:
Radiation therapy
or laser

Treat underlying disorder

ASTHMA

Asthma is characterized by an increased responsiveness of the trachea and bronchi to various stimuli and is manifested by widespread narrowing of the airways that changes in severity. The key feature that distinguishes asthma from other diseases of the airways is the reversibility of the airway obstruction. Conversely, other disorders that have diffuse airway narrowing such as chronic bronchitis, emphysema, or bronchiolitis may have an asthmatic component.

A. The clinical presentation of asthma is a history of episodic dyspnea. The asthma is considered mild in severity when it does not interfere with everyday activities. In some patients, asthma may occur only during exercise. In others, the dyspnea may occur only at night or after exposure to respiratory irritants (such as smoke) or to particular allergens such as cat dander. A small percentage of asthma patients are sensitive to aspirin. These patients often have nasal polyps and an associated sensitivity to tartrazine dye. Asthma may also present with cough as the only complaint. Physical examination may be normal, but often wheezing is present. The presence of intercostal retractions or the use of the accessory muscles of respiration indicates severe disease.

B. When the history is suggestive of asthma but the physical examination is normal, pulmonary function tests (PFTs) can be used to make the diagnosis. The FEV_1 as a percent of vital capacity is reduced to 60 to 70 percent of predicted values in mild disease. If routine PFTs are normal, the diagnosis can be made by exercise or inhalational challenge. These tests are considered positive if wheezing occurs or a decrease of 20 percent or more in the FEV_1 is found after a repeat PFT determination. When the history is highly suggestive, empiric treatment can be started without the demonstration of airway obstruction by spirometry.

C. Arterial blood gases (ABG) should be obtained when a patient is in moderate (FEV_1 percentage at 50 to 60 percent) to severe (FEV_1 percentage below 50 percent) respiratory distress. Hypoxemia is often present when the pulsus paradoxus exceeds 15 mm Hg or when intercostal retractions are noted. A PO_2 value below 65 mm Hg indicates the need for supplemental oxygen. A chest film should be obtained to exclude other diseases such as allergic bronchopulmonary aspergillosis.

D. The initial treatment of mild asthma employs beta-adrenergic agents delivered via the inhalational route. In patients with a bronchitic component, atropine-like agents such as ipratropium bromide are particularly useful. Cromolyn may be used for the subset of patients who have predominantly exercise-induced asthma.

E. Continued symptoms require the addition of oral theophylline derivatives or inhalational steroids. These medications should be continued for several months after symptoms have abated to decrease the likelihood of another exacerbation. PFT can be used to assess whether normal function is restored.

F. Reserve oral steroids for patients with refractory symptoms despite treatment with other medications. Steroids may also be used early on in patients with moderate to severe disease. A commonly used regimen would consist of an initial dose of 30 to 40 mg per day in a single dose. An additional 10 mg may be given at night for patients with severe nocturnal symptomatology. The dose is then tapered once symptoms remit. The average time course of steroid administration is 2 weeks.

References

Bruderman I, Cohen-Aronowski R, Smorzik J. A comparative study of various combinations of ipratropium bromide and metaproterenol in allergic asthma patients. Chest 1983; 83:208.

Eggleston P. Methods of exercise challenge. J Allergy Clin Immunol 1984; 73:666.

Franklin W. Asthma in the emergency room: assessment and treatment. N Engl J Med 1981; 305:826.

McFadden ER. Exercise-induced asthma. Am J Med 1980; 68:471.

Rosenthal R. Inhalation challenge: procedures, indications, techniques. J Allergy Clin Immunol 1979; 64:564.

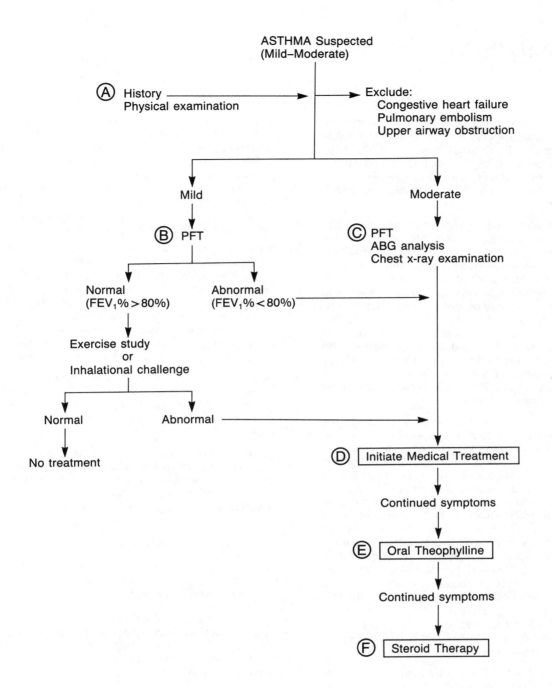

ASTHMA Suspected
(Mild–Moderate)

(A) History ——————→ Exclude:
Physical examination → Congestive heart failure
Pulmonary embolism
Upper airway obstruction

Mild

Moderate

(B) PFT

(C) PFT
ABG analysis
Chest x-ray examination

Normal
(FEV$_1$% > 80%)

Abnormal
(FEV$_1$% < 80%)

Exercise study
or
Inhalational challenge

Normal

Abnormal

No treatment

(D) Initiate Medical Treatment

Continued symptoms

(E) Oral Theophylline

Continued symptoms

(F) Steroid Therapy

SEVERE ASTHMA

A severe asthmatic attack requires arterial blood gas analysis for therapeutic decision making. Both the PO_2 and the PCO_2 vary with the severity of the episode. Initially, the PCO_2 falls, because hyperventilation is used to maintain oxygenation. As the attack progresses, the PO_2 falls further and finally the PCO_2 begins to rise. A rising PCO_2 indicates impending respiratory failure.

A. A complete history and physical examination is difficult to perform in the setting of a severe asthmatic attack. Patients are agitated and have difficulty talking. However, it is usually possible to establish a past history of asthma, determine which medications the patient is taking, and exclude aspiration of a foreign body as a diagnostic possibility. A past history of severe asthma requiring intravenous corticosteroids and intubation suggests that these measures may well be needed again, because severe attacks in the past portend severe recurrences. The presence of intercostal retractions or pulsus paradoxus indicates hypoxemia. There is usually sufficient time to obtain a blood gas analysis, which should be performed before other diagnostic tests.

B. A normal PCO_2 is an ominous sign in a patient with otherwise normal lungs who is experiencing a severe asthmatic attack. Institute vigorous medical treatment immediately in such patients. They require monitoring in an intensive care unit setting and treatment with supplemental oxygen, aerosolized beta-agonists, intravenous aminophylline, and steroids. Avoid administration of aspirin. Initiate treatment with steroids early because of the delayed onset of action (at least 8 hours). Continuous oximetric monitoring is useful to detect sudden changes in oxygenation. However, analyze blood gases periodically to assess the PCO_2 and the status of ventilation. Intubate tiring patients or those with other signs of increasing distress, such as increasing tachycardia, cardiac arrhythmias, or decreasing consciousness. At times it is difficult to determine whether the deterioration is the result of worsening asthma or a complication of the therapy. Avoid excessive use of medications.

C. Persistent elevations of PCO_2 despite vigorous medical therapy indicate respiratory failure; most of these patients require intubation and ventilatory assistance. Initial ventilatory settings include an FIO_2 of 90 percent, tidal volume of 10 ml per kg, and a respiratory rate of approximately 10 breaths per minute. Analyze blood gas from a sample drawn after 10 minutes of ventilatory assistance and adjust the settings as necessary. An arterial line is useful because of the need for multiple blood gas determinations, but the time required for its placement should not interfere with institution of treatment.

D. Persistent hypoxemia in an intubated patient requires vigorous treatment. Optimize the ventilatory status by controlled ventilation after induction of systemic paralysis and sedation. Avoid administration of morphine because of its potential bronchoconstrictor effects. Obtain a chest film to verify placement of the endotracheal tube and exclude the presence of a pneumothorax. Assiduously guard against accidental extubation because of the potential difficulties of emergency reintubation.

E. Treat with bicarbonate those patients who are well oxygenated but who develop a persistent respiratory acidosis in order to maintain their pH above 7.2. If possible, adjust ventilatory settings to allow for a prolonged expiratory phase.

F. Persistent hypoxemia may necessitate general anesthesia. Deep smooth muscle relaxation appears to induce clinical improvement. Some recent studies suggest that PEEP may also be useful in this situation, although it is associated with a high risk of barotrauma.

References

Benatar SR. Fatal asthma. N Engl J Med 1986; 314:423.

Fanta CH, Rossing TH, McFadden ER. Emergency room treatment of asthma. Am J Med 1982; 72:416.

Franklin W. Asthma in the emergency room. Assessment and treatment. N Engl J Med 1981; 305:826.

Karetzky MS. Asthma mortality: an analysis of one year's experience, review of the literature, and assessment of current modes of therapy. Medicine 1975; 54:471.

Scoggin CH, Sahn SA, Petty TL. Status asthmaticus—a nine-year experience. JAMA 1977; 238:1158.

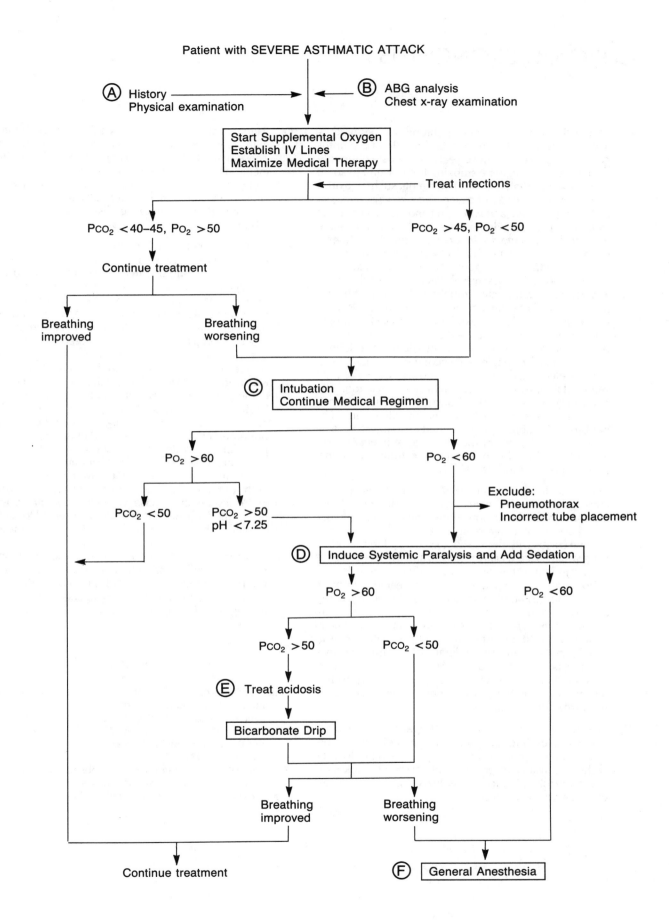

Patient with SEVERE ASTHMATIC ATTACK

(A) History — Physical examination

(B) ABG analysis Chest x-ray examination

Start Supplemental Oxygen
Establish IV Lines
Maximize Medical Therapy

Treat infections

$Pco_2 < 40–45$, $Po_2 > 50$

$Pco_2 > 45$, $Po_2 < 50$

Continue treatment

Breathing improved

Breathing worsening

(C) Intubation
Continue Medical Regimen

$Po_2 > 60$

$Po_2 < 60$

$Pco_2 < 50$

$Pco_2 > 50$
pH < 7.25

Exclude:
Pneumothorax
Incorrect tube placement

(D) Induce Systemic Paralysis and Add Sedation

$Po_2 > 60$

$Po_2 < 60$

$Pco_2 > 50$

$Pco_2 < 50$

(E) Treat acidosis

Bicarbonate Drip

Breathing improved

Breathing worsening

Continue treatment

(F) General Anesthesia

CHRONIC BRONCHITIS

A. Chronic bronchitis is defined as chronic sputum production of more than 250 ml per day for at least 3 months per year over 2 consecutive years. It is most commonly associated with cigarette smoking but is found in some patients after inhalation of toxic agents such as oxides of nitrogen or sulfur. Most patients have mixtures of bronchitis, emphysema, and wheezing and also complain of shortness of breath. Hemoptysis may be found in some patients during acute respiratory infections; bronchogenic carcinoma must be ruled out in these individuals. Affected individuals appear to be chronically ill. Examination of the chest reveals decreased breath sounds and generalized rhonchi throughout. Digital clubbing is not common, but central cyanosis may be noted. Patients with cor pulmonale may exhibit an increased S_2, a right ventricular heave, a right-sided S_3 gallop, hepatojugular reflux, and peripheral, dependent edema. The laboratory examination may reveal secondary erythrocytosis, and the electrocardiogram may show evidence of right ventricular hypertrophy and right axis deviation. The chest film may be normal; however, there is often evidence of increased bronchovascular markings caused by peribronchial fibrosis and retained secretions. Sputum should be evaluated for the presence of infection and, in smokers, should also be sent for cytologic examination during a period of stability.

B. Pulmonary function testing (PFT) reveals decreased flow rates and evidence of increased airway resistance; results indicate airway obstruction. Some patients with mild disease have normal spirometry but have abnormal flow-volume curves with decreased flows at low lung volumes. Lung volumes are usually reduced, and there is evidence of air-trapping with increases in residual volume. Repeat spirometry after the patient has been treated with bronchodilators (usually an inhaled, rapidly acting beta$_2$-agonist); a positive response (more than 20 percent increase in function) indicates that these agents will be of benefit in treatment. Arterial blood gas (ABG) analysis usually reveals mild to moderate hypoxemia and may reveal hypercapnemia as well. Severe CO_2 retention occurs in end-stage disease. Longstanding hypoxemia results in pulmonary hypertension and eventually produces cor pulmonale.

C. The diagnosis may be made with reasonable certainty on the above clinical grounds. The major diagnostic consideration that must be ruled out in a young individual without a history of previous infections or smoking is cystic fibrosis; all such individuals should have sweat chloride measurements.

D. Patients with severe or longstanding chronic bronchitis with associated hypoxemia may develop cor pulmonale. These patients exhibit signs of right ventricular failure, including dependent edema, right ventricular S_3 gallop and heave, and an increased S_2. Clinical findings, ABG analysis and appropriate ECG results, will enable patients with cor pulmonale to be distinguished from those without.

E. Patients with chronic bronchitis have repeated respiratory infectious episodes and require frequent sputum analyses and antibiotic treatments. They should be encouraged to discontinue smoking, since smoking makes treatment more difficult and unlikely to produce positive results. Treatment should be directed toward reducing bronchial wall smooth muscle constriction and mucus production. Theophylline preparations may be used, but side effects increase in frequency at high serum levels; levels must be monitored in these patients. Medications delivered through the inhaled route are becoming the mainstays of treatment. Drugs include beta$_2$-agonists and synthetic anticholinergics. These drugs may be delivered through metered-dose inhalers, but power nebulizers can be used in those patients who have difficulty following instructions or who have coordination problems. Administer continuous low-flow oxygen to those individuals who have resting hypoxemia, with a PO_2 less than 55 mm Hg, or to those who are at this level with exercise, when in the supine position, or during sleep. Steroids should be reserved for patients in whom there is a bronchospastic component to the condition or for those who have been found refractory to other bronchodilator therapies. These agents should not be routinely used; when necessary, they should be given as high-pulse doses and quickly withdrawn. Use diuretics and preload reducing agents in patients with the signs and symptoms of cor pulmonale.

References

American Thoracic Society. Chronic bronchitis, asthma, and pulmonary emphysema. A statement by the Committee on Diagnostic Standards for Nontuberculous Respiratory Diseases. Am Rev Respir Dis 1962; 85:762.

Burrows B. An overview of obstructive lung diseases. Med Clin North Am 1981; 65:455.

Fishman AP. The spectrum of chronic obstructive disease of the airways. In: Fishman AP, ed. Pulmonary diseases and disorders. New York: McGraw-Hill, 1980:458.

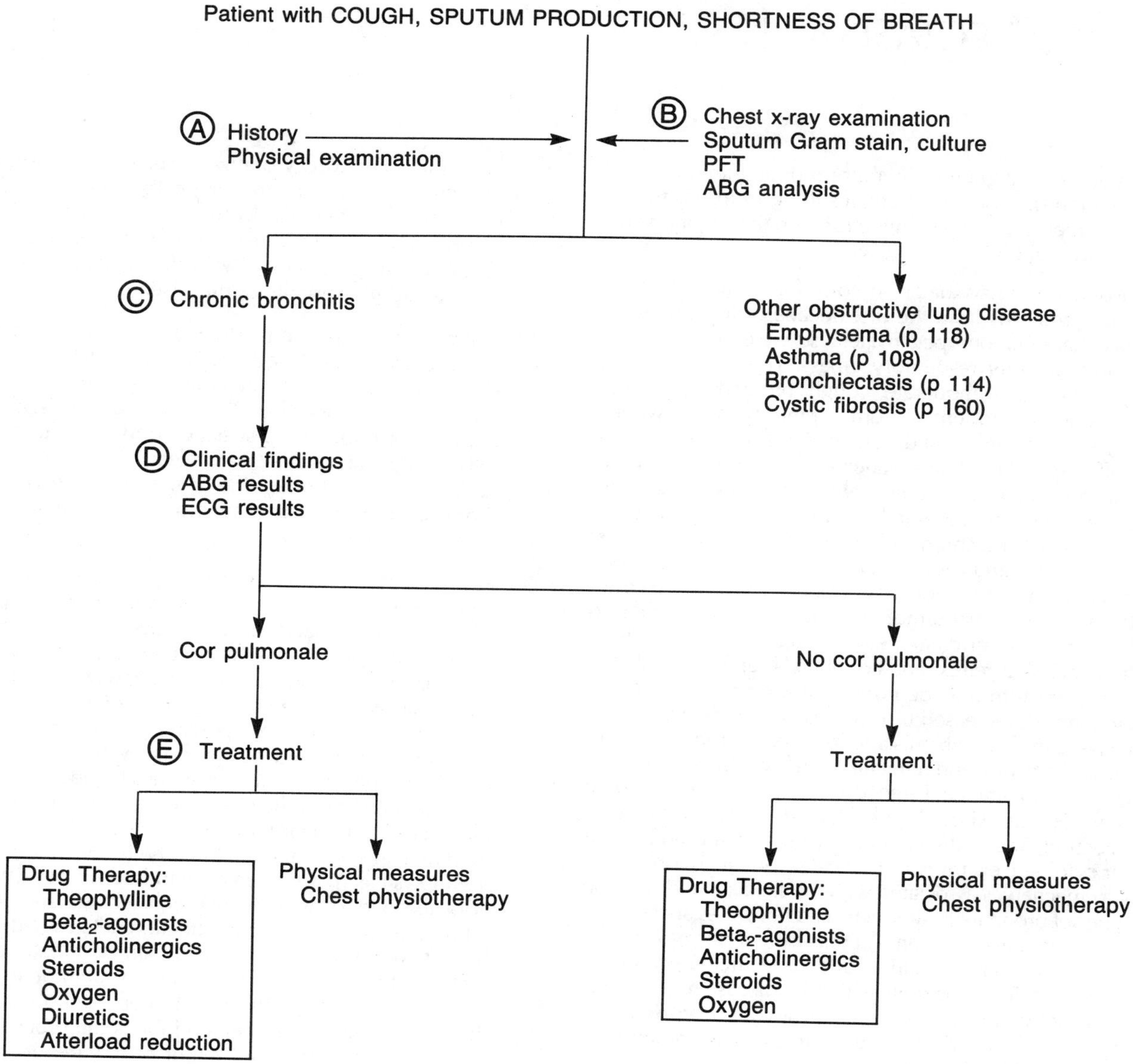

Patient with COUGH, SPUTUM PRODUCTION, SHORTNESS OF BREATH

(A) History
Physical examination

(B) Chest x-ray examination
Sputum Gram stain, culture
PFT
ABG analysis

(C) Chronic bronchitis

Other obstructive lung disease
Emphysema (p 118)
Asthma (p 108)
Bronchiectasis (p 114)
Cystic fibrosis (p 160)

(D) Clinical findings
ABG results
ECG results

Cor pulmonale

No cor pulmonale

(E) Treatment

Treatment

Drug Therapy:
Theophylline
Beta₂-agonists
Anticholinergics
Steroids
Oxygen
Diuretics
Afterload reduction

Physical measures
Chest physiotherapy

Drug Therapy:
Theophylline
Beta₂-agonists
Anticholinergics
Steroids
Oxygen

Physical measures
Chest physiotherapy

BRONCHIECTASIS

Bronchiectasis is a genetically present or acquired irreversible dilatation of bronchial walls resulting from destruction of wall elements, caused by infection, inhalation of noxious gases, or vasculitis.

A. Most patients have had symptoms for many years; some date symptoms from the first decade of life, and many state that symptoms began after a severe episode of pneumonia or other respiratory illness. The most common symptom is a moderate cough productive of large amounts of purulent sputum. Hemoptysis and wheezing is also common, and some patients complain of nasal stuffiness and discharge. Patients with so-called dry bronchiectasis do not produce large amounts of sputum, but more commonly develop hemoptysis. Affected individuals appear to be chronically ill. Examination of the chest reveals rales and rhonchi over the diseased areas. Digital clubbing is common, as is cyanosis in advanced cases. Patients with cor pulmonale may exhibit an increased S_2, a right ventricular heave, a right-sided S_3 gallop, hepatojugular reflux, and peripheral, dependent edema. The chest film may be normal; however, often there is evidence of increased bronchovascular markings caused by peribronchial fibrosis and retained secretions. Parenchymal scarring and retraction can give rise to a "honeycomb" appearance. Large, cystic air spaces may also be seen. Sputum should be evaluated for the presence of infection, and, if the patient is a smoker, should be sent for cytologic examination. Because of the abnormal airway mechanics associated with the saccular and varicose types of bronchiectasis, decreased flow rates are seen on spirometric examination. Patients exhibit decreased maximal voluntary ventilation and have increased airway resistance. Some patients with mild disease have normal spirometry but have abnormal flow-volume curves with decreased flows at low lung volumes. Lung volumes are usually reduced and there is evidence of air-trapping. Repeat spirometry after the patient has been treated with bronchodilators (usually an inhaled, rapidly acting beta$_2$-agonist); a positive response (greater than 20 percent increase in function) indicates that these agents will be of benefit in treatment. Arterial blood gas (ABG) analysis usually reveals mild to moderate hypoxemia, and may reveal hypercapnemia as well. Severe CO_2 retention occurs in end-stage disease. Longstanding hypoxemia results in pulmonary hypertension and eventually produces cor pulmonale.

B. Bronchography establishes the diagnosis of bronchiectasis. Use of this modality in those individuals with the appropriate clinical indications can delineate the cylindrical, saccular, or varicose types of disease. However, bronchography is risky, causes transient reductions in PO_2 and reductions in clearance of secretions, and it increases the possibility of pulmonary infections. CT of the chest may effectively visualize the extent and severity of bronchiectasis without the use of instilled dyes. CT distinguishes between localized and generalized disease and can also visualize mucus impactions and other areas of infiltration. It cannot always distinguish among the three anatomic variants of the disease.

C. The diagnosis may be made with reasonable certainty on the above clinical grounds. The major diagnostic consideration that must be ruled out in a young patient with no history of previous infections is cystic fibrosis; all such individuals should have sweat chloride measurements. Other diagnostic entities that are easily ruled out include Kartagener's syndrome, one of the immotile cilia syndromes, and Swyer-James syndrome or unilateral hyperlucent lung syndrome.

D. Patients with hemoptysis may require surgery or other palliative procedures. The decision to operate depends on the following factors: the frequency and severity of the hemoptysis, whether the bleeding is coming from the bronchiectatic portion of the lung, whether the bronchiectasis is localized to one area of the lung or is widespread, and the postoperative pulmonary function. Bronchoscopy should be done to evaluate the site of bleeding to ensure that it corresponds to the area of bronchiectasis noted on the chest radiograph or CT scan. In rare cases, pulmonary arteriography will be necessary to make this distinction. Surgery is indicated if the hemoptysis is major (greater than 600 ml per day) and is localized to a single area of bronchiectasis, and predicted postoperative pulmonary function determined on the basis of perfusion scanning is adequate (greater than 1 L FEV$_1$). If the predicted postoperative pulmonary function is not adequate, bronchial artery embolization to the vessel feeding the affected lobe is the procedure of choice. If bleeding is not major or is infrequent, then bronchoscopy should still be done, since future bleeding will often come from the same site. However, the decision to operate is not clear-cut. Treatment of associated infections and cough may reduce hemoptysis. Individuals with generalized hemoptysis and mild bleeding should not undergo surgery except under life-threatening conditions, since it is often difficult to know the exact site of bleeding, and these patients with pulmonary hypertension may subsequently bleed from multiple areas.

E. Patients with bronchiectasis are treated with the same modalities as those with chronic bronchitis. These include antibiotics, bronchodilators, and oxygen. Physical measures are often helpful to clear secretions from the airways and reduce the work of breathing. Diuretics and preload reduction should be employed in patients with cor pulmonale.

Patient with COUGH, SPUTUM PRODUCTION, SHORTNESS OF BREATH

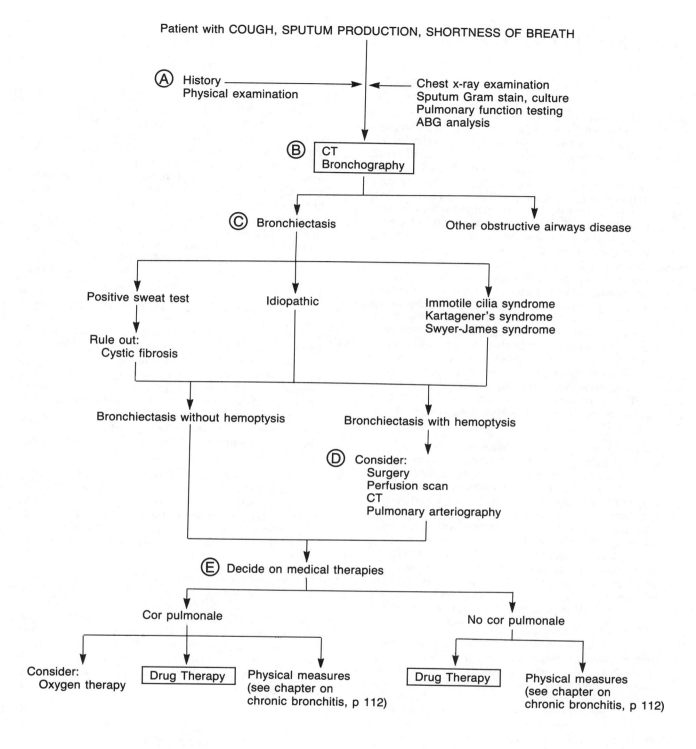

Ⓐ History ——————
Physical examination

Chest x-ray examination
Sputum Gram stain, culture
Pulmonary function testing
ABG analysis

Ⓑ CT
Bronchography

Ⓒ Bronchiectasis

Other obstructive airways disease

Positive sweat test

Idiopathic

Immotile cilia syndrome
Kartagener's syndrome
Swyer-James syndrome

Rule out:
Cystic fibrosis

Bronchiectasis without hemoptysis

Bronchiectasis with hemoptysis

Ⓓ Consider:
Surgery
Perfusion scan
CT
Pulmonary arteriography

Ⓔ Decide on medical therapies

Cor pulmonale

No cor pulmonale

Consider:
Oxygen therapy

Drug Therapy

Physical measures
(see chapter on
chronic bronchitis, p 112)

Drug Therapy

Physical measures
(see chapter on
chronic bronchitis, p 112)

References

Grenier P, Maurice F, Musset D, et al. Bronchiectasis: assessment by thin section CT. Radiology 1986; 161:95.

Luce JM. Bronchiectasis. In: Murray J, Nadel J, eds. Textbook of respiratory medicine. Philadelphia: WB Saunders, 1988: 1107.

Muller NL, Bergin CJ, Ostrow DN, et al. Role of computed tomography in the recognition of bronchiectasis. Am J Radiol 1984; 143:971.

THEOPHYLLINE TOXICITY

Absorption of theophylline is quite variable among individuals. The clinical symptomatology developed by individuals who are theophylline-toxic depends on the absolute serum level as well as the rapidity with which this level was reached. Individuals who reach significantly elevated levels (greater than 50 µg/ml) slowly over long periods of time may have no complaints or only mild complaints of nausea and vomiting. Serum levels that have been maintained within the normal therapeutic range (5 to 20 µg/ml) may suddenly increase to the toxic range (greater than 20 µg/ml) under conditions of fasting or acute illness. On the other hand, patients may develop seizures or have significant cardiac tachyarrhythmias at levels of 30 to 40 µg/ml if this level was reached quickly over hours. Surges in blood level seem to be more likely with the once per day preparations, and this risk may not justify the benefit of increased patient compliance. Acute inflammatory or congestive hepatic disease or congestive heart failure delays metabolism of theophylline by hepatic mechanisms and may elevate serum levels. Measurement of theophylline levels should be obtained: occasionally in stable ambulatory settings, but frequently in individuals who are acutely ill, who have been placed on new drugs that are metabolized by the liver, or in whom dosage regimens are changing.

A. Patients may have no complaints or only minor complaints of gastrointestinal discomfort, including nausea, mild abdominal pain, or vomiting. Cardiac or central nervous system complaints are significant. These include angina pectoris, possibly related to increases in cardiac rate, and dizziness related to tachyarrhythmias and decreases in blood pressure. Patients with and without previous seizure histories may be brought to the hospital in active seizure. Physical examination may be unrevealing or may support the history, with signs of cardiac or central nervous system decompensation. The electrocardiogram may reveal only sinus tachycardia, but may demonstrate abnormal atrial or ventricular tachyarrhythmias, including ventricular tachycardia.

B. Blood should be obtained for rapid determination of theophylline level when a patient with the appropriate symptom complex presents. Toxicity is defined as a theophylline level greater than 20 µg/ml. In general, mild clinical toxicity generally occurs at levels between 20 and 30 µg/ml, moderate toxicity at levels between 31 and 40 µg/ml, and severe toxicity at levels greater than 41 µg/ml. These are arbitrarily defined guidelines, and treatment must be individualized according to the severity of the toxicity no matter what the theophylline level. All patients with toxicity should discontinue theophylline; it may be reinstated later after symptoms disappear and levels decline to the normal range.

C. Assess the degree and severity of toxicity prior to instituting treatment. The variables to be considered in making this judgment include the age of the patient; the presence of illnesses other than pulmonary disease—most importantly cardiac, hepatic, and neurologic disease; the current or potential manifestations of toxicity; the presence of other drugs; and the serum level. In general, relatively asymptomatic patients who are elderly or who have other systemic disease with only moderately high theophylline levels should be considered to be severely toxic. Younger, healthier individuals with few symptoms and levels between 20 and 30 µg/ml may be treated as outpatients. However, if these latter patients have intercurrent illnesses or other factors contributing to toxicity, they may require hospitalization. The definitions of mild, moderate, or severe toxicity are therefore combinations of chemical levels and clinical symptoms.

D. In asymptomatic patients or patients with nausea and vomiting, any tablets or capsules of the drug should be removed from the GI tract with either ipecac and induced vomiting or with orally administered activated charcoal. The decision of which of these agents to use depends on the patient's age, mental status, and other cardiorespiratory factors. Treat young patients with normal mental status and cardiorespiratory function with ipecac; treat elderly patients with decreased gag reflexes or patients with angina pectoris or cardiac dysrhythmias with activated charcoal and admit them to hospital. Monitor theophylline levels daily.

E. Patients with gastrointestinal symptoms or who have sinus tachycardia should receive activated charcoal and be monitored in an intensive care unit setting. The tachycardia need not be treated since it will remit as the level of theophylline decreases. Levels of theophylline should be monitored several times daily over the initial 2 days.

F. Treat seizure activity, cardiac tachyarrythmias, and angina in standard fashion and rapidly reduce the serum level of theophylline. Such treatment may require endotracheal intubation. Orally administered charcoal in doses of 30 g should be given every 2 hours until levels are reduced by 50 percent. Charcoal hemoperfusion is rarely necessary and should be reserved for patients in whom levels are extremely high and orally administered charcoal is working slowly.

References

Helliwell M, Berry D. Theophylline poisoning in adults. Br Med J 1979; 2:114.

Karlinsky JB. The use of theophylline: a review. American College of Chest Physicians Clinical Challenge 1986; 4:1.

Weinberger M, Hendeles L, Ahrens R. Pharmacologic management of reversible obstructive airways disease. Med Clin North Am 1981; 65:579.

CLINICAL SYMPTOMS OF THEOPHYLLINE TOXICITY

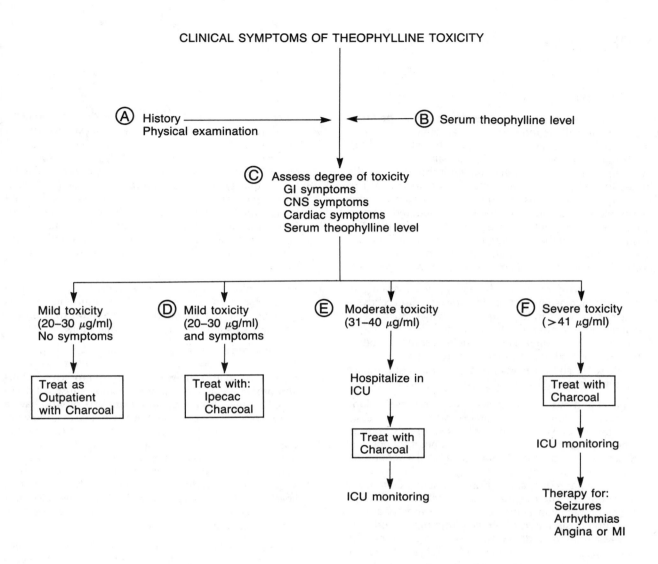

EMPHYSEMA

Emphysema is a destructive lung disease in which the number of alveolar walls is reduced. The causative mechanism is thought to be excess amounts of elastolytic activity in lung parenchyma, which proteolyzes alveolar wall elastin. This activity is released from activated polymorphonuclear cells recruited to the lung by components of cigarette smoke. The major lung protease responsible for inactivating these elastases, alpha$_1$-protease inhibitor, is also rendered inactive by components of cigarette smoke. Over many years the elastic tissue network of the lung becomes more compliant, air-trapping increases, and air spaces greatly increase in size, although the total number of air spaces significantly declines.

A. The major symptom of emphysema is progressive dyspnea with increasing exertion. In end-stage disease, dyspnea occurs with mild forms of activity, and patients cannot perform normal activities of daily life. A long history of smoking can usually be elicited; sputum production may or may not be found. Very young patients with emphysema should have levels of alpha$_1$-antiprotease inhibitor measured.

B. Physical findings associated with severe disease include the classic barrel chest appearance, wasting of accessory muscles of ventilation, decreased breath sounds, hyper-resonance to percussion, distant heart sounds, and evidence of cor pulmonale, including jugular venous distention, a prominent S$_2$, an enlarged, tender liver with hepatojugular reflux, and peripheral edema. Cyanosis is not common. The diagnosis can be made with a high degree of specificity at the bedside if the appropriate history and constellation of physical findings are present; however, mild to moderate emphysema may not be clinically apparent. The diagnosis of emphysema may be made with certainty only from histologic examination of lung parenchyma.

C. There are no classic roentgenographic findings diagnostic of emphysema. Compatible findings include overdistended large lungs with flattened diaphragms seen on the lateral view. Attenuation of peripheral vascular shadows may be seen. The cardiac silhouette may appear smaller than usual due to hyperaeration of the adjacent lung tissue. The pulmonary artery shadows may appear enlarged; this finding suggests the presence of pulmonary hypertension. Edges of bullae may be seen.

D. Electrocardiographic findings consistent with emphysema include right axis deviation, evidence of right ventricular hypertrophy with large R waves in the anterior precordial leads, large S waves laterally, and P pulmonale evident in the inferior limb leads. In patients with chest pain or findings suggesting congestive heart failure, perform cardiac ultrasonography or gated blood pool scans to measure left ventricular function.

E. Spirometric findings are consistent with airflow obstruction. The FVC (forced vital capacity) is reduced as is the FEV$_1$. The ratio of FEV$_1$/FVC is less than 75 percent. Midmaximal flows are also reduced. Lung volume studies usually reveal an increased RV (residual volume) and FRC (functional residual capacity). Because the RV is increased more than the vital capacity is reduced, TLC (total lung capacity) is usually elevated. The single breath diffusing capacity is also reduced (because emphysema is a destructive lung disease), resulting in reduced alveolar complexity (alveolar surface area). Pulmonary exercise testing indicates that ventilation is limiting, and patients usually evidence a reduced VO$_2$ per kg body weight.

F. Arterial blood gases usually demonstrate hypoxemia without carbon dioxide retention until the FEV$_1$ is reduced below 1 L, when CO$_2$ retention may ensue. The pH is usually within the normal range.

G. The work-up allows exclusion of cardiac causes of dyspnea such as chronic congestive heart failure or cardiomyopathy and also allows exclusion of chronic bronchitis and bronchiectasis, two other common causes of dyspnea. Patients who are currently smokers or who have a history of smoking and who have evidence of airflow obstruction, hyperinflated lungs, and no CO$_2$ retention will probably have emphysema. Levels of alpha$_1$-antiprotease should be measured in young nonsmoking patients with significant amounts of pulmonary dysfunction and other findings compatible with emphysema. Levels should be above 80 ng/ml. Reductions below this level suggest the diagnosis of alpha$_1$-antiprotease deficiency, accounting for the disease.

H. Since most patients have elements of chronic bronchitis and wheezing along with emphysema, treatment is centered around relieving bronchospasm and decreasing pulmonary secretions. Theophylline and a beta$_2$ selective adrenergic aerosolized preparation should be employed if the patient exhibits evidence of reversibility of airway obstruction after bronchodilation on pulmonary function testing. These agents may be used on a trial basis even if formal testing does not indicate improvement. Steroids should be used only as a last resort. Low-flow oxygen should be prescribed if the patient is hypoxemic at rest or has an exercise or sleep PO$_2$ of less than 55 mm Hg. Continuous low-flow oxygen has been shown to increase exercise tolerance and may improve survival in patients with severe disease. Diuretics may be used in those patients with cor pulmonale, and antibiotics should be added in individuals with bronchitis due to bacterial infection. Some patients may receive benefit from pulmonary rehabilitation designed to improve performance of the respiratory muscles. Patients with diaphragmatic fatigue and CO$_2$ retention may also benefit from external ventilatory support devices such as pneumobelts, or negative pressure devices that allow respiratory muscle rest. These devices can be used during sleep.

Patient with WORSENING DYSPNEA ON EXERTION

(A) History ⟶ ⟵ (C) Chest x-ray examination

(B) Physical examination ⟶ (D) ECG

(E) Pulmonary function testing

(F) Arterial blood gas on room air

Normal studies   Abnormal studies

Pulmonary Exercise Test

Other obstructive airway disease

Suggests cardiac disease   Suggests pulmonary disease

Cardiac work-up

(G) Diagnosis of emphysema

Smoking-related emphysema   Alpha₁-antiprotease deficiency

Alpha₁-antiprotease Replacement

(H) Treatment:
   Bronchodilators
   Oxygen
   Steroids
   Diuretics
   Antibiotics

Additional Treatment Modalities:
Pulmonary Rehabilitation
Negative-Pressure Ventilators

References

Snider GL, Kleinerman J, Thurlbeck WM, Bengali Z. The definition of emphysema: report of a National Heart, Lung, and Blood Institute, Division of Lung Diseases, workshop. Am Rev Respir Dis 1985; 132:182.

Snider GL. Chronic bronchitis and emphysema. In: Murray J, Nadel J, eds. Textbook of respiratory medicine. Philadelphia: WB Saunders, 1988:1069.

RESPIRATORY FAILURE

Etiologies of respiratory failure are multiple and varied. Decisions regarding respiratory failure center around judging whether the failure is acute or chronic, the rate at which the underlying disorder and related failure are improving or worsening, whether drugs are etiologically involved, and whether the initial presentation is severe enough to warrant immediate intubation and ventilatory support. In general, these decisions are made on clinical grounds in association with the findings of the chest x-ray examination and arterial blood gas analysis. It is necessary to know the alveolar-arterial oxygen difference, $(A-a)DO_2$, which may be calculated after calculating the alveolar oxygen tension (PAO_2) via the following alveolar-air equation: $PAO_2 = FIO_2(713) - 1.25(PACO_2)$. If a blood gas is obtained with the patient breathing room air, the alveolar oxygen tension will equal $150 - 1.25 (PACO_2)$. If the $PACO_2$ is found to equal 60 mm Hg, then the alveolar oxygen tension will equal $150 - 1.25(60)$ or 75 mm Hg. If the oxygen tension is 50 mm Hg, the alveolar-arterial difference is $75 - 50$ or 25 mm Hg, indicating a severe pulmonary problem; the normal difference is less than 12 mm Hg. If the alveolar-arterial oxygen difference is normal but the patient is hypoxemic, the cause of respiratory failure is most probably neuromuscular, possibly drug-related.

A. In general, patients with respiratory failure will be either apneic or extremely dyspneic. In both cases a complete history is difficult to obtain. Family or friends accompanying the patient may provide history of drug ingestion or foreign-body aspiration, or a history of prior problems with heart or lung disease. The physical examination generally reveals an extremely agitated, dyspneic patient. While a blood gas sample is being drawn, measure the blood pressure and evaluate the cardiac rhythm by ECG. The initial examination focuses on revealing the severity and etiology of the failure. Patients may be cyanotic. The presence of murmurs, cardiac gallops, and pulmonary rales suggests cardiac failure; the presence of high-pitched wheezes suggests an asthmatic crisis; rhonchi and voluminous sputum and fever suggest respiratory infection; neurologic findings may suggest stroke, myasthenia, or Guillain-Barré syndrome. There may be signs of trauma or bleeding.

B. An arterial blood gas (ABG) analysis is the initial test performed. A chest x-ray examination may confirm suspicions of tension penumothorax, respiratory infection, or cardiac failure. The ECG may confirm suspicions of myocardial infarction and/or provide evidence of cardiac arrhythmia.

C. If the initial ABG analysis indicates acute, severe respiratory failure with acidosis with or without associated hypotension or hypertension, or cardiac rhythm abnormalities, immediate intubation is warranted. The pH abnormalities may be corrected, and further evaluation of the patient may be safely done.

D. If the patient is in respiratory failure by ABG analysis (PCO_2 greater than 50 mm Hg) but does not have respiratory acidosis and is otherwise clinically stable, immediate intubation is not necessary. The value of the $(A-a)DO_2$ may indicate lung disease, and the chest film and associated clinical findings may confirm the diagnosis of chronic obstructive pulmonary disease and chronic respiratory failure. In these patients, the underlying lung disease and any acute new problem may be safely treated. The patient may require diuretics for increased cor pulmonale, antibiotics for bronchitis or pneumonia, or further work-up for a possible pulmonary embolus. Pulmonary rehabilitation with night-time ventilation may be indicated.

E. The patient who does not require immediate intubation but is unstable, with rising PCO_2 and falling pH, should undergo further evaluation in an intensive care unit setting. If the patient has a known diagnosis and information is available regarding responses to previous episodes, treatment with bronchodilators, antibiotics, cardiotonic agents, and fluids may be safely begun.

F. If a diagnosis of lung disease is not known but is suggested by the $(A-a)DO_2$ value, perform simple bedside spirometry to make a distinction between obstructive and restrictive lung disease. A normal $(A-a)DO_2$ with low lung volumes and the appropriate clinical findings suggests that the restrictive defect is caused by neuromuscular disease. Increased $(A-a)DO_2$ with low lung volumes suggests restrictive lung disease, whereas increased $(A-a)DO_2$ with reduced flows suggests obstructive lung disease.

G. When a preliminary diagnosis has been made, treatment may begin. Treatments may include steroids for patients with severe asthmatic attacks, or for those with interstitial pneumonia, antibiotics and chest tubes. Patients who have worsening or unresponsive disease may still require intubation and mechanical ventilation.

References

Johanson WG Jr, Peters JI. Respiratory failure. In: Murray JF, Nadel JA, eds. Textbook of respiratory medicine. Philadelphia: WB Saunders, 1988: 1973–2054.

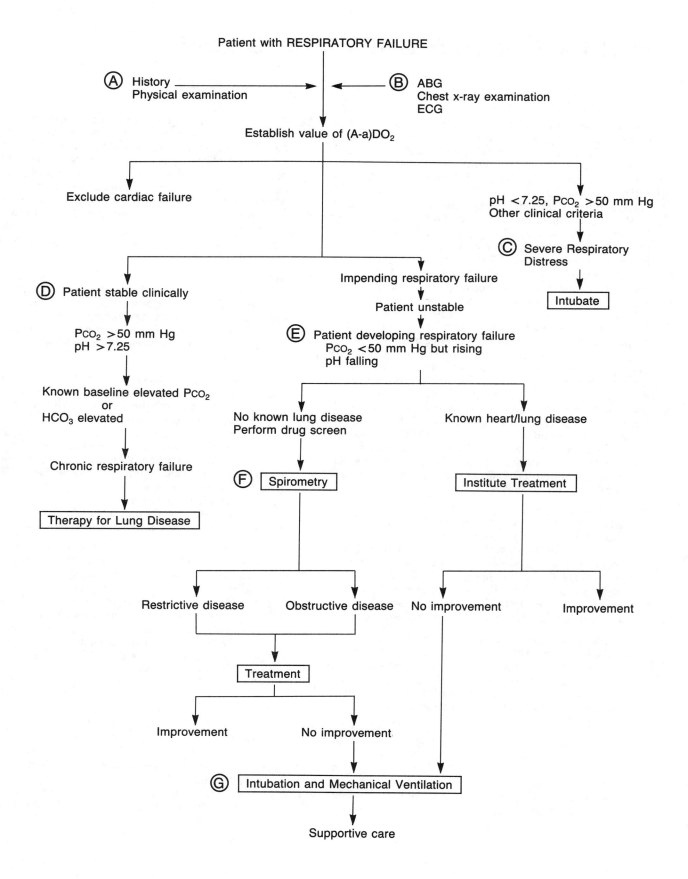

Patient with RESPIRATORY FAILURE

Ⓐ History / Physical examination

Ⓑ ABG / Chest x-ray examination / ECG

Establish value of (A-a)DO$_2$

Exclude cardiac failure

pH <7.25, Pco$_2$ >50 mm Hg / Other clinical criteria

Ⓒ Severe Respiratory Distress

Intubate

Ⓓ Patient stable clinically

Pco$_2$ >50 mm Hg / pH >7.25

Known baseline elevated Pco$_2$ / or / HCO$_3$ elevated

Chronic respiratory failure

Therapy for Lung Disease

Impending respiratory failure

Patient unstable

Ⓔ Patient developing respiratory failure / Pco$_2$ <50 mm Hg but rising / pH falling

No known lung disease / Perform drug screen

Known heart/lung disease

Ⓕ Spirometry

Institute Treatment

Restrictive disease   Obstructive disease   No improvement   Improvement

Treatment

Improvement   No improvement

Ⓖ Intubation and Mechanical Ventilation

Supportive care

ADULT RESPIRATORY DISTRESS SYNDROME

The adult respiratory distress syndrome (ARDS) is acute respiratory failure presenting as noncardiogenic pulmonary edema. The primary defect of this disorder is increased alveolar-capillary permeability that results in alveolar and interstitial edema. Despite modern therapy, the mortality from ARDS is greater than 50 percent. Many disorders have been linked to the development of ARDS. The most common cause of ARDS is gram-negative sepsis; other infectious etiologies include other bacterial and viral pneumonias, pneumonias caused by *Pneumocystis carinii* and *Legionella,* and miliary tuberculosis. Other causes of ARDS include aspiration of gastric contents (Mendelson's syndrome), ethylene glycol or hydrocarbon ingestion, near-drowning, traumatic or hemorrhagic shock, fat or amniotic fluid emboli, lung contusion, nonthoracic trauma, head injury, increased intracranial pressure, pancreatitis, drug overdose from heroin, methadone, propoxyphene, or barbiturates, or paraquat ingestion. Smoke inhalation, prolonged ventilation with high concentrations of oxygen, uremia, cardiopulmonary bypass, disseminated intravascular coagulation, massive blood transfusion, transfusion reaction, radiation pneumonitis, high altitude exposure, and Goodpasture's syndrome also have been found in association with ARDS. Diagnostic criteria for ARDS include: (1) presence of a condition known to cause ARDS, (2) a chest film showing diffuse bilateral infiltrates, (3) a pulmonary artery capillary wedge pressure equal to 12 mm Hg or less, and (4) an arterial blood gas PaO_2 of 50 mm Hg or less with FiO_2 of 60 percent or greater.

A. Most patients presenting with ARDS have a severe medical, surgical, or obstetric problem that is unrelated to the lung. Pulmonary involvement develops over the course of a few hours to a few days. A careful review of recent events discloses most of the disorders associated with ARDS. Clinical findings are nonspecific in ARDS. Tachypnea and tachycardia are almost universally present, and auscultation of the lungs may reveal scattered rales and rhonchi. Jugular venous distention is not present.

B. There are no specific laboratory tests for ARDS. An arterial blood gas (ABG) analysis will demonstrate hypoxia and hypocapnia; hypoxemia is likely to persist despite administration of oxygen and assisted ventilation. Additional laboratory evaluation focuses on identifying a potential infectious etiology. Electrocardiography identifies possible acute myocardial infarction.

C. The severity of the initial presentation depends on the etiology of the underlying disorder. The arterial PO_2 is used to assess the severity of the illness and to guide management. Intubate patients who are in respiratory failure despite supplemental oxygen and start assisted ventilation. Vasopressors may be necessary for those in shock.

D. Abnormal radiographic findings may not appear on chest films until 12 to 24 hours after the onset of clinical symptoms. Early findings consist of bilateral, ill-defined patchy infiltrates. Unlike cardiogenic pulmonary edema, cardiomegaly and pleural effusion are usually absent, as are Kerley B lines and pulmonary vascular redistribution. As ARDS progresses, the radiographic pattern evolves into homogenous and confluent infiltrates. The radiographic findings of pulmonary edema in ARDS are nonspecific and cannot be distinguished from those of cardiogenic pulmonary edema.

E. In patients with probable noncardiogenic pulmonary edema who are unstable (hypotension, poor oxygenation) and in those with uncertain diagnoses place a Swan-Ganz catheter to assess the pulmonary capillary wedge pressure. An elevated wedge pressure greater than 12 mm Hg is indicative of a cardiogenic cause for the pulmonary edema.

F. There are no specific effective treatments for ARDS. The mainstay of therapy is general medical supportive care and treatment of the underlying disorder. The use of corticosteroids has not been found to be useful. Initially patients with ARDS should be placed on 100 percent oxygen, and the concentration should be reduced to 60 percent when possible to avoid the development of oxygen toxicity. Add positive end-expiratory pressure (PEEP) to assisted ventilation in an attempt to decrease the oxygen concentration requirement. Since high levels of PEEP may result in decreased cardiac output, the level of PEEP, FiO_2, and cardiac output must be carefully titrated.

G. The course of ARDS depends on the severity of lung injury and the underlying disorder. Patients with minimal lung damage and no other major organ failure may be extubated after 4 to 5 days, whereas some patients with more serious disease may require 4 to 8 weeks of assisted ventilation. Focus on the prevention and treatment of associated medical problems that occur with high frequency in patients in intensive care units (e.g., nosocomial infections, upper gastrointestinal hemorrhage, renal failure, and poor nutrition).

References

Brandsetter RD. The adult respiratory distress syndrome. Heart Lung 1986; 15:155.

Matthay MA. The adult respiratory distress syndrome. New insights into diagnosis, pathophysiology, and treatment. West J Med 1989; 150:187.

ADULT RESPIRATORY DISTRESS SYNDROME Suspected

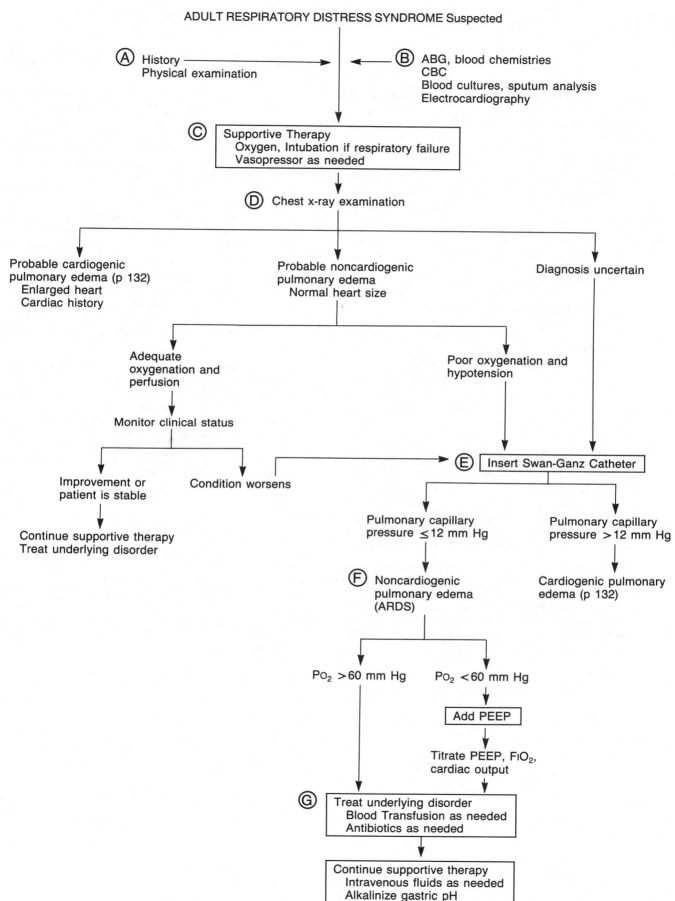

Ⓐ History
Physical examination

Ⓑ ABG, blood chemistries
CBC
Blood cultures, sputum analysis
Electrocardiography

Ⓒ Supportive Therapy
Oxygen, Intubation if respiratory failure
Vasopressor as needed

Ⓓ Chest x-ray examination

Probable cardiogenic
pulmonary edema (p 132)
Enlarged heart
Cardiac history

Probable noncardiogenic
pulmonary edema
Normal heart size

Diagnosis uncertain

Adequate
oxygenation and
perfusion

Poor oxygenation and
hypotension

Monitor clinical status

Improvement or
patient is stable

Condition worsens

Continue supportive therapy
Treat underlying disorder

Ⓔ Insert Swan-Ganz Catheter

Pulmonary capillary
pressure ≤12 mm Hg

Pulmonary capillary
pressure >12 mm Hg

Ⓕ Noncardiogenic
pulmonary edema
(ARDS)

Cardiogenic pulmonary
edema (p 132)

PO_2 >60 mm Hg

PO_2 <60 mm Hg

Add PEEP

Titrate PEEP, FIO_2,
cardiac output

Ⓖ Treat underlying disorder
Blood Transfusion as needed
Antibiotics as needed

Continue supportive therapy
Intravenous fluids as needed
Alkalinize gastric pH

123

WEANING FROM MECHANICAL VENTILATION

The decision to begin weaning a patient from a mechanical ventilator is usually made because of improvement in the underlying disease process that prompted the need for mechanical ventilation. The underlying disease process may or may not involve the lung. When there is significant lung disease, the process is more difficult, but the weaning procedures are the same with a few modifications. In general, weaning requires patience and supportive personnel. The key determinant is whether the patient's respiratory status can support independent ventilation.

A. Measurements of lung mechanics provide rough guidelines to indicate whether pulmonary function has improved sufficiently to allow weaning to proceed. These criteria include inspiratory force greater than −20 cm H_2O, tidal volume (TV) greater than 5 ml per kg, vital capacity (VC) greater than 10 ml per kg, and a resting minute ventilation of less than 10 L per minute. If a patient does not fulfill all the criteria, a weaning trial may still be initiated, with the patient watched carefully and the weaning process accomplished slowly.

B. Problems such as acidosis, fever, hypophosphatemia, hypocalcemia, or hypomagnesemia may contribute to poor lung mechanics and should be corrected. Severe anemia decreases oxygen transport to the tissues and should be corrected before a weaning trial is instituted. Thyroid function tests should be obtained in patients with generalized weakness. Patients who were chronically hypercarbic prior to intubation should be ventilated at a lower minute ventilation in order to approximate their baseline blood gas determinations more closely. Attempts should be made to provide adequate nutrition; low carbohydrate supplementations should be employed (decreased metabolic production of carbon dioxide).

C. The method of weaning varies considerably from one institution to another. We generally prefer to use T-piece weaning rather than intermittent mandatory ventilation (IMV). However, this decision depends on the availability of personnel to monitor the weaning process. T-piece weaning requires more extensive monitoring. Oxygen saturation is closely monitored with an ear oximeter.

Weaning is begun with a T-piece, and the vital signs are carefully followed over a 15-minute interval. If the patient remains comfortable, weaning is continued for another 15 minutes, a blood gas measurement is repeated, and the patient is placed back on the ventilator. If the blood gases remain favorable, the patient is allowed to remain off the ventilator for progressively longer intervals. Weaning is best attempted during the day, when the patient's mental status can be assessed and support personnel are more readily available. Moreover, adequate rest facilitates the weaning process. Patients who tolerate 4 to 8 hours of T-piece weaning are generally ready for extubation.

D. Some patients with good respiratory mechanics rapidly develop hypoxemia during weaning. If this is the result of highly collapsible airways, add continuous positive airway pressure (CPAP) or low levels of positive end-expiratory pressure (PEEP), which may speed the weaning process.

E. Failure to wean over 2 to 3 weeks indicates the need for a prolonged weaning process, and a tracheostomy must be performed. The best time to perform tracheostomy is uncertain, although the risk of laryngeal injury increases with prolonged intubation. Tracheostomy improves patient comfort, facilitates removal of secretions, removes the problem of accidental extubation, and allows the weaning process to continue over a long period of time (months).

References

Luce JM, Pierson DT, Hudson LD. Intermittent mandatory ventilation. Chest 1981; 79:678.

Petty TL. IMV vs IMS. Chest 1975; 67:630.

Sahn S, Lakshminarayan S, Petty TL. Weaning from mechanical ventilation. JAMA 1976; 235:2208.

Stauffer JL, Olsen DE, Petty TL. Complications and consequences of endotracheal intubation and tracheostomy. Am J Med 1981; 70:65.

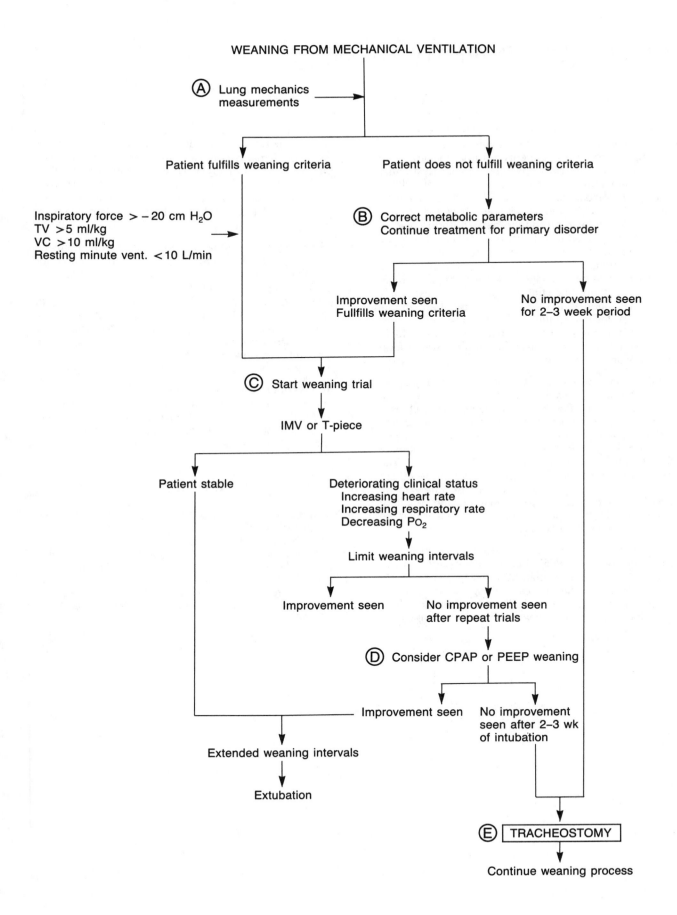

WEANING FROM MECHANICAL VENTILATION

(A) Lung mechanics
measurements

Patient fulfills weaning criteria

Patient does not fulfill weaning criteria

Inspiratory force > – 20 cm H$_2$O
TV >5 ml/kg
VC >10 ml/kg
Resting minute vent. <10 L/min

(B) Correct metabolic parameters
Continue treatment for primary disorder

Improvement seen
Fullfills weaning criteria

No improvement seen
for 2–3 week period

(C) Start weaning trial

IMV or T-piece

Patient stable

Deteriorating clinical status
Increasing heart rate
Increasing respiratory rate
Decreasing P$_{O_2}$

Limit weaning intervals

Improvement seen

No improvement seen
after repeat trials

(D) Consider CPAP or PEEP weaning

Improvement seen

No improvement
seen after 2–3 wk
of intubation

Extended weaning intervals

Extubation

(E) TRACHEOSTOMY

Continue weaning process

HIGH-FREQUENCY VENTILATION

High-frequency ventilators are experimental devices to be used only in adults with ventilatory failure under certain defined circumstances. These patients must have failed a trial of conventional volume-cycled ventilation and must either have significant non-compliant, stiff lungs, be at risk for barotrauma or have barotrauma, or have bronchopleural fistulae with chest tubes. This modality has also been used to ventilate patients undergoing upper airway endoscopy or otolaryngologic procedures. Patients with bronchopleural fistulae requiring conventional mechanical ventilation may lose a large portion of the delivered volume through the fistulae. These patients are ideally suited for a trial of high-frequency ventilation, since these devices deliver extremely small volumes (often 10 to 20 ml per breath) at a high rate (10 Hz, 600 cycles per minute); consequently, airway pressure and air leak are low. The mechanism by which high-frequency ventilation exchanges gases at the alveolar level is not known, and its efficacy has yet to be firmly established.

A. Adult patients with respiratory failure from any cause should always be placed on conventional volume-cycled ventilators initially. Physiologic guidelines to be achieved for patients placed on mechanical ventilation include the following: a respiratory rate of 10 to 15 per minute, a vital capacity greater than 15 ml per kg, a PO_2 greater than 65 mm Hg, and a pH between 7.38 and 7.42. The peak airway pressure should be less than 30 to 40 cm H_2O. Patients are sedated or sometimes (rarely) paralyzed if they cannot be synchronized to the ventilator and should be thus maintained until it is clear that the underlying disease process is improving.

B. If increasing FIO_2 and/or high levels of positive end-expiratory pressure (PEEP) become necessary to maintain the PO_2 at greater than 60 mm Hg, worsening of the underlying disease process or appearance of a new process has taken place. Under these circumstances, lung compliance will have decreased and the airway pressure necessary to maintain vital capacity will have substantially increased. The risk of barotrauma increases in this situation. It may become impossible to maintain oxygenation, even at an FIO_2 of 1.0 with a PEEP greater than 25 cm H_2O. In this case, or if the patient sustains a pneumothorax or develops a bronchopleural fistula and requires unilateral or bilateral chest tubes, consider high-frequency ventilation.

C. High-frequency ventilation should be instituted only by trained personnel who must be routinely available for problems. The patient may be begun at a rate of 200 to 300 breaths per minute at a volume of 3 to 6 ml at an oxygen concentration of 100 percent. It is necessary to analyze arterial blood gases at frequent intervals to assess the adequacy of oxygenation and ventilation. The patient does not need to make ventilatory efforts; the amount of leakage through chest tubes will decline since the airway pressure will be low.

D. If the patient does not improve, modifications may be made to the ventilatory regimen to eliminate stacking or to add airway support (PEEP) at a lower ventilatory rate. Patients should be switched back to conventional ventilation as soon as possible.

References

Bohn DJ, Miyasaka K, Marchak BE, et al. Ventilation by high-frequency oscillation. J Appl Physiol Respirat Environ Exercise Physiol 1980; 48:710.

Crawford M, Rehder K. High-frequency small-volume ventilation in anesthetized humans. Anesthesiology 1985; 62:298.

Gallagher TJ, Boysen PG, Davidson DD, Miller JR, Leven SB, et al. High-frequency percussive ventilation compared with conventional mechanical ventilation. Crit Care Med 1989; 17:364.

HIGH-FREQUENCY VENTILATION

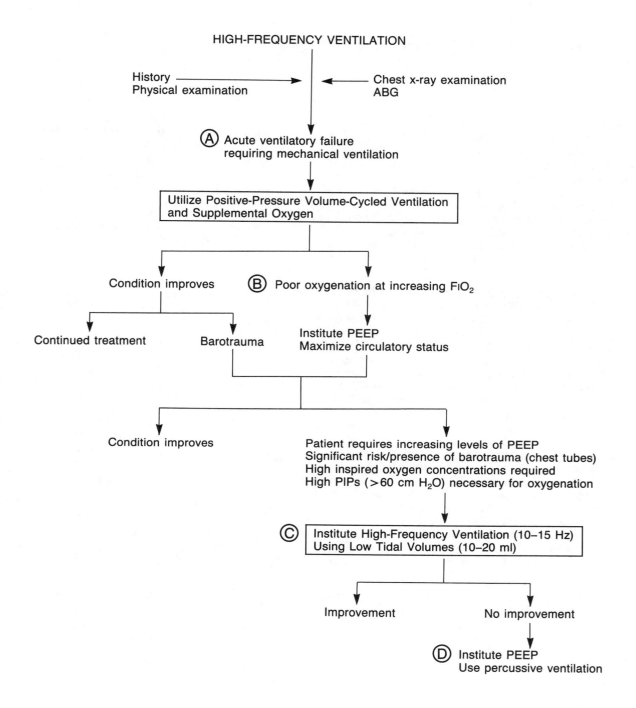

History ——————→ ←—————— Chest x-ray examination
Physical examination   ABG

(A) Acute ventilatory failure
requiring mechanical ventilation

Utilize Positive-Pressure Volume-Cycled Ventilation
and Supplemental Oxygen

Condition improves   (B) Poor oxygenation at increasing FIO_2

Continued treatment   Barotrauma   Institute PEEP
Maximize circulatory status

Condition improves   Patient requires increasing levels of PEEP
Significant risk/presence of barotrauma (chest tubes)
High inspired oxygen concentrations required
High PIPs (>60 cm H_2O) necessary for oxygenation

(C) Institute High-Frequency Ventilation (10–15 Hz)
Using Low Tidal Volumes (10–20 ml)

Improvement   No improvement

(D) Institute PEEP
Use percussive ventilation

PULMONARY REHABILITATION

Pulmonary rehabilitation requires a multidisciplinary approach to stabilizing and reversing the psychological and physiologic abnormalities associated with chronic lung disease. It has been used primarily for patients with chronic obstructive pulmonary disease and includes support from physicians, respiratory therapists, exercise physiologists, nutritionists, psychologists, psychiatrists, and social workers. There is no convincing evidence that pulmonary rehabilitation alters the progression of chronic lung disease or ultimate survival, but it does improve quality of life, exercise tolerance, and may improve the mechanical efficiency of the respiratory musculature.

A. In general, patients who have severe chronic obstructive lung disease are candidates for pulmonary rehabilitation, although less affected individuals are more likely to benefit. These patients are extremely dyspneic during the activities of daily living and may have difficulty with dressing, performing his or her toilet, and even eating. Some patients may require night-time mechanical ventilation. Pulmonary function testing reveals the FEV_1 to be less than 1 L, and it is usually less than 0.8 L. Patients may be maintained on home supplemental oxygen. Candidates for pulmonary rehabilitation should be well studied with regard to bronchoreversibility to assess the need for theophylline preparations and corticosteroids. Evaluate sputum to ensure the absence of infectious bronchitis, and assess cardiac function (echocardiography, nuclear scanning) to determine whether unsuspected cardiac disease is contributing to the dyspnea. Patients may undergo pulmonary exercise testing to determine the oxygen consumption, which should improve as a result of the rehabilitation program. Patients should also discontinue smoking before entering into the program.

B. Therapy with oral and aerosolized bronchodilators (theophylline preparations, beta-agonists) should be continued even if the patient does not have reversible disease as measured by PFT, since tests are performed at only one point in time. Corticosteroids should not be used unless there is a clear indication, such as an acute episode of asthmatic bronchitis. Use antibiotics in patients with chronic bronchitis whose airways are colonized with organisms. Use oxygen in all individuals whose baseline resting PO_2 is less than 55 mm Hg or whose night-time supine PO_2 is below this level. Oxygen should also be used in individuals with a hematocrit of more than 55 percent and/or evidence of pulmonary hypertension. Oxygen may be delivered by several routes, including the direct intratracheal route, which may reduce the work of breathing. Portable oxygen delivery systems should be employed to encourage patient mobility. Diuretics may be useful in patients who exhibit signs of right ventricular failure.

C. The above-mentioned measures may be supplemented with breathing exercises that stress diaphragmatic breathing during exhalation. Mild aerobic exercise that stresses activities useful to daily life also promote cardiovascular conditioning. Inspiratory resistive training devices may help to condition accessory ventilatory muscles, although this is still unproven. Provide patient education and nutritional and psychosocial support to improve outlook and overall emotional state.

References

Hodgkin JE, Zorn EG, Connors GL, eds. Pulmonary rehabilitation: Guidelines to success. Boston: Butterworths, 1984.

Make BJ. Pulmonary rehabilitation: myth or reality? Clin Chest Med 1986; 7:519.

Petty TL. Pulmonary rehabilitation. Am Rev Respir Dis 1980; 122(part 2):159.

Sahn SA, Nett LM, Petty TL. Ten year follow-up of a comprehensive rehabilitation program for severe COPD. Chest 1980; 77(Suppl):311.

PULMONARY REHABILITATION

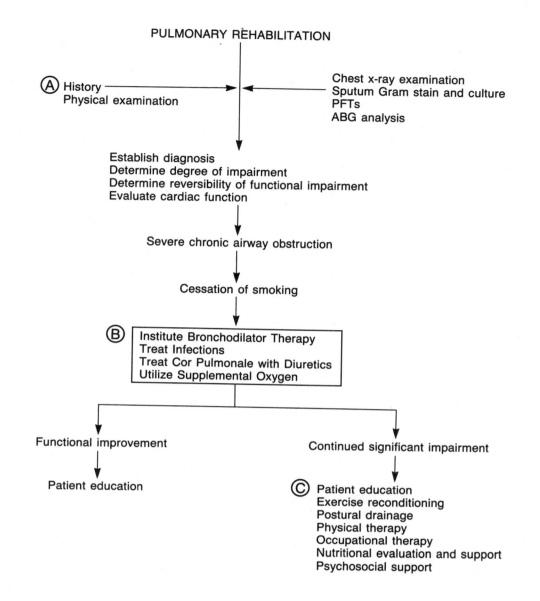

A History ——— Physical examination

Chest x-ray examination
Sputum Gram stain and culture
PFTs
ABG analysis

Establish diagnosis
Determine degree of impairment
Determine reversibility of functional impairment
Evaluate cardiac function

Severe chronic airway obstruction

Cessation of smoking

B Institute Bronchodilator Therapy
Treat Infections
Treat Cor Pulmonale with Diuretics
Utilize Supplemental Oxygen

Functional improvement

Patient education

Continued significant impairment

C Patient education
Exercise reconditioning
Postural drainage
Physical therapy
Occupational therapy
Nutritional evaluation and support
Psychosocial support

THROMBOEMBOLIC AND PULMONARY VASCULAR DISEASE

Acute Pulmonary Edema
High-Altitude Pulmonary Edema
Cor Pulmonale
Primary Pulmonary Vascular Disease
Hemodynamically Stable Pulmonary Embolus

Hemodynamically Significant Pulmonary
   Embolus
Fat Embolism
Amniotic Fluid Embolism
Veno-Occlusive Disease
Septic Pulmonary Embolism

ACUTE PULMONARY EDEMA

Acute pulmonary edema is caused either by severe increases in pulmonary venous pressure (hydrostatic edema), usually due to diseases of the heart, or by conditions which increase the permeability (permeability edema) of the pulmonary vasculature to protein, water, and other solutes. Both conditions produce increases in total lung water and reductions in gas exchange and may result in respiratory failure.

A. Patients may give a history consistent with acute myocardial infarction with a rapid deterioration of pulmonary function or a history of slowly worsening shortness of breath. Shortness of breath may appear in the setting of respiratory infection or recent surgery or after exposure to certain narcotic drugs. Physical examination usually reveals respiratory distress with a rapid respiratory rate and frothy sputum. The patient may be cyanotic. Examination of the heart may reveal the presence of atrial and ventricular gallops, abnormal cardiac rhythm, rales on lung examination, and peripheral edema.

B. In all patients, immediately take an arterial blood sample for analysis to determine adequacy of gas exchange. When conditions permit, obtain a chest radiograph. Other important studies include an ECG, measurement of electrolyte concentrations, and determination of renal function. If the history is consistent with acute myocardial infarction, perform cardiac enzyme measurements.

C. If the patient is cyanotic, has frothy sputum, rales, and gallops, with thready pulse and hypotension, make a tentative diagnosis of pulmonary edema prior to performing chest radiography and blood work. Obtain arterial blood, monitor the electrocardiogram, and intubate and oxygenate the patient. Treat severe CO_2 retention and acidosis with controlled ventilation; however, it should not be routinely necessary to correct acidosis with infusions of sodium bicarbonate. When the patient has been stabilized, obtain routine blood studies.

D. If the patient is not in fulminant edema, judgments must be made about whether the patient has cardiogenic or noncardiogenic pulmonary edema and regarding the severity of the disease. The chest film usually demonstrates the typical bat wing appearance of pulmonary edema; the cardiac silhouette will be enlarged if the patient has hydrostatic pulmonary edema, but may be normal if the patient has permeability pulmonary edema. Pleural effusions may be present. The typical chest film appearance may not be seen if the patient has severe obstructive airway disease.

E. If the patient is suspected of having pulmonary edema but the chest film is not typical, or if the chest film is typical but the heart is not enlarged, a Swan-Ganz right heart catheter must be placed to measure the pulmonary capillary wedge pressure (PCWP) to make the diagnosis. If the PCWP is greater than 15 mm Hg, the patient has cardiogenic pulmonary edema. If the PCWP is less than 12 mm Hg and the heart is not enlarged, then the probable diagnosis is permeability pulmonary edema, perhaps due to sepsis.

F. Once the diagnosis has been made, severity can be assessed on the basis of whether CO_2 retention is present. Patients with CO_2 retention have a poorer prognosis than those without this finding. The presence of respiratory or metabolic acidosis implies severe disease. Intubate and treat these patients with diuretics and preload reduction, to the extent that blood pressure and urine output do not suffer.

G. Patients with normal or low PCWP and an illness consistent with pulmonary edema probably have permeability edema (adult respiratory distress syndrome). Diastolic dysfunction of the heart must also be ruled out. Patients with adult respiratory distress syndrome usually require prolonged mechanical ventilation (days to weeks) coupled with medical management designed to minimize associated problems such as nutritional deficits, gastric bleeding, nosocomial infections, and barotrauma. In some cases, the capillary endothelium will regenerate over this time.

H. Patients with typical clinical findings, but an atypical chest film, may have elevated PCWP and atypical pulmonary edema. Once the diagnosis has been made, treat these patients similarly to patients with cardiogenic pulmonary edema.

References

Murray JF. Acute pulmonary injury in sepsis. In: Sande MA, Root RK, eds. Contemporary issues in infectious disease. Vol 4. New York: Churchill Livingstone, 1985:105.

O'Quinn R, Marini JJ. Pulmonary artery occlusion pressure: Clinical physiology, measurement, and interpretation. Am Rev Respir Dis 1983; 128:319.

Pistolesi M, Miniati M, Milne ENC, Giuntini C. The chest roentgenogram in pulmonary edema. Clin Chest Med 1985; 6:315.

Staub NC. Pulmonary edema. Physiol Rev 1974; 54:678.

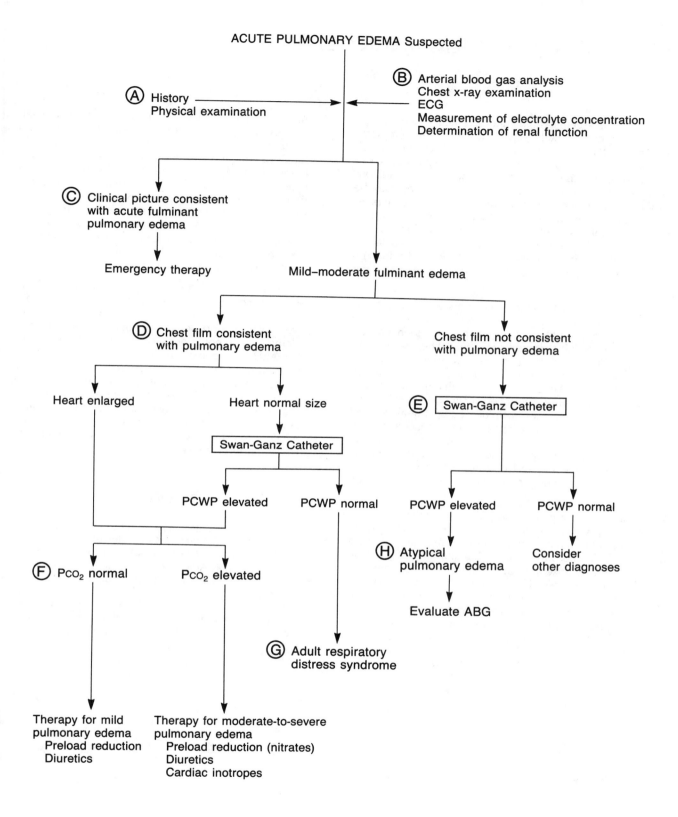

ACUTE PULMONARY EDEMA Suspected

(A) History
Physical examination

(B) Arterial blood gas analysis
Chest x-ray examination
ECG
Measurement of electrolyte concentration
Determination of renal function

(C) Clinical picture consistent
with acute fulminant
pulmonary edema

Emergency therapy

Mild–moderate fulminant edema

(D) Chest film consistent
with pulmonary edema

Chest film not consistent
with pulmonary edema

Heart enlarged

Heart normal size

Swan-Ganz Catheter

(E) Swan-Ganz Catheter

PCWP elevated

PCWP normal

PCWP elevated

PCWP normal

(F) Pco₂ normal

Pco₂ elevated

(H) Atypical
pulmonary edema

Consider
other diagnoses

Evaluate ABG

(G) Adult respiratory
distress syndrome

Therapy for mild
pulmonary edema
Preload reduction
Diuretics

Therapy for moderate-to-severe
pulmonary edema
Preload reduction (nitrates)
Diuretics
Cardiac inotropes

HIGH-ALTITUDE PULMONARY EDEMA

The rapidity of ascent to high altitude is the major determining factor of clinical pathology in this syndrome. Problems that arise include acute mountain sickness, high-altitude pulmonary edema, high-altitude cerebral edema, and other hematologic-thrombotic problems. Although these conditions depend largely on individual susceptibility, they may be avoided by slow ascents and limitation of exercise until physiologic adaptation has occurred. Coexisting cardiac or pulmonary problems, although not predisposing to the development of altitude-related illness, may exacerbate any of these conditions. In individuals who have lived at high altitudes, altitude-related illnesses may develop upon reascent from sea level.

A. Both patients with acute mountain sickness and those with high-altitude pulmonary edema give a history of rapid ascent to altitude. Those with acute mountain sickness complain of severe frontal headache, evening lassitude, and vomiting. Headache may wane but reappear with any physical exertion. Respiratory distress is usually not present. Although patients with high-altitude pulmonary edema may have been at altitude before without difficulty, they now complain of exertional weakness and marked dyspnea, and may also have headache, orthopnea, and frothy sputum, and they may be cyanotic. If patients are severely hypoxemic, they may exhibit mental status changes. Physical examination may only reveal tachycardia in those individuals with acute mountain sickness.

B. Patients with high-altitude pulmonary edema may be febrile as well as tachycardic with end-inspiratory rales. Sputum examination rules out the possibility of pneumonia. Arterial blood gas (ABG) analysis reflects mild to severe hypoxemia, and a chest x-ray examination demonstrates the infiltrates of pulmonary edema without cardiomegaly, a picture mirroring adult respiratory distress syndrome (ARDS). These laboratory and radiologic studies may not be available at altitude, however, so the diagnosis is usually based on clinical findings.

C. Altitude reduction may be required for acute mountain sickness, but patients with this disorder may recover at altitude with bedrest alone. The decision to reduce altitude in a patient with acute mountain sickness must be based on the degree and intensity of symptoms, since hypoxemia is not usually a major feature of this condition. Furosemide has been used with success to reduce symptoms in patients with acute mountain sickness, as has acetazolamide. Acetazolamide (250 mg twice daily, beginning the day before ascent) is now used as a preventive therapy for mountain sickness, although the mechanism by which it works is not yet known.

D. The mainstays of therapy for high-altitude pulmonary edema are oxygen administration and reduction in altitude. Diuretics may also afford some improvement. Further treatment for patients with high-altitude pulmonary edema who do not improve is similar to that for patients with ARDS. Morphine and CPAP may be used as adjunctive therapy to reduce extravascular lung water. Patients may require mechanical ventilation but usually do well and may return to altitude upon recovery. Upon return to altitude, physical exercise should be avoided, since it increases pulmonary artery pressure, which may result in increased extravascular lung water in a lung that is still recovering from injury.

References

Fred HL, Schmidt AM, Bates T, Hecht HH. Acute pulmonary edema at altitude. Circulation 1962; 25:929.

Hackett PH. Mountain sickness: prevention, recognition and treatment. New York: American Alpine Club, 1980.

Houston CS. Acute pulmonary edema of high altitude. N Engl J Med 1960; 263:478.

Larson EB, Roach RC, Schoene RB, Hornbein TF. Acute mountain sickness and acetazolamide: clinical efficacy and effect on ventilation. JAMA 1982; 248:328.

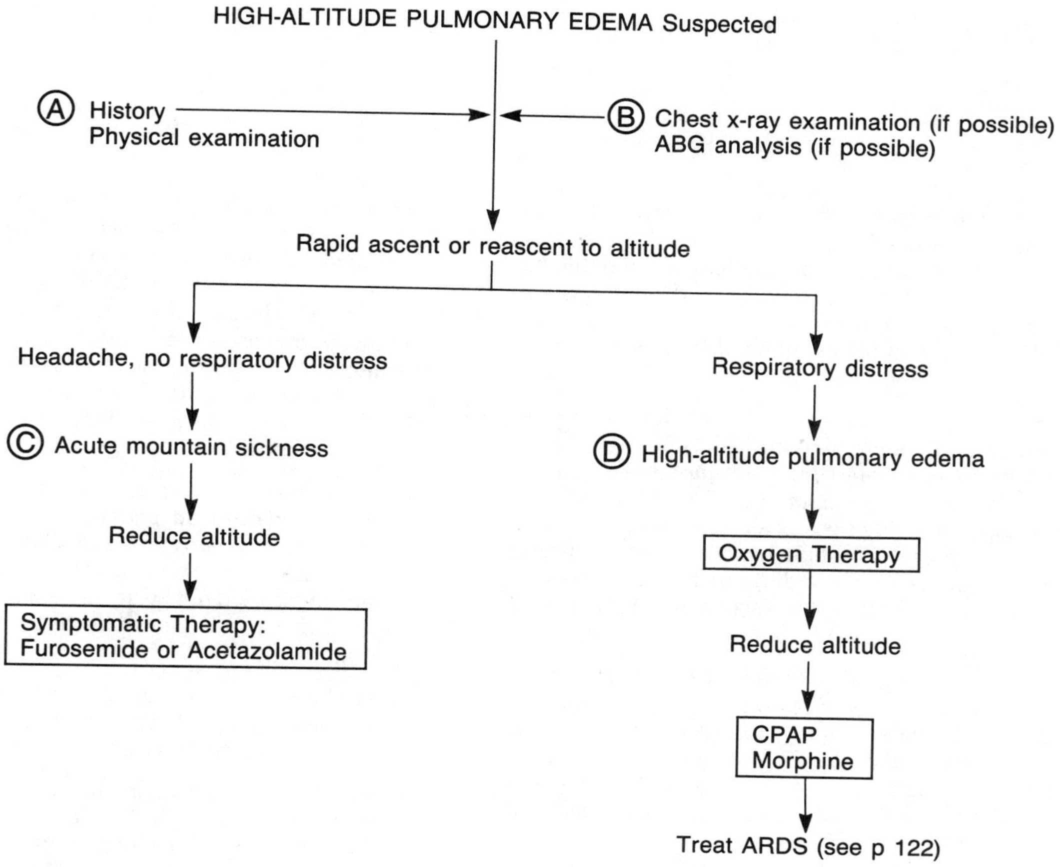

HIGH-ALTITUDE PULMONARY EDEMA Suspected

(A) History
Physical examination

(B) Chest x-ray examination (if possible)
ABG analysis (if possible)

Rapid ascent or reascent to altitude

Headache, no respiratory distress

(C) Acute mountain sickness

Reduce altitude

Symptomatic Therapy:
Furosemide or Acetazolamide

Respiratory distress

(D) High-altitude pulmonary edema

Oxygen Therapy

Reduce altitude

CPAP
Morphine

Treat ARDS (see p 122)

COR PULMONALE

Cor pulmonale is enlargement of the right ventricle or failure that results from increases in pulmonary vascular resistance due to primary or secondary pulmonary vascular disease. It must be differentiated from primary failure of the right ventricle resulting from ischemic, valvular, and other specific cardiac diseases. Right ventricle failure can also result from congenital abnormalities of the pulmonary circulation, such as stenosis of the pulmonary artery.

A. Patients may be asymptomatic or complain of mild to severe dyspnea on exertion. Usually the disease is characterized by a slow progression of symptoms over months to years. Physical examination reveals evidence of overt heart failure, including signs of elevated venous pressure with jugular venous distention, hepatic enlargement, and peripheral edema. Other findings include right ventricular heave or increase in the second pulmonic sound (P_2).

B. Right ventricular enlargement can be suspected on a lateral chest film when the cardiac silhouette encroaches on the retrosternal airspace. A biphasic P wave present on the inferior leads of the ECG suggests right atrial enlargement. An echocardiogram demonstrates increased right ventricular wall thickness and any associated left ventricular abnormalities.

C. Large and prolonged increases in pulmonary vascular resistance and pressures result in right ventricle enlargement and failure. This may be caused by a primary vascular problem (primary pulmonary hypertension) or loss of vascular bed secondary to pulmonary embolism or venocclusive disease. Hypoxemia resulting from pulmonary parenchymal diseases or from disorders of ventilation cause reflex vasoconstriction and elevations in pulmonary vascular pressures.

D. Biventricular failure suggests the presence of a primary cardiac problem such as a cardiomyopathy. Isolated failure of the right ventricle does not result in left ventricular failure.

E. Chronic bronchitis and emphysema are common causes of elevated pulmonary vascular pressures and right ventricle failure. Patients with these disorders usually have a long history of respiratory problems. However, chronic bronchitis may cause episodes of right ventricle failure early in the course of the disease. These patients have profound ventilation perfusion mismatching, which results in hypoxia and reflex vasoconstriction, particularly during disease exacerbations. Patients with emphysema or restrictive lung diseases develop right ventricle failure during the final stages of their illness. In the absence of severe parenchymal disease the possibility of a sleep disorder with nocturnal hypoxemia should be considered.

F. Treatment consists of oxygen therapy for hypoxemia, diuresis for fluid overload, and the use of beta-agonists and theophylline derivatives for bronchospasm. Digitalis is not indicated in isolated right heart failure. Elevations in hematocrit need not be treated unless they are marked (>55). The hematocrit often decreases after oxygen therapy is initiated.

G. When the PO_2 is less than 55 mm Hg on room air, give supplement oxygen therapy to raise the PO_2 above 65 mm Hg. This therapy has been shown to prolong survival.

H. Recent progress has been made with unilateral lung transplantation. It is indicated in young, otherwise healthy patients with isolated end-stage pulmonary disease.

References

Marmor AT, Mijiritsky Y, Plich M, Frenkle A, Front D. Improved radionuclide method for assessment of pulmonary artery pressure in COPD. Chest 1986; 89:64.

Mathur PN, Powles P, Pugsley SO, McEwan MP, Campbell EJM. Effect of digoxin on right ventricular function in severe chronic air flow obstruction. Ann Intern Med 1981; 95:283.

Schrijen F, Uffholtz H, Polu YM, Poincetol F. Pulmonary and systemic hemodynamic evolution in chronic bronchitis. Am Rev Respir Dis 1978; 117:25.

Yamaoka S, Yonekura Y, Koide H, Ohi M, Kuno K. Non-invasive method to assess cor pulmonale in patients with chronic obstructive lung disease. Chest 1987; 92:10.

COR PULMONALE Suspected

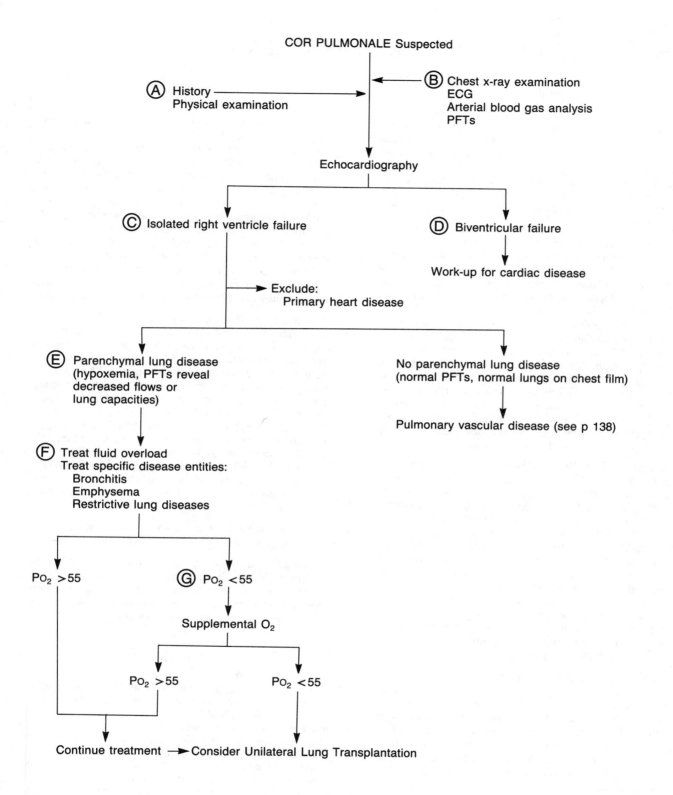

Ⓐ History
Physical examination

Ⓑ Chest x-ray examination
ECG
Arterial blood gas analysis
PFTs

Echocardiography

Ⓒ Isolated right ventricle failure

Ⓓ Biventricular failure

Work-up for cardiac disease

Exclude:
Primary heart disease

Ⓔ Parenchymal lung disease
(hypoxemia, PFTs reveal
decreased flows or
lung capacities)

No parenchymal lung disease
(normal PFTs, normal lungs on chest film)

Pulmonary vascular disease (see p 138)

Ⓕ Treat fluid overload
Treat specific disease entities:
Bronchitis
Emphysema
Restrictive lung diseases

$Po_2 > 55$

Ⓖ $Po_2 < 55$

Supplemental O_2

$Po_2 > 55$

$Po_2 < 55$

Continue treatment ⟶ Consider Unilateral Lung Transplantation

PRIMARY PULMONARY VASCULAR DISEASE

Primary pulmonary hypertension is a slowly progressive disease of unknown etiology causing chronic dyspnea and usually resulting in death. Primary pulmonary hypertension is seen predominantly in females (5:1, female-to-male ratio). A subgroup of patients with pulmonary hypertension have chronic pulmonary embolic disease. Pulmonary hypertension is also associated with cirrhosis and with the use of oral contraceptive medications.

A. Primary pulmonary hypertension presents with symptoms of dyspnea on exertion. Some patients complain of angina-like symptoms that are not responsive to sublingual nitroglycerin. Other patients may have syncopal episodes. Raynaud's phenomena may be present. Occasionally, early cases are identified by discovering enlargement of pulmonary arteries on routine chest films. Physical examination reveals a narrowly split S_2 with an increased P_2. A right ventricular gallop and evidence of tricuspid insufficiency may be noted if right ventricular dilation has occurred. Pulmonary function tests often reveal normal or slightly reduced flows and lung capacities; the diffusing capacity for carbon monoxide (DLCO) is also reduced. The ECG may reveal evidence of right ventricular enlargement, right axis deviation, right bundle branch block, and supraventricular arrhythmias.

B. Patients with pulmonary hypertension secondary to parenchymal lung disease usually have a distinctive history, physical examination and chest x-ray abnormalities, and pulmonary function tests usually yield abnormal results. Patients with emphysema or chronic bronchitis have obstructive airway physiology, and patients with interstitial fibrosis have reduced lung capacity. A small percentage of patients with pulmonary fibrosis can present with dyspnea, reduced diffusing capacity for carbon monoxide, and normal chest films. High-resolution CT scanning may reveal abnormalities consistent with interstitial fibrosis. In these patients enlargement of the pulmonary arteries is not a prominent feature; this lack of enlargement serves to eliminate primary pulmonary vascular disease as a diagnostic consideration.

C. Pulmonary hypertension is confirmed by right ventricle catheterization. A level of mean pulmonary artery pressures greater than 30 mm Hg is considered abnormal. Right ventricle catheterization is also useful to exclude intracardiac shunt (oxygen step-up) and diseases of the left ventricle (pulmonary capillary wedge pressure measurement). Some authorities recommend open-lung biopsy to exclude other diseases, but this approach is controversial.

D. Patients with occult pulmonary embolism can present with pulmonary hypertension. In most patients with pulmonary emboli, the emboli resolve and intravascular flow is restored. However, in a small percentage of cases, the emboli fail to resolve, and increased pulmonary vascular pressures ensue. In such cases, the patient may recall episodes of marked worsening of the dyspnea that occurs during embolic episodes. In other cases, however, the symptoms are indistinguishable from those seen in primary pulmonary hypertension. Although lung scans detect the presence of old pulmonary emboli, this procedure must be used with caution in patients with very high pulmonary artery pressures because scanning can result in refractory hypoxemia and hypotension, which are caused by occlusion of microvessels with technetium. Pulmonary angiography is required to confirm the diagnosis of chronic pulmonary emboli. Pulmonary vascular pressures can be measured during this procedure.

E. The degree of elevation of the pulmonary arterial pressures does not correlate well with survival. Increased right atrial pressure and decreased right cardiac index are poor prognostic signs. Systemic vasodilator therapy may reduce pulmonary vascular pressure. A battery of drugs may be tried for efficacy during a vasodilator study performed during right ventricle catheterization. Drugs that may be used include direct smooth muscle relaxants (hydralazine), calcium channel blocker (nifedipine), converting enzyme inhibitors (captopril), beta-adrenergic agonists (isoproterenol), vasodilator prostaglandins (prostacyclin), and alpha-adrenergic blockers (phentolamine). These agents must be used with extreme caution because they can cause refractory hypotension resulting in death.

F. In young patients with advanced pulmonary vascular disease, consider heart-lung transplantation.

G. Use anticoagulants in patients with evidence of emboli. Consider embolectomy to remove proximal emboli that do not respond to anticoagulation. In patients who are poor surgical candidates, balloon angioplasty has been used to open obstructed vessels.

References

Bengtsson L, Henze A, Holmgren A, Bjork VO. Thrombendarterectomy in chronic pulmonary embolism. Scand J Thor Cardiovasc Surg 1986; 20:67.

Fishman AJ, Moser KM, Fedullo PF. Perfusion lung scans vs pulmonary angiography in evaluation of suspected primary pulmonary hypertension. Chest 1983; 84:679.

Jamieson SW, Baldwin J, Stinson EB, et al. Clinical heart-lung transplantation. Transplantation 1984; 37:81.

Rich S, Levy PS. Characteristics of surviving and nonsurviving patients with primary pulmonary hypertension. Am J Med 1984; 76:573.

Rounds S, Hill NS. Pulmonary hypertensive disease. Chest 1984; 85:394.

PRIMARY PULMONARY VASCULAR DISEASE Suspected

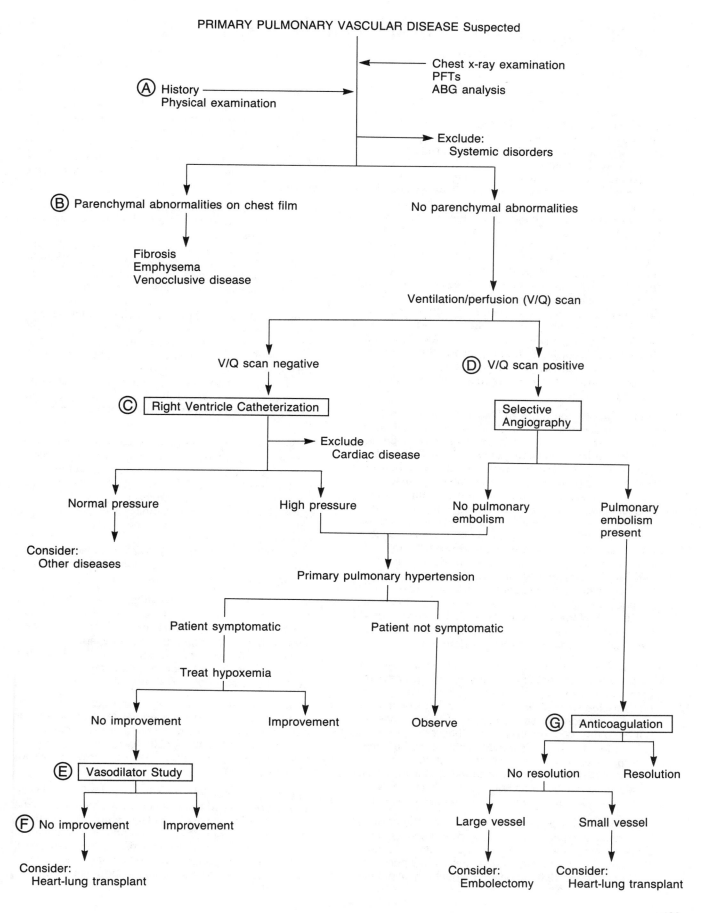

HEMODYNAMICALLY STABLE PULMONARY EMBOLUS

A. The diagnosis of pulmonary embolism is frequently based on a high degree of clinical suspicion. This condition occurs in a diverse clinical spectrum, from the classic presentation of acute pleuritic chest pain, shortness of breath, and hemoptysis in a previously healthy young woman taking oral contraceptives to mental confusion in an elderly bedridden patient. Predisposing factors for pulmonary embolism include immobility due to recent surgery, illness, stroke, travel, congestive heart failure or low cardiac output state, and familial hypercoagulable states such as protein C deficiency (hypercoagulable state may also be present in patients with nephrotic syndrome), and oral contraceptive use in women. Most patients with pulmonary embolism have nonspecific physical findings. The most common symptoms are dyspnea and pleuritic chest pain, occurring in 80 percent and 60 percent of patients, respectively. The most common physical findings on examination are tachypnea and tachycardia, occurring in 80 percent and 50 percent of patients. Hemoptysis, mostly in the form of blood-streaked sputum, occurs in approximately one-third of patients.

B. Routine blood chemistries and blood counts are not useful for the diagnosis of pulmonary embolism, although they are useful to determine the baseline coagulation status and to establish other diagnoses. Chest films are frequently normal in patients with pulmonary embolism; the combination of infiltrate and volume loss may indicate pulmonary infarction. The most common electrocardiographic findings are nonspecific atrial and ventricular ectopy. The electrocardiographic pattern of acute cor pulmonale (S_1-Q_3), if present, would suggest the diagnosis. A chest x-ray examination and electrocardiography are also used to exclude diseases with similar presentation, such as acute myocardial infarction, pneumonia, and congestive heart failure. Arterial blood gas (ABG) analysis is useful to estimate the significance of the embolism; however, it cannot be used to exclude the diagnosis; as many as 6 percent of patients with embolism may have a normal PO_2.

C. Obtain a perfusion lung scan with at least six views in all patients suspected of pulmonary embolism. Perfusion lung scan has a very high sensitivity; a normal scan virtually excludes the diagnosis. However, because it lacks specificity, a positive scan, except in a few situations, requires further confirmation with other tests. Perfusion lung scans are generally reported as demonstrating a low, intermediate, or high probability for pulmonary embolism. If performed in combination with the perfusion scan, ventilation lung scan improves the specificity of the test. For many others, the diagnosis remains uncertain.

D. A low-probability perfusion lung scan typically involves subsegmental defects; however, the consequences of untreated pulmonary embolism dictate further evaluation. Patients with low- to intermediate-probability perfusion lung scan have a 10 to 50 percent probability of pulmonary embolism. If pulmonary embolism is found, patients in whom anticoagulation is contraindicated should be considered for vena cava interruption. Pulmonary arteriography should be performed in these patients to confirm the diagnosis. Patients not at increased risk of anticoagulation require additional tests to determine the presence of thrombosis.

E. Approximately 90 percent of pulmonary emboli originate from the pelvis or deep veins in the lower extremities. The diagnosis of deep-vein thrombosis in patients suspected of pulmonary embolism clearly establishes the need for anticoagulation therapy, and further testing with pulmonary angiography is not necessary. Contrast venography is the standard for the diagnosis of deep-vein thrombosis. It is, however, an invasive test and may cause allergic reactions and thrombophlebitis in some patients. Impedance plethysmography is a noninvasive test with high sensitivity and specificity for the diagnosis of deep-vein thrombosis. In most situations, impedance plethysmography has been found to be a reliable test in place of contrast venography. Recently, two-dimensional ultrasonographic study of the deep venous system has been gaining acceptance as another noninvasive diagnostic test.

F. A high-probability perfusion scan typically involves multiple segments or lobar involvement; this evidence, along with a high clinical suspicion in a patient without preexisting heart or lung diseases, virtually establishes the diagnosis. Anticoagulation in this category of patient is reasonable if the risk of hemorrhage is judged to be low, although some authorities recommend angiography to confirm the presence of thromboembolic disease. Patients with contraindications to anticoagulation such as intracranial lesions, recent gastrointestinal hemorrhage, or surgery must be further evaluated.

G. In the absence of contraindication, initiation of heparin therapy should not be delayed until the diagnosis of pulmonary embolism is firmly established. Anticoagulation should commence with intravenous heparin for a duration of 7 to 10 days. Oral warfarin should then be added to achieve the desired anticoagulation effects for a total treatment duration of 3 to 6 months.

H. Pulmonary arteriography is considered the "gold-standard" of diagnostic procedures for pulmonary embolism. However, it carries a complications rate of approximately one death per 200 to 500 patients. It often is required prior to the placement of an inferior vena cava filter (IVC filter).

I. The Kimray-Greenfield filter is an umbrellalike device that can be inserted percutaneously into the inferior vena cava. It blocks the passage of large emboli to the lungs. It is used as a prophylaxis to prevent pulmonary emboli in patients in whom anticoagulation is contraindicated. It is also used in patients with recurrent pulmonary emboli due to failure of anticoagulation treatment.

PULMONARY EMBOLISM Suspected in Patient with STABLE VITAL SIGNS

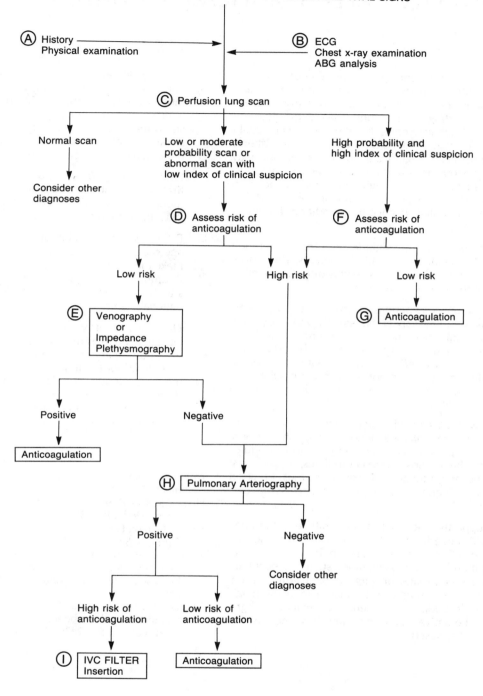

References

Dobkin J, Reichel J. Pulmonary embolism: diagnosis and treatment. Cardiol Clin 1987; 5:577.

Heim CR, DesPrez RM. Pulmonary embolism: a review. Adv Intern Med 1986; 31:187.

Hirsh J, Genton E, Hull R. Venous thromboembolism. New York: Grune & Stratton, 1981.

Kramer FL, Teitelbaum G, Merli GJ. Panvenography and pulmonary angiography in the diagnosis of deep venous thrombosis and pulmonary thromboembolism. Radiol Clin North Am 1986; 24:397.

Sasahara AA, Sharma GVRK, Barsamian EM, Schoolman M, Cella G. Pulmonary thromboembolism: diagnosis and treatment. Arch Intern Med 1983; 249:2945.

HEMODYNAMICALLY SIGNIFICANT PULMONARY EMBOLUS

In otherwise healthy patients, pulmonary emboli generally do not cause significant hemodynamic changes unless at least 60 percent of the pulmonary vascular bed is involved. Patients with pre-existing heart or lung diseases may have inadequate hemodynamic reserves so that smaller emboli could produce significant hemodynamic derangements. Patients with hemodynamically significant pulmonary emboli may present with syncope, hypotension, or altered mental status. Anterior chest pain similar to angina pectoris may occur in some patients. The diagnosis and treatment of this condition must be rapidly established since this condition, if untreated, is highly fatal.

A. Many hemodynamically significant pulmonary emboli occur in hospitalized, critically ill patients. The history and physical examination may readily differentiate other causes of these acute symptoms.

B. Acute pulmonary hypertension may occur in patients with massive pulmonary embolism. The ECG may show right heart strain pattern of S_1–Q_3 and right axis deviation. The ECG and chest films can also be used to exclude acute myocardial infarction with cardiogenic shock, tension pneumothorax, and pericardial tamponade. The ECG may also be used to diagnose pericardial effusion.

C. Patients with unstable vital signs should be admitted to the intensive care unit for treatment and monitoring. Supportive therapy must be instituted prior to procedures to confirm the diagnosis. Intravenous fluids, oxygen, pressor agents, and intubation, if necessary, must be given to ensure adequate blood pressure and tissue oxygenation.

D. Once supportive therapy has been initiated, start treatment with heparin for patients in whom there are no contraindications to anticoagulation. Patients with contraindications to anticoagulation, such as recent intracranial hemorrhage or surgery, pericarditis, recent gastrointestinal hemorrhage, or other major hemorrhagic risks, should undergo emergent pulmonary arteriography and alternative definitive therapy if pulmonary embolism is diagnosed.

E. The clinical status of patients receiving heparin must be reassessed after 1 hour of supportive therapy to identify those who do not respond. In unstable patients, emergency pulmonary arteriography establishes the diagnosis so that thrombolytic therapy can be considered. In stable patients, continue heparin therapy, and perform nonemergent pulmonary arteriography.

F. Once the diagnosis of pulmonary embolism is confirmed, continue anticoagulation therapy for 3 to 6 months, and consider placement of an inferior vena cava (IVC) filter if the patient re-embolizes while on therapy.

G. Patients who cannot be stabilized with supportive therapy should have emergent pulmonary arteriography to make the diagnosis. Although not yet definitively proven, thrombolytic therapy is generally advocated for this situation. Consider an IVC filter, and continue anticoagulants.

H. Unstable patients with absolute contraindications to anticoagulation must receive drastic therapy urgently to survive. Pulmonary embolectomy is rarely performed and is reserved for the few patients who do not respond to the usual supportive and specific treatments. The procedure carries a mortality rate in excess of 50 percent but may be life-saving for the few who need it. IVC filters are generally inserted during the procedure.

References

Dobkin J, Reichel J. Pulmonary embolism: diagnosis and treatment. Cardiol Clin 1987; 5:577.

Heim CR, Des Prez RM. Pulmonary embolism: a review. Adv Intern Med 1986; 31:187.

Hirsh J, Genton E, Hull R. Venous thromboembolism. New York: Grune & Stratton, 1981.

Kramer FL, Teitelbaum G, Merli GJ. Panvenography and pulmonary angiography in the diagnosis of deep venous thrombosis and pulmonary thromboembolism. Radiol Clin North Am 1986; 24:397.

Sasahara AA, Sharma GVRK, Barsamian EM, Schoolman M, Cella G. Pulmonary thromboembolism: diagnosis and treatment. Arch Intern Med 1983; 249:2945.

PULMONARY EMBOLISM Suspected in a Patient with HEMODYNAMICALLY UNSTABLE VITAL SIGNS

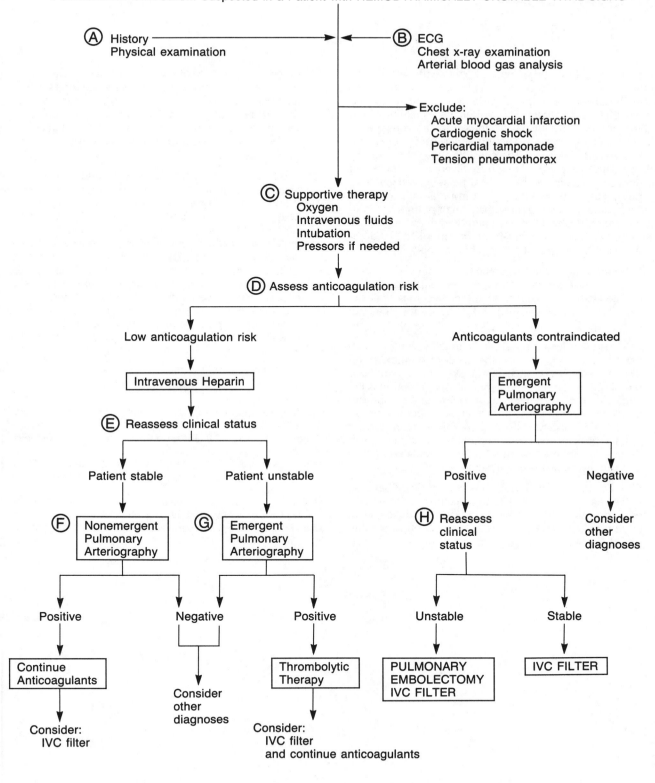

FAT EMBOLISM

The syndrome of fat embolization begins with severe trauma that causes fractures of the long bones, particularly the femur. The incidence of this disorder in this situation is approximately 1 to 5 percent. The emboli are widely distributed, but symptoms usually involve the central nervous system and the respiratory system. The initial clinical features consist of fever and confusion. The chest film may show a hazy infiltrate. This may progress to diffuse alveolar infiltrates and hypoxemia with a widened alveolar-arterial oxygen gradient. The pulmonary abnormalities result from fat-induced local capillary damage. The exact mechanism of pulmonary injury is unclear. Although it has been proposed that injury results from release of free fatty acids from the embolized fat, injury may result from neutral fat or other factors.

A. Pulmonary fat embolism can be detected in a significant proportion of patients who die after major trauma associated with fractures. The syndrome becomes clinically evident usually between 12 and 72 hours after the traumatic injury.

B. Hypoxemia is a cardinal sign of clinically significant fat embolism. It may precede the onset of pulmonary infiltrates. This occurrence may result in the erroneous presumption that thrombotic pulmonary embolism is the etiologic event. Although pulmonary thromboembolism is not uncommon in the post-traumatic setting, it usually occurs 2 to 3 days following the injury, a time period past the peak incidence of fat embolism. In addition, with thrombotic pulmonary embolism the associated signs of fat embolism are usually absent.

C. The diagnosis of fat embolism is often difficult because of the lack of definitive diagnostic features. The associated findings provide the key to making the diagnosis of fat embolism. These include fever, confusion, skin petechiae, and fat globules in the urine or in clotted blood. The presence of several of the associated findings of fat embolism strongly supports the diagnosis. For example, although relatively uncommon (occurring in less than 20 percent of patients), skin petechiae offer convincing evidence for fat embolism. The petechiae may be found on the conjunctiva, retina, neck, and upper trunk.

D. The treatment of fat embolism syndrome remains controversial. Rapid immobilization of long bone fractures is important in preventing embolic events. A variety of treatments have been tried without clearcut success. Among these are alcohol infusion, heparin, low-molecular–weight dextran, clofibrate, and others. The survival of the patient depends mainly on supportive care, such as oxygen administration and mechanical ventilation with positive end-expiratory pressure (PEEP) as required. Most investigators still advocate the use of short-term high-dose steroids. The anti-inflammatory action of the drug may reduce the severity of the illness. Specific therapies may become available once the pathogenesis of the capillary leak is elucidated.

References

Gossling HR, Donohue TA. The fat embolism syndrome. JAMA 1979; 241:2740.

Guenter CA, Braun TE. Fat embolism syndrome. Chest 1981; 79:143.

Lahiri B, Wallack RZ. The early diagnosis and treatment of fat embolism syndrome: a preliminary report. J Trauma 1977; 17:956.

Moylan JA, Evenson MA. Diagnosis and treatment of fat embolism. Ann Rev Med 1977; 28:85.

Riska EB, Myllynen P. Fat embolism in patients with multiple injuries. J Trauma 1982; 22:891.

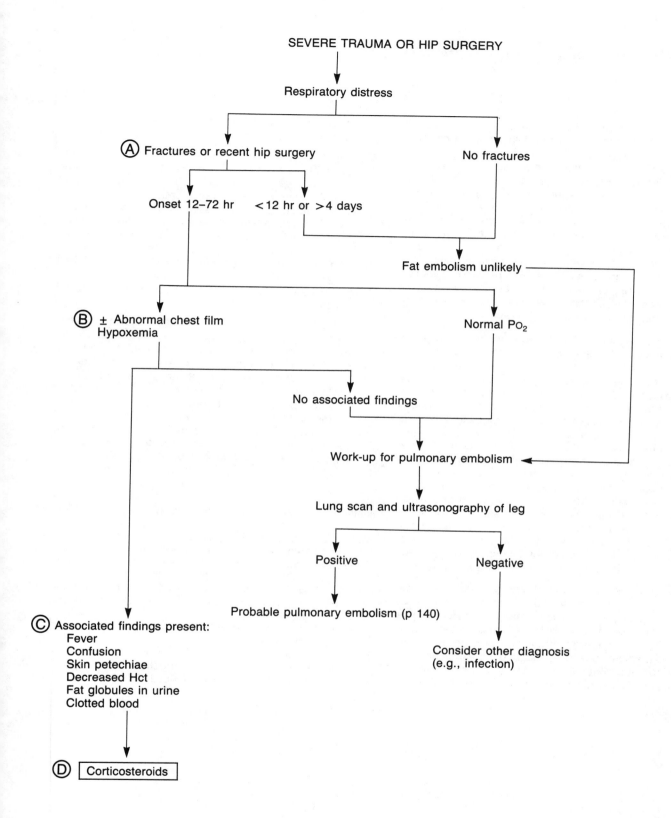

SEVERE TRAUMA OR HIP SURGERY

Respiratory distress

Ⓐ Fractures or recent hip surgery

No fractures

Onset 12–72 hr   < 12 hr or > 4 days

Fat embolism unlikely

Ⓑ ± Abnormal chest film
Hypoxemia

Normal PO₂

No associated findings

Work-up for pulmonary embolism

Lung scan and ultrasonography of leg

Positive   Negative

Probable pulmonary embolism (p 140)

Consider other diagnosis
(e.g., infection)

Ⓒ Associated findings present:
Fever
Confusion
Skin petechiae
Decreased Hct
Fat globules in urine
Clotted blood

Ⓓ Corticosteroids

AMNIOTIC FLUID EMBOLISM

Amniotic fluid embolism is a rare catastrophic event that occurs during or soon after labor and delivery and occasionally during cesarean section. This condition is caused by the embolization of amniotic fluid containing cellular elements and other debris such as lanugo hair and vernix into the maternal pulmonary circulation. Occasionally the onset of the syndrome may be delayed after cesarean delivery, presumably due to a gradual release of trapped amniotic fluid in the uterine veins immediately after delivery. This disturbance results in profound alternation of maternal hemodynamics and oxygenation. In the United States, the incidence of the condition has been estimated to be approximately one case per 30,000 deliveries. Despite modern cardiopulmonary resuscitative measures, the overall mortality rate of this condition exceeds 80 percent.

A. The diagnosis of amniotic fluid embolism is made on clinical grounds. Because of the acuteness and rarity of the condition, the medical history is not particularly useful in the diagnosis. Most reported cases involve multiparous women with an average age of 32 years. The use of uterine stimulants during labor, the presence of an intrauterine contraceptive device throughout pregnancy, pregnancy termination by hypertonic solution or operative procedure, and cesarean section delivery have also been associated with this event. The classic presentation occurs during a hard labor with the sudden onset of dyspnea, cyanosis, and hypotension, often accompanied by pulmonary edema. In many cases, cardiorespiratory arrest occurs within minutes of the initial symptoms. The major differential diagnoses include hemorrhagic shock, septic shock, acute myocardial infarction, hemodynamically significant pulmonary thromboembolism, and aspiration of acidic gastric contents (Mendelson's syndrome).

B. Owing to the rapid onset of the signs and symptoms, the diagnosis of amniotic fluid embolism must often be made presumptively while treatment is initiated. The patient must be stabilized before diagnostic steps can be taken. Use intravenous fluids and pressors to sustain blood pressure and circulation, and intubation and ventilation with 100 percent oxygen to ensure tissue oxygenation. When the patient survives the initial insult, insert a Swan-Ganz catheter to monitor the hemodynamic status.

C. Diagnostic tests can be initiated once the patient is stabilized. The presence of pulmonary edema is demonstrated with chest films. Examination of the buffy coat of blood withdrawn through the central venous or Swan-Ganz catheter may reveal amniotic fluid debris, which establishes the diagnosis. Recent studies, however, have found a small number of fetal squamous cells in the pulmonary artery of virtually all pregnant women studied. Therefore, although confirming the presence of fetal squamous cells in wedged pulmonary capillary blood is a necessary step, it is not sufficient evidence for the diagnosis of this syndrome.

D. Overall, less than 20 percent of patients survive the initial event. Among survivors, almost all develop disseminated intravascular coagulopathy accompanied by the usual clinical and laboratory manifestations, with bleeding from the uterine surfaces and needle puncture sites, prolongation of the prothrombin and activated partial thromboplastin times, thrombocytopenia and hypofibrinogenemia. Management of coagulopathy includes packed red blood cell replacement and factor replacement with cryoprecipitate. The role of heparin in this condition has not been established.

References

Finley BE. Acute coagulopathy in pregnancy. Med Clin North Am 1989; 73:723.

Mulder JI. Amniotic fluid embolism: an overview and case report. Am J Obstet Gynecol 1985; 152:430.

Peterson EP, Taylor HB. Amniotic fluid embolism: an analysis of 40 cases. Obstet Gynecol 1970; 35:787.

Price TM, Baker VV, Cefalo RC. Amniotic fluid embolism: three case reports with a review of the literature. Obstet Gynecol Surv 1985; 40:462.

Sperry K. Amniotic fluid embolism: to understand an enigma. JAMA 1986; 255:2183.

Steiner PE, Lushbaugh CC. Maternal pulmonary embolism by amniotic fluid as a cause of obstetric shock and unexpected deaths in obstetrics. JAMA 1986; 255:2187.

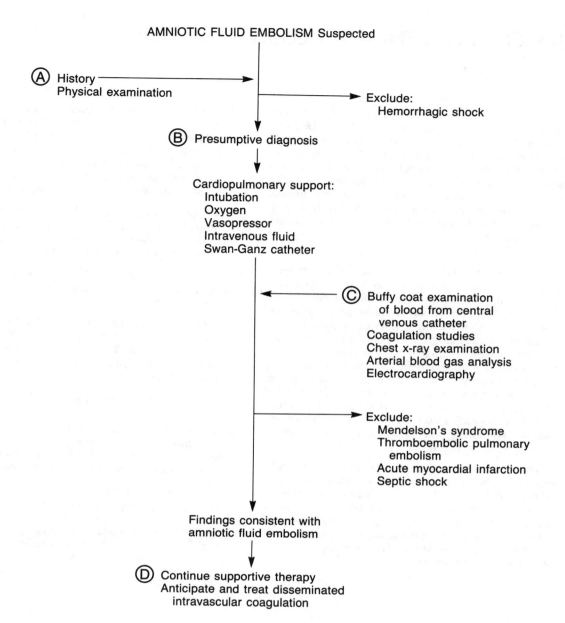

AMNIOTIC FLUID EMBOLISM Suspected

(A) History
Physical examination

Exclude:
  Hemorrhagic shock

(B) Presumptive diagnosis

Cardiopulmonary support:
  Intubation
  Oxygen
  Vasopressor
  Intravenous fluid
  Swan-Ganz catheter

(C) Buffy coat examination
    of blood from central
    venous catheter
  Coagulation studies
  Chest x-ray examination
  Arterial blood gas analysis
  Electrocardiography

Exclude:
  Mendelson's syndrome
  Thromboembolic pulmonary
    embolism
  Acute myocardial infarction
  Septic shock

Findings consistent with
amniotic fluid embolism

(D) Continue supportive therapy
Anticipate and treat disseminated
  intravascular coagulation

PULMONARY VENO-OCCLUSIVE DISEASE

Pulmonary veno-occlusive disease is a rare disorder characterized by narrowing or obstruction of small veins by cellular proliferation of the intima and eventual fibrosis. In approximately 50 percent of cases, the arteries are also involved. The etiology of the disorder is unknown but may occur after viral infections or as part of an immunologic disorder. In some cases, the onset of veno-occlusive disease follows therapy for malignant neoplasms. The chest film abnormality of interstitial edema differentiates this entity from primary pulmonary hypertension.

A. The occlusion of small veins results in marked elevations in pulmonary artery pressures. The signs and symptoms of pulmonary hypertension are usually present. Patients often experience progressive dyspnea, palpitations, and episodes of lightheadedness. Physical findings include a right ventricular heave, a loud pulmonic closure sound (P_2), and a right ventricular S_4. The chest film reveals right ventricular enlargement and enlarged pulmonary arteries; parenchymal findings include a haziness consistent with interstitial pulmonary edema and Kerley B lines. Lung scans do not reveal evidence of pulmonary emboli. Echocardiography helps exclude cardiogenic causes of pulmonary hypertension and interstitial edema, such as mitral stenosis.

B. Mediastinal fibrosis may result from granulomatous infections such as histoplasmosis or tuberculosis and produce obstruction of the superior vena cava. In some cases, the fibrosis is limited to the posterior mediastinum and may selectively obstruct pulmonary veins, leading to pulmonary hypertension and pulmonary venous congestion. This picture closely resembles that of the veno-occlusive syndrome.

C. Right ventricle catheterization reveals marked elevations in pulmonary artery pressures. The wedge pressure is variable but may be normal because the catheter is usually positioned to reflect pressures in large pulmonary veins, which are not obstructed. In some cases, wedge pressures may be increased; in these cases, high pressures probably do reflect involvement of large veins.

D. The diagnosis is based on the characteristic clinical and laboratory findings. Whether tissue confirmation is required is a difficult judgment that depends on the exact clinical presentation and the risks of biopsy.

E. The diagnosis can be definitively established by lung biopsy. The risk of this procedure is increased because of the markedly elevated pulmonary vascular pressures.

F. Treatment for this disorder is controversial. There are no controlled studies demonstrating the efficacy of any particular approach. There are case reports showing improvement after either anticoagulation or azathioprine administration.

References

Chawla SK, Kittle CF, Faber LP, Jensik RJ. Pulmonary veno-occlusive disease. Ann Thorac Surg 1976; 22:249.

Lombard CM, Churg A, Winokur S. Pulmonary veno-occlusive disease following therapy for malignant neoplasms. Chest 1987; 92:871.

Sanderson JE, Spiro SG, Hendry AT, Turner-Warwick M. A case of pulmonary veno-occlusive disease responding to azathioprine. Thorax 1977; 32:140.

Wagenvoort CA, Wagenvoort N, Takahashi T. Pulmonary veno-occlusive disease: involvement of pulmonary arteries and review of the literature. Hum Pathol 1985; 16:1033.

VENO-OCCLUSIVE DISEASE Suspected

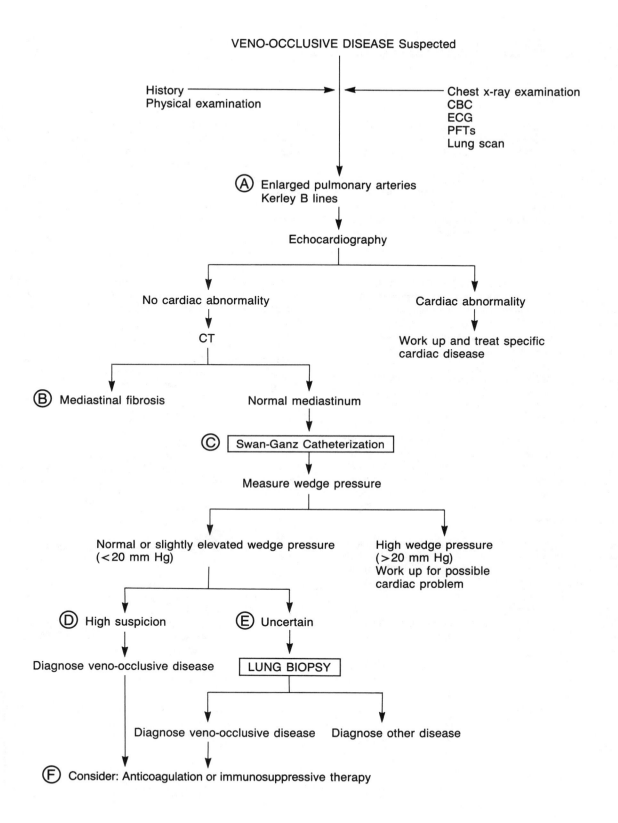

History ——————→ ←—————— Chest x-ray examination
Physical examination   CBC
                                        ECG
                                        PFTs
                                        Lung scan

Ⓐ Enlarged pulmonary arteries
   Kerley B lines

Echocardiography

No cardiac abnormality   Cardiac abnormality

CT   Work up and treat specific
                                                cardiac disease

Ⓑ Mediastinal fibrosis   Normal mediastinum

Ⓒ │ Swan-Ganz Catheterization │

Measure wedge pressure

Normal or slightly elevated wedge pressure   High wedge pressure
(<20 mm Hg)   (>20 mm Hg)
                                                    Work up for possible
                                                    cardiac problem

Ⓓ High suspicion   Ⓔ Uncertain

Diagnose veno-occlusive disease   │ LUNG BIOPSY │

                    Diagnose veno-occlusive disease   Diagnose other disease

Ⓕ Consider: Anticoagulation or immunosuppressive therapy

SEPTIC PULMONARY EMBOLISM

Septic pulmonary emboli are caused by infected clots originating from systemic veins or the right side of the heart. When lodged in the pulmonary arteries, they may result in pulmonary infarction, abscess formation, and other complications. Septic emboli occur in the setting of intravenous drug abuse, or in the setting of phlebitis and suppurative processes involving the pelvic veins, head and neck, or lower extremities. They result from iatrogenic causes such as infected indwelling intravenous catheters. The management goal is to control the source of infection and to treat pulmonary complications.

A. The symptoms of septic pulmonary emboli—dyspnea, tachypnea, and pleuritic chest pain—are common findings. Fever, shaking chills, and a toxic appearance of the patient indicate an underlying infectious process. Septic pulmonary emboli in intravenous drug abusers are typically due to tricuspid valve endocarditis; empyema may be found in half of these patients. Examination of the lower extremities and all indwelling intravenous catheter sites must be carefully performed. In patients with septic pelvic phlebitis, the pelvic examination may reveal extreme tenderness of the uterine or ovarian areas.

B. Initiate appropriate antibiotics promptly once blood and pleural fluids have been obtained for cultures. The predominant organism is likely to be *Staphylococcus aureus*, followed by streptococci, gram-negative bacteria such as *Klebsiella*, *Pseudomonas*, *Escherichia coli*, and *Proteus*. Multiple organisms may be found in some patients with endocarditis.

C. Chest films are usually abnormal. In one study, almost half of the patients had diffuse bilateral nodules in various stages of cavitation, and pulmonary infiltrates were seen in virtually all patients. Chest CT is highly sensitive and specific in identifying cavitating nodules and subpleural septic infarcts. Perfusion lung scan has high sensitivity. A negative lung scan excludes the presence of emboli, but a positive lung scan lacks the specificity of the CT scan.

D. The origin of the septic emboli must be determined in order to control the infection. The tricuspid valve is the most likely site in intravenous drug abusers. Echocardiography detects the presence of valvular vegetation or mural thrombus. Patients with recent history of abortion, delivery, or other pelvic manipulation may have involvement of the uterine or ovarian veins. Suspected infected intravenous catheters must be removed.

E. Tricuspid valve endocarditis caused by *Staphyloccus* frequently responds to antibiotic therapy alone. The role of anticoagulants has not been established. Patients who do not respond or those who develop complications such as hemoptysis while receiving antibiotic therapy should have the infected valve excised. Exsanguinating hemoptysis may occur in this setting.

F. Antibiotics along with anticoagulants usually are adequate to treat septic phlebitis in the lower extremities. In patients with contraindications to anticoagulants, the involved veins should be excised.

References

Griffith GL, Maull KI, Sachatello CR. Septic pulmonary embolization. Surg Gynecol Obstet 1977; 144:105.

Huang RM, Naudich DP, Lubat E, Schinella R, Garay SM, McCauley DI. Septic pulmonary emboli: CT-radiographic correlation. Am J Roentgenol 1989; 153:41.

MacMillan JC, Milstein SH, Samson PC. Clinical spectrum of septic pulmonary embolism and infarction. Thorac Cardiovasc Surg 1978; 75:670.

O'Donnell AE, Pappas LS. Pulmonary complications of intravenous drug abuse: experience at an inner-city hospital. Chest 1988; 94:251.

Osei C, Berger HW, Nicholas P. Septic pulmonary infarction: clinical and radiographic manifestations in 11 patients. Mt Sinai J Med 1979; 46:145.

Weinberg G, Pasternak BM. Upper-extremity suppurative thrombophlebitis and septic pulmonary emboli. JAMA 1978; 240:1519.

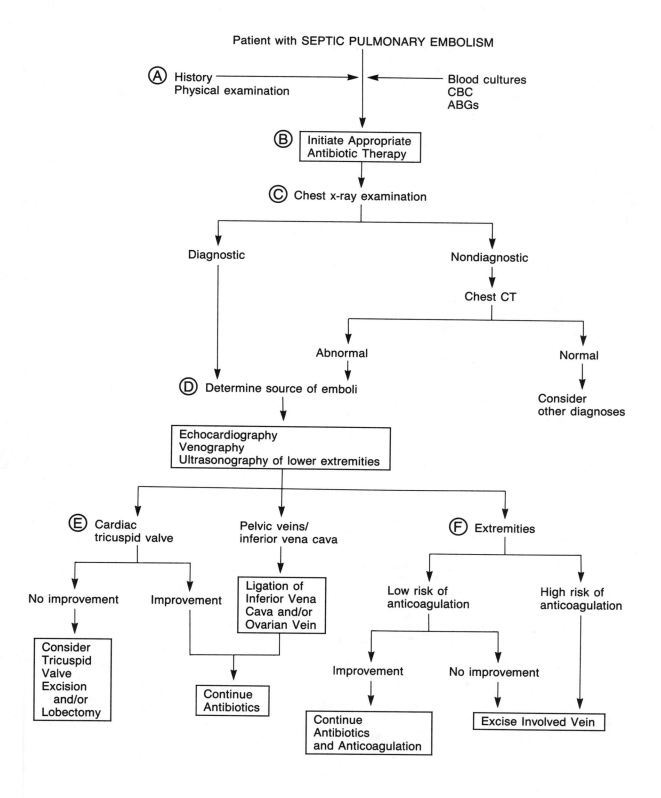

Patient with SEPTIC PULMONARY EMBOLISM

(A) History ——————→ ←—————— Blood cultures
Physical examination   CBC
                                    ABGs

(B) Initiate Appropriate
    Antibiotic Therapy

(C) Chest x-ray examination

Diagnostic   Nondiagnostic

                                    Chest CT

                        Abnormal   Normal

(D) Determine source of emboli   Consider
                                    other diagnoses

Echocardiography
Venography
Ultrasonography of lower extremities

(E) Cardiac   Pelvic veins/   (F) Extremities
    tricuspid valve inferior vena cava

No improvement   Improvement   Ligation of   Low risk of   High risk of
                               Inferior Vena   anticoagulation   anticoagulation
                               Cava and/or
                               Ovarian Vein

Consider   Improvement   No improvement
Tricuspid
Valve
Excision   Continue
and/or   Antibiotics
Lobectomy   Continue
                                        Antibiotics   Excise Involved Vein
                                        and Anticoagulation

CONGENITAL LUNG DISEASE

Bronchopulmonary Sequestration
Bronchogenic Cyst
Arteriovenous Malformation
Cystic Fibrosis
Marfan's Syndrome

BRONCHOPULMONARY SEQUESTRATION

Bronchopulmonary sequestration is an area of lung parenchyma with no airway connection to the bronchial system. Sequestrations receive blood supplied by an aberrant artery from the aorta or its branches and are usually drained by pulmonary veins. Intralobar sequestrations share a common pleura with normal lung; extralobar sequestrations have a separate pleura. Sequestration is a relatively rare anomaly that usually occurs alone; however, in approximately 10 percent of cases it is accompanied by other congenital abnormalities such as diaphragmatic hernias. In some cases, sequestration may be an acquired defect. In either case, cystic degeneration and fibrosis occurs in the sequestered lung.

A. Approximately one-third of cases are detected during childhood. Most patients present with a history of recurrent episodes of fever, cough, and pneumonia. Treat active infection with antibiotics and exclude tuberculosis. In some patients, the abnormality is found on routine chest films.

B. The radiographic findings are variable. Usually a mass density is found in the posterior basilar segments of the lower lobe. Calcification may be present. Other patterns include cystic areas, with or without single or multiple air-fluid levels. Sequestrations occur most commonly in the posterior segment of the lower lobe. A radiographic density in this area should suggest the diagnosis, particularly when cystic elements are also present. In the past, bronchography was performed as part of the diagnostic evaluation. This procedure usually demonstrated normal bronchi displaced by the involved area of lung. In rare cases, the contrast entered the abnormal bronchi of the sequestration. The role of bronchography is now limited because similar information can be obtained from noninvasive studies.

C. The patient should undergo CT scanning. The scan may suggest another diagnosis or, in some cases, provide definitive evidence of sequestration by visualization of the anomalous artery. However, the arteries tend to be small and are easily missed on CT scans.

D. Bronchoscopy is usually performed during the evaluation of a mass or localized density in the lung. It is most useful in excluding other processes such as bronchogenic carcinoma or foreign body aspiration. Since many sequestrations do not communicate with the bronchial tree, bronchoscopic examination is almost always unremarkable. An MRI examination of the chest should be performed if the clinical course and radiographic appearance of the lesion suggest sequestration. An MRI scan can visualize the abnormal artery, although the small size of the abnormal artery limits sensitivity. In addition, it is not yet certain whether the demonstration of an abnormal artery by MRI obviates the need for angiography.

E. Aortic angiography is necessary to completely define the anatomy prior to surgical resection of the sequestration. Intraoperative hemorrhage is a significant risk during resection.

F. Sequestrations are usually removed surgically because of the possibility of recurrent infections or malignant degeneration.

References

Chan CK, Hyland RH, Gray RR, Jones DP, Hutcheon MA. Diagnostic imaging of intralobar bronchopulmonary sequestration. Chest 1988; 93:189.

Miller PA, Williamson BRJ, Minor GR, Buschi AJ. Pulmonary sequestration: visualization of the feeding artery by CT. J Comput Assist Tomogr 1982; 6:828.

Oliphant L, McFadden RG, Carr TJ, Mackenzie DA. Magnetic resonance imaging to diagnose intralobar pulmonary sequestration. Chest 1987; 91:500.

Savic B, Birtel FJ, Tholen W, Funke HD, Knoche R. Lung sequestration: report of seven cases and review of 540 published cases. Thorax 1979; 34:96.

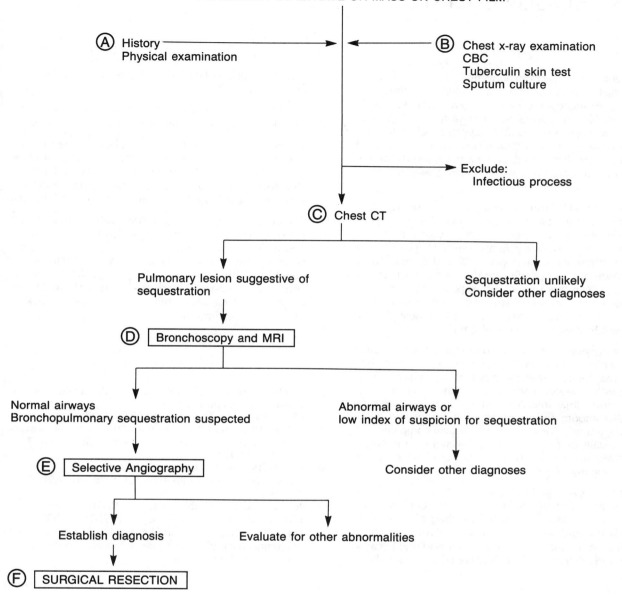

PERSISTENT INFILTRATE OR MASS ON CHEST FILM

Ⓐ History
Physical examination

Ⓑ Chest x-ray examination
CBC
Tuberculin skin test
Sputum culture

Exclude:
Infectious process

Ⓒ Chest CT

Pulmonary lesion suggestive of
sequestration

Sequestration unlikely
Consider other diagnoses

Ⓓ Bronchoscopy and MRI

Normal airways
Bronchopulmonary sequestration suspected

Abnormal airways or
low index of suspicion for sequestration

Ⓔ Selective Angiography

Consider other diagnoses

Establish diagnosis

Evaluate for other abnormalities

Ⓕ SURGICAL RESECTION

BRONCHOGENIC CYST

Bronchogenic cysts arise from abnormal budding or branching of the tracheobronchial tree as it develops from the primitive foregut. Bronchogenic cysts that are formed early in development have a residual attachment to the trachea or esophagus, whereas those formed later in development are intrapulmonary and may communicate with the bronchial tree. The cysts are thin-walled, contain clear, serous, or mucoid material, and are lined with ciliated, pseudostratified epithelium.

A. The patient with bronchogenic cysts may be asymptomatic or have symptoms when the cysts become infected or when they compress pulmonary or mediastinal structures. Symptomatic patients commonly present with cough, chest pain, hemoptysis, and dyspnea. These symptoms are nonspecific and do not aid in diagnosis. Rarely, patients may present with superior vena caval syndrome or upper airway obstruction. Bronchogenic cysts found in the paraesophageal location may cause dysphagia, weight loss, or abdominal pain.

B. A well-defined, solitary, round or oval density, usually confined to a lower lobe, can be seen on the chest film. Cysts may be homogenous in density but may also contain air-fluid levels when they communicate with the tracheobronchial tree. Mediastinal bronchogenic cysts are also smooth and round and may be located in the middle, posterior, or superior mediastinal compartments. They usually do not communicate with the tracheobronchial tree; hence they do not contain air-fluid levels and are frequently asymptomatic.

C. CT scanning aids in the diagnosis and evaluation of the size of the lesion and its relation to adjacent structures. CT imaging helps differentiate bronchogenic cysts from neoplasms and vascular structures. The attenuation coefficients of bronchogenic cysts are variable because of the variable nature of the fluid contained within them.

Percutaneous needle aspiration of the cysts may be performed using CT guidance.

D. Cysts located in the paraesophageal region may be further defined by barium swallow or esophagoscopy.

E. The treatment of patients with bronchogenic cysts is controversial. Many studies suggest that all cysts should be resected because of the risk of eventual complications. However, other studies indicate that asymptomatic patients may be followed clinically using serial CT studies.

F. Symptomatic patients with bronchogenic cysts should undergo resection. Resection is also the treatment of choice when the diagnosis is in doubt. There are case reports of bronchogenic cysts treated by percutaneous needle aspiration and complete drainage. Infected bronchogenic cysts should be treated with antibiotics prior to needle aspiration or surgery to decrease the risk of postoperative empyema.

References

Coselli MP, de Ipolyi P, Bloss RS, Diaz RF, Fitzgerald JB. Bronchogenic cysts above and below the diaphragm: report of eight cases. Ann Thorac Surg 1987; 44:491.

Kirwan WO, Walbaum PR, McCormack RJM. Cystic intrathoracic derivatives of the foregut and their complications. Thorax 1973; 28:424.

Mendelson DS, Rose JS, Efremidis SC, Kirschner PA, Cohen BA. Bronchogenic cysts with high CT numbers. AJR 1983; 140:463.

Pugatch RD, Faling LJ, Robbins AH, Spira R. CT diagnosis of benign mediastinal abnormalities. AJR 1980; 134:685.

Schwartz AR, Fishman EK, Wang KP. Diagnosis and treatment of a bronchogenic cyst using transbronchial needle aspiration. Thorax 1986; 41:326.

BRONCHOGENIC CYST Suspected

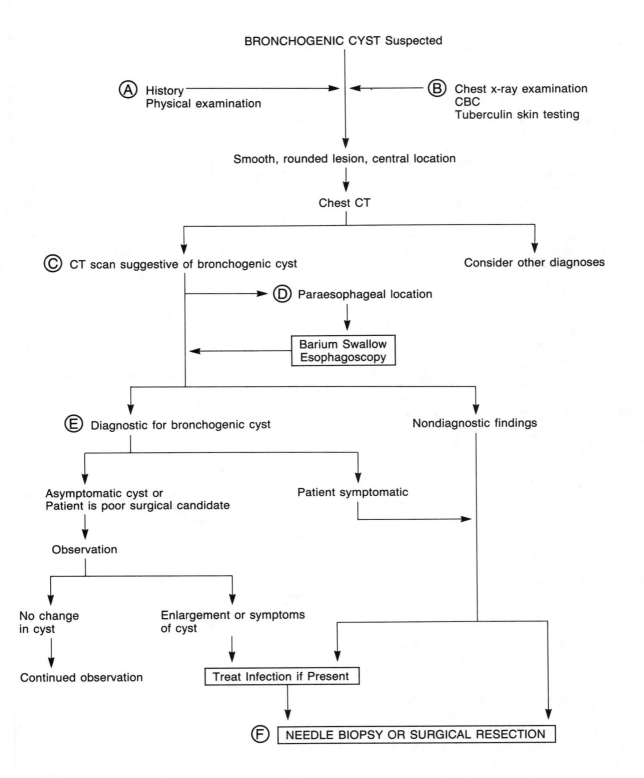

Ⓐ History
Physical examination

Ⓑ Chest x-ray examination
CBC
Tuberculin skin testing

Smooth, rounded lesion, central location

Chest CT

Ⓒ CT scan suggestive of bronchogenic cyst

Consider other diagnoses

Ⓓ Paraesophageal location

Barium Swallow
Esophagoscopy

Ⓔ Diagnostic for bronchogenic cyst

Nondiagnostic findings

Asymptomatic cyst or
Patient is poor surgical candidate

Patient symptomatic

Observation

No change
in cyst

Enlargement or symptoms
of cyst

Continued observation

Treat Infection if Present

Ⓕ NEEDLE BIOPSY OR SURGICAL RESECTION

ARTERIOVENOUS MALFORMATION

The common causes of right-to-left shunting in the lung include arteriovenous congenital malformations (AVMs), hepatic cirrhosis, mitral stenosis, trauma, actinomycosis, and metastatic carcinoma of the thyroid. Half of all patients with congenital malformations have AVMs elsewhere (Osler-Weber-Rendu disease or hereditary hemorrhagic telangiectasia [HHT]); the other half have AVMs limited to the lung.

A. Patients may be asymptomatic and lesions may be detected incidentally on chest radiographs taken for different reasons. Symptoms, if present, are rarely evident until midlife, when patients will complain of dyspnea on exertion. Dyspnea may worsen when the patient is in the upright position and improve when the patient reclines (platypnea), and it may persist even when he or she receives oxygen. Hemoptysis is the second most common symptom but is rarely massive. Neurologic symptoms are also common. These range from headaches, tinnitus, and seizures to completed cerebrovascular accidents. Patients with HHT may bleed from any telangiectatic lesion. The findings of the physical examination may be completely normal except for the presence of multiple skin telangiectasias. Older patients may be cyanotic and have clubbing of the fingers; audible flow murmurs may be heard over some pulmonary AVMs upon examination of the thorax.

B. Although the chest film may be within normal limits, more commonly it demonstrates single or multiple rounded, multilobulated masses in the lower lung zones. Feeding vessels emanating from the hilum may be evident. The arterial blood gas (ABG), obtained with the patient breathing room air, reveals hypoxemia and a widened $(A-a)DO_2$. Laboratory studies may reveal polycythemia, secondary to the low PO_2, and other studies will be within normal limits. Pulmonary function tests ensure the absence of any mechanical abnormality that might cause arterial desaturation; the diffusing capacity for carbon monoxide will be reduced.

C. CT of the thorax verifies the number, position, and size of the lesions seen on the chest film. If the patient is older than 40 years of age and smokes, or if the lesions are new, a work-up should be instituted for neoplastic disease of the lungs or elsewhere. Sputum cytologic analysis should be performed, and if the patient is acutely ill, septic pulmonary embolic disease should be ruled out.

D. In order to make the diagnosis of a right-to-left shunt, place the patient on 100 percent oxygen for 20 minutes and perform an ABG analysis. If no shunt is present other than the normal anatomic shunts present at birth, the value of PO_2 measured will be greater than 600 mm Hg. If the value is less than 600 mm Hg, pulmonary parenchymal disease such as chronic obstructive pulmonary disease must be ruled out. Through the use of the shunt equation, it is possible to calculate the percentage of cardiac output that is being shunted from the right side. In one study of ten patients, the shunt was found to average 44 percent of the cardiac output.

E. Intracardiac shunt may be ruled out by means of cardiac ultrasonography and a bubble study, which allow the diagnosis of septal defects. If findings of these tests are equivocal, cardiac catheterization is necessary to rule out intracardiac shunt completely.

F. Intrapulmonic shunts are unequivocally demonstrated by means of pulmonary angiography.

G. Percutaneous angiographic treatment may then be undertaken if the shunts are few and small in diameter, if the shunt fraction is large enough that the patient is symptomatic, if the shunts are known to be enlarging, or if for other reasons the patient is not a surgical candidate. Balloon occlusion of the affected feeder vessel must be done prior to embolization (with balloons or metal coils or springs) to ensure that pulmonary hypertension does not occur. If pulmonary hypertension is not a problem, embolization can proceed. Surgical resection of a single AVM can also be performed if angiographic embolization cannot be done. Some investigators believe that all patients with HHT and AVMs can be treated. However, treatment of asymptomatic shunts is not generally performed.

References

Gula G, Nakvi A, Radley-Smith R, Yacoub M. The spectrum of pulmonary arteriovenous fistulae: clinico-pathological correlations. Thorac Cardiovasc Surg 1981; 29:51.

Harrow EM, Beach PM, Wise JR, et al. Pulmonary arteriovenous fistula: preoperative evaluation with a Swan-Ganz catheter. Chest 1978; 73:92.

Hatfield DR, Fried AM. Therapeutic embolization of diffuse pulmonary arteriovenous malformations. Am J Roentgenol 1981; 137:861.

Terry PB, White RI, Barth KH, Kaufman SL, Mitchell SE. Pulmonary arteriovenous malformations: physiologic observations and results of therapeutic balloon embolization. N Engl J Med 1983; 308:1197.

White RI, Mitchell SE, Barth KH, et al. Angioarchitecture of pulmonary arteriovenous malformations: an important consideration before embolotherapy. Am J Radiol 1983; 140:681.

ARTERIOVENOUS MALFORMATION Suspected

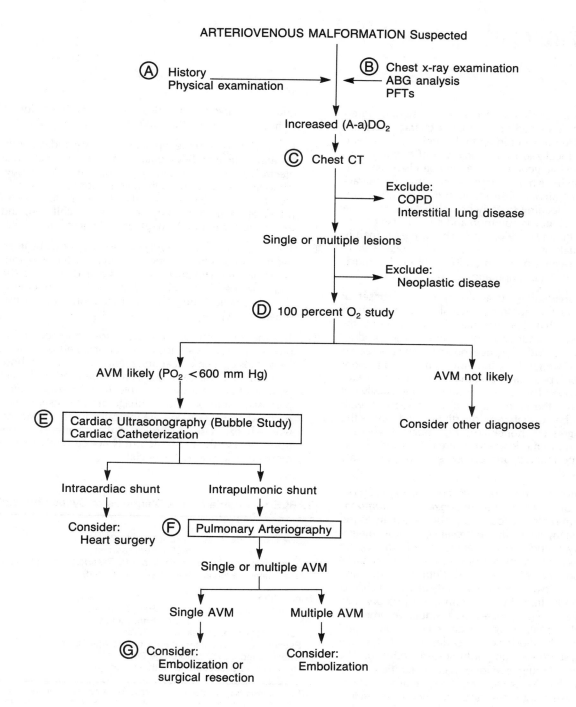

Ⓐ History
Physical examination

Ⓑ Chest x-ray examination
ABG analysis
PFTs

Increased (A-a)DO₂

Ⓒ Chest CT

Exclude:
COPD
Interstitial lung disease

Single or multiple lesions

Exclude:
Neoplastic disease

Ⓓ 100 percent O₂ study

AVM likely (PO₂ <600 mm Hg)

AVM not likely

Consider other diagnoses

Ⓔ Cardiac Ultrasonography (Bubble Study)
Cardiac Catheterization

Intracardiac shunt

Intrapulmonic shunt

Consider:
Heart surgery

Ⓕ Pulmonary Arteriography

Single or multiple AVM

Single AVM

Multiple AVM

Ⓖ Consider:
Embolization or
surgical resection

Consider:
Embolization

CYSTIC FIBROSIS

Cystic fibrosis is an autosomal recessive disease of children and young to middle-aged adults that is characterized by defects of chloride transport in epithelial cells. The genetic defect has been localized to the long arm of chromosome 7, and the responsible gene has recently been isolated. The disease is protean in its manifestations and is mainly characterized by chronic airway obstruction and unrelenting pulmonary infections leading to early bronchiectasis. Exocrine pancreatic insufficiency is common and has adverse consequences for growth and development. The disease is mainly found in individuals of northern and central European extraction and has a frequency of one in 2,500 live births. It is much rarer in Black and Asian populations.

A. Affected individuals give a history of early onset of respiratory tract symptoms punctuated by episodes of productive cough and pneumonias. Bronchitic symptoms may progress to continuous cough and sputum production associated with dyspnea on exertion, decreased appetite, and weight loss. Individuals may also present with nasal polyposis or abdominal pain and right lower quadrant masses. The physical examination is usually not helpful during the early stages of the disease. Breath sounds may be normal or mildly diminished, but as the disease progresses, rhonchi and high-pitched wheezes may be heard. In moderate-to-severe disease, the lungs become hyperinflated, and evidence of cor pulmonale may be found.

B. Sputum is usually viscid and may contain *Staphylococcus aureus* or *Haemophilus influenzae*. *Pseudomonas aeruginosa* may also be found early but is usually found later, after many years, in the presence of bronchiectasis. Typically, *Pseudomonas* is of the mucoid variety, but other strains are becoming more common. Other gram-negative rods may also be found. Pulmonary function testing reveals airway obstruction. Early disease is characterized by reductions in maximum midexpiratory flow rates. As the disease progresses, residual volume and residual volume/total lung capacity ratios increase, and the single-breath diffusing capacity decreases. In the later stages of disease, all lung volumes are reduced. The alveolar-arterial difference for oxygen is significantly increased and the Po_2 is reduced. Oxygenation worsens as the disease progresses, and may be severe in the recumbent position or during sleep. Eventually, Pco_2 begins to increase, which signifies end-stage disease.

C. The chest x-ray examination usually indicates hyperinflation. Mucus impaction is also a common finding, as are peripheral rounded densities. Evidence of bronchiectatic airways may be seen on the plain film. Eventually, subpleural blebs or cysts develop, the pulmonary arteries enlarge, and peripheral vasculature disappears.

D. Computed tomography is appropriate when the chest film is not consistent with the diagnosis of cystic fibrosis or when the condition is suspected because of appropriate history and physical examination in a young adult. This modality may illustrate bronchiectatic airways or mucus impaction that are not seen on the plain film.

E. In individuals with the typical pulmonary and gastrointestinal clinical findings, obtain a measurement of sweat electrolytes by the pilocarpine iontophoresis technique. Although the values of sodium and chloride in sweat increase with age, levels of sweat chloride greater than 60 mEq/L are diagnostic of cystic fibrosis in children, and levels greater than 80 mEq/L are diagnostic in adults.

F. The diagnosis of cystic fibrosis is also supported by intermediate sweat chloride levels in atypical presentations of the disease. The diagnosis may be made if two of the major or one of the major and one of the minor criteria shown in Table 1 are present. Criteria must involve two separate organ systems.

G. Treatment is centered around controlling infection, improving airway clearance of secretions, and preventing weight loss. The medical treatments are similar to those for bronchiectasis. Antibiotics must be used for longer periods of time during acute infectious episodes. Chest percussion and postural drainage are also useful. Aerosolized bronchodilators are indicated for those patients who wheeze. Use of steroids in these patients is controversial and their chronic use is not currently recommended. Exercise is beneficial.

TABLE 1 Criteria for the Diagnosis of Cystic Fibrosis*

Major Criteria
  Sweat chloride levels: >60 mEq/L (<20 yr)
                          >80 mEq/L (adults)
  Chronic obstructive lung disease with *Pseudomonas* infection
  Unexplained azoospermia (biopsy confirmed)

Minor Criteria
  Sweat chloride levels: >40 mEq/L (<20 yr)
                          >60 mEq/L (adults)
  Family history of classic cystic fibrosis
  Exocrine pancreas insufficiency before age 20 yr
  Unexplained COPD before age 20 yr
  Unexplained azoospermia (without biopsy)

*The diagnosis may be made in the presence of two major or one major and one minor criteria. Criteria must involve two separate organ systems.

References

Davis PB, ed. Cystic fibrosis. Sem Respir Med 1985; 6:243.
Friedman PJ, Hardwood IR, Ellenbogen PH. Pulmonary cystic fibrosis in the adult: early and late radiologic findings with pathologic correlation. Am J Radiol 1981; 136:1131.
Rosenstein BJ, Langbaum TS. Diagnosis. In: Taussig LM, ed. Cystic fibrosis. New York: Thieme-Stratton, 1984:85.
Taussig LM. Cystic fibrosis: an overview. In: Taussig LM, ed. Cystic fibrosis. New York: Thieme-Stratton, 1984:1.

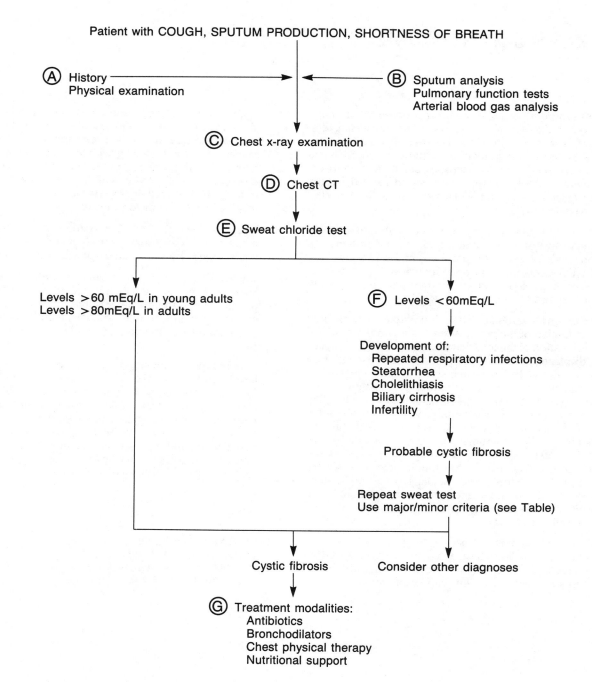

Patient with COUGH, SPUTUM PRODUCTION, SHORTNESS OF BREATH

Ⓐ History
Physical examination

Ⓑ Sputum analysis
Pulmonary function tests
Arterial blood gas analysis

Ⓒ Chest x-ray examination

Ⓓ Chest CT

Ⓔ Sweat chloride test

Levels >60 mEq/L in young adults
Levels >80mEq/L in adults

Ⓕ Levels <60mEq/L

Development of:
Repeated respiratory infections
Steatorrhea
Cholelithiasis
Biliary cirrhosis
Infertility

Probable cystic fibrosis

Repeat sweat test
Use major/minor criteria (see Table)

Cystic fibrosis

Consider other diagnoses

Ⓖ Treatment modalities:
Antibiotics
Bronchodilators
Chest physical therapy
Nutritional support

MARFAN'S SYNDROME

Marfan's syndrome is a rare, autosomal dominant (usually) inherited disorder of connective tissue primarily affecting elastic tissue. New mutations cause between 5 and 25 percent of cases. At present, it cannot be diagnosed in utero. It is a cause of early sudden death in athletes, and there is no specific treatment. Multiple connective tissues are affected, but the cardiovascular, skeletal, and ocular systems are the most clinically important systems.

A. Diagnosis is based on the presence of abnormalities in at least two of the three above-mentioned systems. Patients may present with problems of visual acuity due to a dislocated lens or myopia, spontaneous pneumothorax, or dyspnea on exertion, or they may be completely asymptomatic.

B. The physical examination reveals multiple abnormalities. Examination of the ocular system (slit lamp) may reveal a dislocation of the lens that is usually limited to superior displacement. Increase in the axial globe length may cause myopia. Patients will commonly have arachnodactyly, which may be documented by the thumb sign (thumb projects beyond the ulnar edge of the clenched hand), or the wrist sign (thumb and little finger overlap when wrapped around the opposite wrist). Patients may also have dolichostenomelia (extremely long limbs, arm span greater than height) and may have pectus excavatum, high palate, hyperextensible joints, and scoliosis. Examination of the cardiovascular system reveals signs of mitral valve prolapse and aortic root dilatation. Mitral and/or aortic regurgitation may be present as evidenced by systolic murmurs.

C. Chest x-ray examination may reveal cardiac enlargement, widening of the aortic root, and bullous emphysema. Pulmonary function tests may indicate residual volume increases that are consistent with emphysema.

D. Patients with homocystinuria may present with ocular changes, osteoporosis, and vascular disease (thrombotic episodes), features which resemble those found in Marfan's syndrome. Patients with homocystinuria usually have inferior displacement of the lens and have increased excretion of sulfhydryl-containing compounds in the urine (positive cyanide-nitroprusside test). These patients may be treated by dietary means.

E. The diagnosis of Marfan's syndrome may usually be made on clinical grounds. Family members of such patients should be evaluated to provide counseling.

F. Patients should undergo imaging of the aortic root by means of echocardiography, dye-enhanced CT scanning, or MRI. When the diameter of the root exceeds 6 cm, graft replacement should be considered. Spontaneous pneumothoraces should be treated by the usual means (see p 176).

G. Careful monitoring including repeat evaluations of ocular, skeletal, and cardiovascular systems should be performed at least yearly. Evaluations should include repeat imaging studies of the aorta. Ongoing management includes the use of beta-blockers to reduce cardiac work, the use of prophylactic antibiotics for any procedures or dental work, and the institution of an nonisometric aerobic exercise program for cardiovascular fitness. Lens dislocations should be treated with surgery if necessary.

References

Woerner EM, Royalty K. Marfan syndrome: what you need to know. Postgrad Med 1990; 87:229.
Wood JR, Bellamy D. Pulmonary disease in patients with Marfan syndrome. Thorax 1984; 39:780.

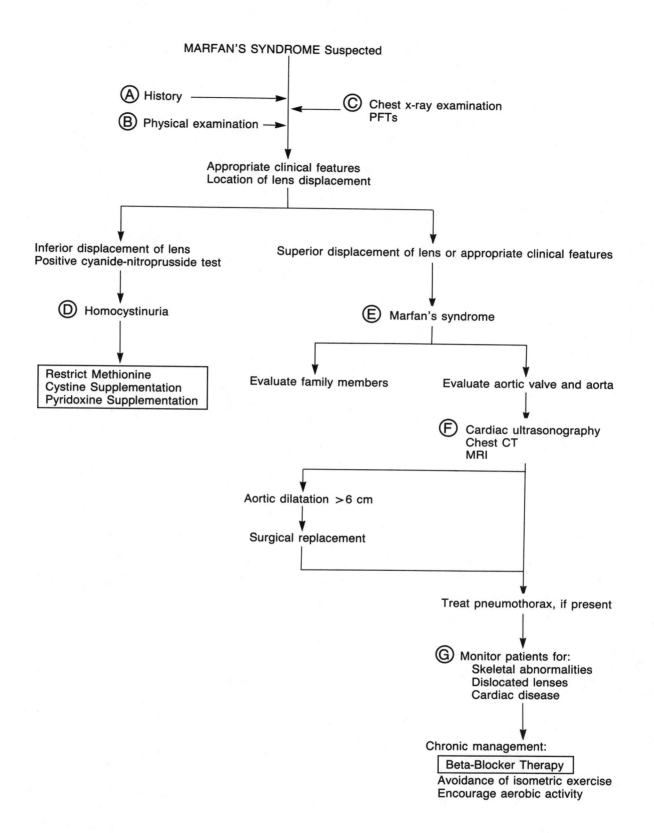

MARFAN'S SYNDROME Suspected

(A) History

(B) Physical examination

(C) Chest x-ray examination
PFTs

Appropriate clinical features
Location of lens displacement

Inferior displacement of lens
Positive cyanide-nitroprusside test

Superior displacement of lens or appropriate clinical features

(D) Homocystinuria

(E) Marfan's syndrome

Restrict Methionine
Cystine Supplementation
Pyridoxine Supplementation

Evaluate family members

Evaluate aortic valve and aorta

(F) Cardiac ultrasonography
Chest CT
MRI

Aortic dilatation >6 cm

Surgical replacement

Treat pneumothorax, if present

(G) Monitor patients for:
Skeletal abnormalities
Dislocated lenses
Cardiac disease

Chronic management:

Beta-Blocker Therapy
Avoidance of isometric exercise
Encourage aerobic activity

NEUROMUSCULAR, CHEST WALL, AND PLEURAL DISEASE

Diaphragmatic Paralysis
Acute Neuromuscular Disease
Sleep-Breathing Disorders

Lung Contusion
Kyphoscoliosis
Spontaneous Pneumothorax

DIAPHRAGMATIC PARALYSIS

Diaphragmatic paralysis may be unilateral or bilateral. The cause of the paralysis is usually idiopathic but may result either from conditions that affect the phrenic nerves directly or from muscle diseases that affect diaphragm function. Conditions that affect the phrenic nerves include surgical phrenic nerve crush formerly used for partial treatment of tuberculosis; cold injury to the phrenic nerves during cold-induced cardioplegia; polio; and other infectious diseases usually of viral origin. Diseases that affect diaphragm muscles include phosphorylase deficiency and McArdle's syndrome.

A. Patients usually complain of progressive shortness of breath without cough or sputum production. If patients have a concomitant history of cigarette smoking it may be difficult to separate abnormalities due to pulmonary airway or parenchymal dysfunction from those due to respiratory muscle (diaphragm) dysfunction.

B. The physical examination may be entirely normal. In the case of bilateral diaphragm paralysis, diaphragm excursions are severely reduced, but this may be difficult to appreciate.

C. When the chest film is entirely within normal limits, abnormalities of pulmonary function provide the correct clues that lead to the diagnosis. Lung volumes may appear small and one or both hemidiaphragms may be elevated, suggesting the diagnosis. If this is the only abnormal finding, perform pulmonary function tests.

D. Pulmonary function testing reveals decreases in lung volumes, particularly in vital capacity, without concomitant reduction in flow rates, thus suggesting a diagnosis of restrictive, neuromuscular disease. If pulmonary function performed in the upright and recumbent positions is normal, rule out cardiac causes of dyspnea.

E. Analysis of arterial blood may be normal, except for decreases in PCO_2, which indicate hyperventilation, or PO_2 may be reduced in severe disease when PCO_2 is increased and patients are in respiratory distress. If the analysis is consistent with V/Q mismatch, the patient most likely has pulmonary disease but neuromuscular disease cannot be ruled out. Treat these patients for airway disease and retest; if improvement occurs, the work-up need be carried out no further. If the analysis is consistent with alveolar hypoventilation or is normal, perform specific diaphragm muscle testing.

F. An evaluation of diaphragm function includes measurements of transdiaphragmatic pressure through placement of esophageal (intrapleural) and gastric balloons. Measure esophageal and gastric pressures throughout the respiratory cycle with the patient in both upright and supine positions. Also record the maximal pressure generated by the diaphragm. The normal maximal transdiaphragmatic pressure is greater than 100 cm H_2O, the normal maximal pressure generated by the diaphragm is also greater than 100 cm H_2O, and the gastric and esophageal pressure tracings are out of phase by 180 degrees. When the diaphragm is paralyzed, maximal pressures are severely reduced and may be zero; partial paralysis produces values between zero and 100 cm H_2O. In addition, the gastric and esophageal pressures become aligned in phase since the diaphragm is floppy and does not contract. These findings allow the diagnosis of partial-to-complete dysfunction of the diaphragm. If evaluation of diaphragm function is normal, rule out cardiac causes of dyspnea.

G. The sniff test, performed under fluoroscopy, allows visualization of diaphragmatic movement. Paralysis of one or both hemidiaphragms results in little to no movement of the affected side when the patient sniffs. This test is not 100 percent reliable, but may assist in diagnosing the affected side.

H. Electromyography, performed through either external detection leads or through an esophageal lead, allows differentiation of phrenic nerve dysfunction from diaphragm muscle dysfunction. If an externally stimulated impulse delivered through the phrenic nerve from stimulation at the neck can be detected at the level of the diaphragm, but no muscle contraction occurs, then the problem is one of the muscle. If no impulse can be detected, then a phrenic nerve problem is quite likely although muscle may still be abnormal.

References

Bergofsky EH. Respiratory failure in disorders of the respiratory cage. Am Rev Respir Dis 1979; 119:643.

De Troyer A, Pride NB. The respiratory system in neuromuscular disorders. In: Roussous C, Macklem PT, eds. The thorax. (Lung biology in health and disease, Volume 29, Part B). New York: Marcel Dekker, 1985:1089.

Glenn WWL, Hogan JF, Phelps ML. Ventilatory support of the quadriplegic patient with respiratory paralysis by diaphragm pacing. Surg Clin North Am 1980; 60:1055.

Greene W, L'Heureux P, Hunt CE. Paralysis of the diaphragm. Am J Dis Child 1975; 129:1402.

Spiteri MA, Mier AK, Brophy CJ, Pantin CFA, Green M. Bilateral diaphragm weakness. Thorax 1985; 40:631.

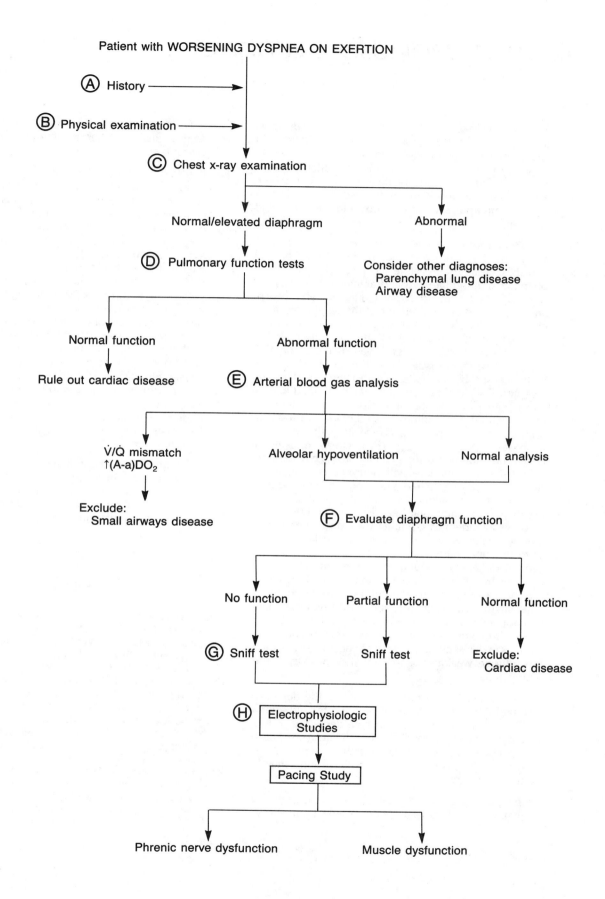

Patient with WORSENING DYSPNEA ON EXERTION

(A) History

(B) Physical examination

(C) Chest x-ray examination

Normal/elevated diaphragm — Abnormal

(D) Pulmonary function tests

Abnormal → Consider other diagnoses:
Parenchymal lung disease
Airway disease

Normal function — Abnormal function

Rule out cardiac disease

(E) Arterial blood gas analysis

$\dot{V}/\dot{Q}$ mismatch
$\uparrow$(A-a)DO$_2$ — Alveolar hypoventilation — Normal analysis

Exclude:
Small airways disease

(F) Evaluate diaphragm function

No function — Partial function — Normal function

(G) Sniff test — Sniff test — Exclude:
Cardiac disease

(H) Electrophysiologic Studies

Pacing Study

Phrenic nerve dysfunction — Muscle dysfunction

167

ACUTE NEUROMUSCULAR DISEASE

A. The baseline history, physical examination, and diagnostic work-up permit diagnosis of one of the four main causes of acute neuromuscular diseases. These conditions are Guillain-Barré syndrome, myasthenia gravis, botulism, and organophosphate poisoning. Other conditions that can result in neuromuscular impairment include multiple sclerosis, polio, and the postpolio syndrome.

B. *Guillain-Barré syndrome* is an acute inflammatory ascending polyneuropathy that involves the abdominal and chest wall muscles before affecting the laryngeal and pharyngeal musculature. It is characterized by progressive weakness leading to dyspnea, difficulty with speech, and cough. Initial involvement of the respiratory muscles results in tachypnea only, but progressive weakness eventually causes decreases in vital capacity (VC) and in the maximal pressure developed by the diaphragm (Pdi_{max}). *Myasthenia gravis* is a disease of motor endplates caused by antibodies against the acetylcholine receptor of skeletal muscle. It is usually limited to ocular or bulbar muscles but may also affect the muscles of respiration. Anticholinesterase therapy can result in improvement in respiratory muscle strength, producing increases in VC and Pdi_{max}. Thymectomy, myasthenic crisis, and cholinergic crisis can all produce respiratory failure. *Botulism* interferes with neuromuscular transmission, and respiratory failure is common in this condition. Usual symptoms include visual blurring, slurred speech, dysphagia, vomiting, diarrhea, dyspnea, and dizziness. Findings include ptosis, pupillary abnormalities, ocular muscle weakness, and skeletal muscle weakness. Onset of respiratory failure may be slow and insidious. *Organophosphate* compounds induce respiratory muscle paralysis by inhibiting acetycholinesterase at the motor end-plate. Commonly used drugs include edrophonium, physostigmine, prostigmine, and pyridostigmine. Many organophosphate insecticides also produce the syndrome. Laryngospasm is commonly found in association with excessive secretions, bronchoconstriction, respiratory muscle weakness, and central respiratory center depression.

C. Once a diagnosis is established, assess the degree of respiratory impairment. Simple spirometry and arterial blood gas analysis will demonstrate decreases in lung volumes, and increased Pco_2 indicates respiratory failure. Use supplemental oxygen in hypoxemic patients even if the Pco_2 is elevated. All initial studies may be normal.

D. If the initial arterial blood gas analysis and measurement of vital capacity is normal, perform repeat bedside VC measurements often, on a regular schedule, until it becomes clear whether respiratory impairment is developing.

E. If the degree of impairment is mild to moderate with increases in Pco_2 of 10 mm Hg or less, with only minor changes in pH, frequent measurements of VC and blood gases are necessary to assess the rapidity of ventilatory decompensation. If there is any question of interpretation, use the maximum inspiratory pressure (Pdi_{max}) to assess diaphragmatic function. When the Pdi_{max} decreases to less than 50 cm H_2O, diaphragmatic failure is imminent. Patients with diaphragmatic failure or those with rising Pco_2 or a VC decreasing to less than 15 ml per kg of body weight should be intubated and placed on assisted or controlled ventilation until the primary disease improves. The margin for decompensation is lower in those patients with underlying chronic lung disease and limited pulmonary reserve. Those patients in whom VC and blood gases remain stable over several days may require exogenous oxygen to maintain Po_2 greater than 55 mm Hg but may not develop severe CO_2 retention or diaphragmatic failure. These patients may be followed by retesting on a daily schedule until the primary disease improves.

F. If the initial assessment of the patient is indicative of severe respiratory impairment with CO_2 retention, acidosis, hypoxemia, and a reduction in the vital capacity of 50 percent or more of the predicted value, consider mechanical ventilation.

References

Bergofsky EH. Respiratory failure in diseases of the thoracic cage. Am Rev Respir Dis 1979; 119:643.

Cashman NR, Maselli R, Wollman RL, et al. Late denervation in patients with antecedent paralytic poliomyelitis. N Engl J Med 1987; 317:7.

De Troyer A, Pride NB. The respiratory system in neuromuscular disorders. In: Roussous C, Macklem PR, eds. The thorax. (Lung biology in health and disease, Vol 29, Part B). New York: Marcel Dekker, 1985:1089.

Glenn WWL, Hogan JF, Phelps ML. Ventilatory support of the quadriplegic patient with respiratory paralysis by diaphragm pacing. Surg Clin North Am 1980; 60:1055.

Kaminski MJ, Young RR. Neuromuscular and neurologic diseases affecting respiration. In: Roussous C, Macklem PR, eds. The thorax. (Lung biology in health and disease, Volume 29, Part B) New York: Marcel Dekker, 1985:1023.

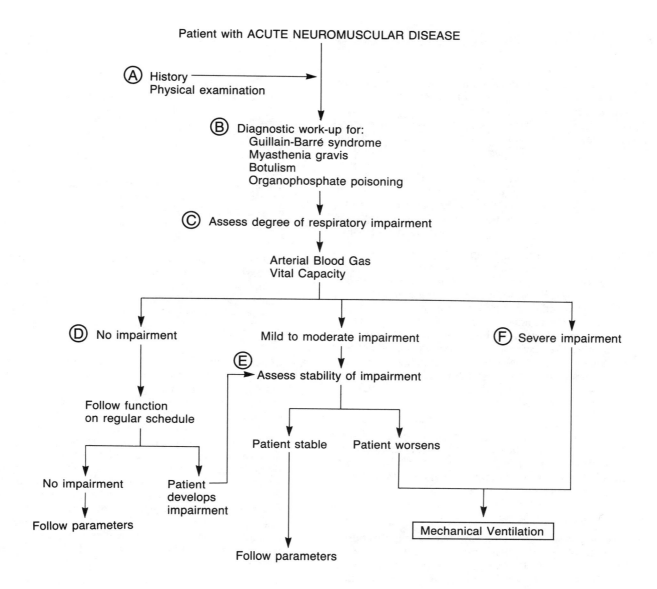

Patient with ACUTE NEUROMUSCULAR DISEASE

(A) History
Physical examination

(B) Diagnostic work-up for:
Guillain-Barré syndrome
Myasthenia gravis
Botulism
Organophosphate poisoning

(C) Assess degree of respiratory impairment

Arterial Blood Gas
Vital Capacity

(D) No impairment

Mild to moderate impairment

(F) Severe impairment

Follow function
on regular schedule

(E) Assess stability of impairment

No impairment

Patient
develops
impairment

Follow parameters

Patient stable

Patient worsens

Follow parameters

Mechanical Ventilation

SLEEP-BREATHING DISORDERS

A. Although most individuals snore, some have snoring episodes interrupted by periods of apnea, which may be witnessed by bedmates. Patients complain of interrupted sleep; daytime somnolence is a common sequela, and behavioral abnormalities including memory deficits and poor judgment sometimes result. Some individuals fall asleep during activities such as driving or operating machinery and are severely injured. Occasionally, individuals complain of morning headache and incontinence. The findings of the physical examination may range from completely normal with only mild obesity to findings of cor pulmonale and systemic hypertension.

B. Arterial blood gases obtained during the daytime while the patient is awake may be normal or may reveal hypoxemia with hypercapnemia. The chest film may be normal or may provide additional evidence of pulmonary hypertension and cor pulmonale. On the basis of the history, physical examination, and the above screening tests, patients may be grouped into one of the following four categories: Those who are asymptomatic and do not have witnessed apnea, those who are symptomatic but do not have witnessed apnea, those who are asymptomatic but have witnessed apnea, and those who are symptomatic and have witnessed apnea.

C. Patients who are asymptomatic or have no symptoms other than snoring without observed apneas do not require polysomnography. For these patients, an ENT examination rules out nasal narrowing; advise them to avoid alcohol or other sedatives that depress upper airway muscle activity and to lose weight if they are obese. They should be observed while sleeping to determine if apneas are occurring.

D. Individuals who snore and have other symptoms but are without observed apneas should undergo a screening nap study. A nap study includes temporal recordings of oxygen saturation using ear or finger oximetry, and of the heart rate and rhythm. If the nap study is negative, these patients require an ENT examination to rule out the presence of nasal pathology. A positive nap study confirms the presence or absence of apneas, and also allows one to determine whether oxygen desaturation and arrhythmias are occurring. Individuals in whom nap studies yield positive results should be treated as an asymptomatic patient with apnea.

E. Those individuals who are symptomatic or have positive nap studies and those individuals (both symptomatic and asymptomatic) with witnessed apnea should undergo full polysomnography. This test includes the monitors listed above as well as EEG monitoring to ensure that these findings are occurring during sleep. In addition, monitor the breathing pattern and conduct submental and tibialis electromyography. A negative polysomnogram indicates that no apneas are occurring during sleep and allows identification of associated conditions such as narcolepsy, nocturnal myoclonus, and phase-shift syndromes.

F. A positive polysomnogram allows classification of apneas into one of three patterns: pure obstructive sleep apnea, pure central sleep apnea, or a mixed pattern combining central and obstructive features. Obstructive sleep apnea is characterized by apneas associated with increasing diaphragmatic excursions and eventual onset of flow; central apnea is characterized by periods of no respiratory muscle movement and no airflow; and mixed patterns have apneas that have both these patterns.

G. Obstructive sleep apnea (OSA) is the most common abnormal breathing pattern. These individuals should undergo ENT evaluation to rule out upper airway narrowing caused by micrognathia or retrognathia, macroglossia, or adenotonsillar hypertrophy. CT of the trachea allows measurement of tracheal size during full inspiration and expiration; it is sometimes possible to make these measurements during sleep.

H. Evaluate individuals with mixed features of both obstructive and central apneas for neuromuscular disease, congestive heart disease, and other metabolic diseases that cause periodic ventilation. When these conditions have been ruled out, submit patients for a full ENT evaluation. The obstructive component of this condition should be treated (see I).

I. Consider surgical treatment if any clear remediable anatomic pathologic condition is found such as a jaw deformity. Uvulopalatopharyngoplasty results in short-term improvement in about 50 percent of those that undergo the procedure; long-term benefits are not clear. Other procedures are not recommended. Medical therapy includes the use of continuous nasal positive pressure with or without oxygen supplementation. The amount of nasal pressure necessary to effect reductions in apneas should be determined during a nap study. Further, if use of low-flow oxygen is contemplated, evaluate patients to make sure that breathing will not be compromised by worsening CO_2 retention. Drugs that may be used to increase respiratory muscle tone during sleep include the tricyclic antidepressants and progesterone. Long-term benefits from these drugs have not been documented.

J. Individuals with mixed apneas who do not benefit from treatment of the obstructive component and those who have primarily central patterns should be treated for any associated medical condition that produces periodic breathing. If sleep-related apneas continue, consider electrophrenic stimulation (when available) in young, otherwise healthy patients with central alveolar hypoventilation. Mechanical ventilation applied through a nose mask or tracheostomy should be used as a last resort when everything else has failed and the condition is life-threatening.

References

Ancoli IS. Epidemiology of sleep disorders. Clin Geriatr Med 1989; 5:347.

Aubert-Tulkens G, Culee C, Rodenstein DO. Cure of sleep apnea syndrome after long-term nasal continuous positive airway pressure therapy and weight loss. Sleep 1989; 12:216.

Macaluso RA, Reams C, Gibson WS, Vrabec DP, Matragrano A. Uvulopalatopharyngoplasty: postoperative management and evaluation of results. Ann Otol Rhinol Laryngol 1989; 98:502.

Phillipson EA. Sleep apnea. Med Clin North Am 1982; 23:2314.

Stradling JR, Phillipson EA. Breathing disorders during sleep. Quart J Med 1986; 58:3.

SNORING, DAYTIME SOMNOLENCE, BEHAVIORAL PROBLEMS, OBSERVED APNEA

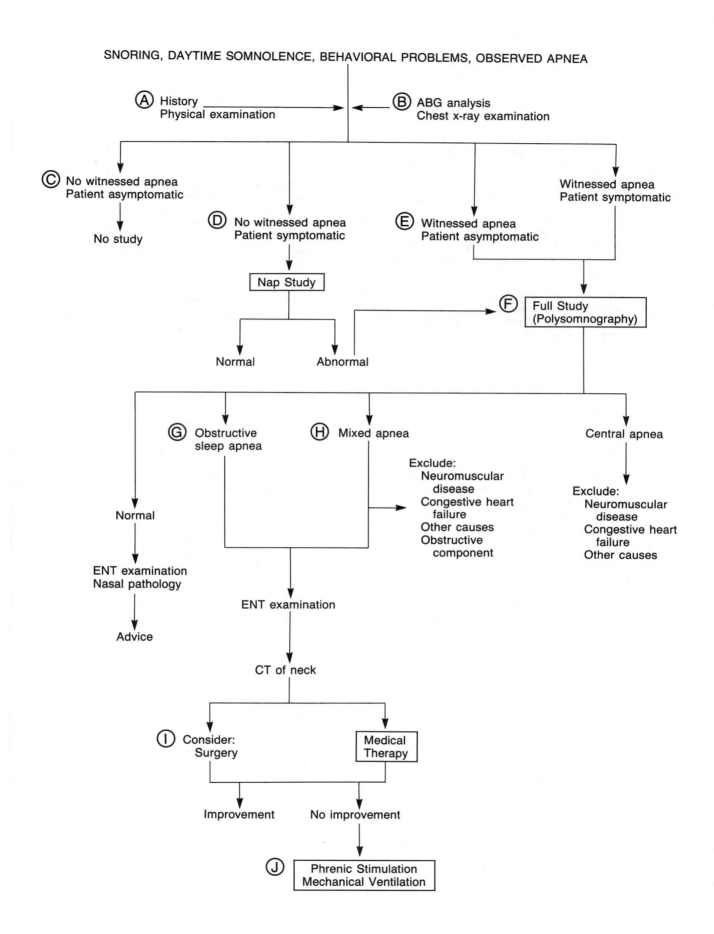

LUNG CONTUSION

Blunt trauma to the chest may result in injury to the lung. A sudden, large, positive intrathoracic pressure results in a lung compression/decompression injury with rupture of capillaries. Histologically, intra-alveolar hemorrhage, interstitial edema, and atelectasis are seen. The appearance of a radiographic infiltrate in the area of the injury or directly opposite (contrecoup) suggests the possibility of lung contusion. Significant blunt trauma often produces fractured ribs, which are associated with a pleural effusion. The possibility of additional related injuries (e.g., rupture of the diaphragm or esophagus) should always be considered.

A. The presence of an infiltrate is evidence of a possible lung contusion. The possibility of associated injuries must be addressed. Flail chest is characterized by paradoxic respiratory movements in the presence of rib fractures. Fractures of anterior thoracic ribs have a greater effect on chest wall stability than fractures of lateral ribs. When the first three ribs are fractured, consider the possibility of an associated tracheobronchial fracture.

B. Pleural effusions are common after chest trauma. Thoracentesis should be performed; the presence of hemothorax requires insertion of a chest tube for drainage and monitoring of additional bleeding. Bleeding may come from systemic or pulmonary vessels. Bleeding from pulmonary vessels tends to be self-limited. Drainage of blood is necessary to reduce the risk of fibrothorax, particularly if pleural damage has occurred. Experimental data in animal studies indicate that blood in a normal pleural space is reabsorbed without a fibrogenic pleural reaction.

C. Pneumothorax is also a frequent complication of lung contusion occurring in adults with rib fractures. A small pneumothorax (5 to 10 percent) can be observed, but large amounts of air should be removed by a chest tube or a one-way valve device (Heimlich valve).

D. Only multiple rib fractures resulting in chest wall instability require treatment. These patients require intubation and mechanical ventilation.

E. Infiltrates associated with lung contusions usually appear soon after injury and resolve rapidly (1 to 3 days). Most infiltrates are visible within 1 hour of injury. A deviation from this pattern suggests another process, such as aspiration pneumonia or pulmonary embolism. Infiltrates tend to be localized to the area of the trauma rather than diffusely present throughout the lung.

F. Intubation and mechanical ventilation are necessary if respiratory failure develops. Lung contusion usually resolves rapidly, and patients can be rapidly weaned provided that no other pulmonary problems are present.

References

Dougall AM, Paul ME, Finley RJ, et al. Chest trauma: current mortality and morbidity. J Trauma 1977; 17:547.

Parham AM, Yarbrough DR, Redding JS. Flail chest syndrome and pulmonary contusion. Arch Surg 1978; 113:900.

Richardson JD, Adams L, FLint LM. Selective management of flail chest and pulmonary contusion. Ann Surg 1982; 196:481.

Shackford SR, Virgilio RW, Peters RM. Selective use of ventilatory therapy in flail chest injury. J Thorac Cardiovasc Surg 1981; 81:194.

Shin B, McAslan TC, Hankins JR, Ayella RJ, Cowley RA. Management of lung contusion. Am Surg 1979; 45:168.

Trinkle JK, Furman RW, Hinshaw MA, Bryant LR, Griffen WO. Pulmonary contusion: pathogenesis and effect of various resuscitative measures. Ann Thorac Surg 1973; 16:568.

Wilson JM, Boren CH, Peterson SR, Thomas AN. Traumatic hemothorax: is decortication necessary? J Thorac Cardiovasc Surg 1979; 77:489.

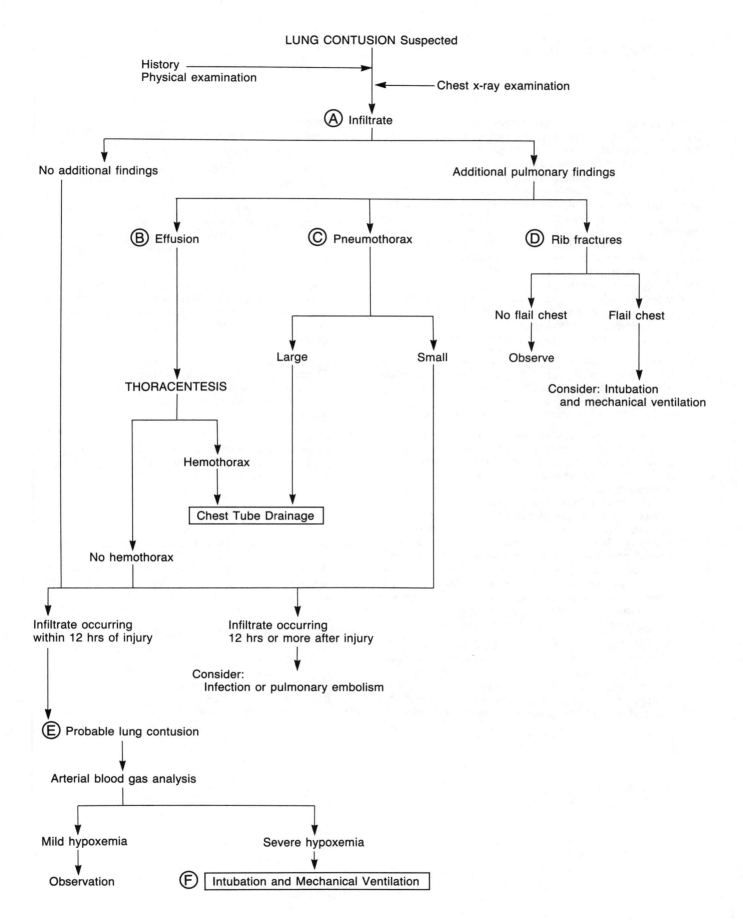

LUNG CONTUSION Suspected

History ⎯⎯⎯⎯⎯⎯⎯⎯
Physical examination

Chest x-ray examination

Ⓐ Infiltrate

No additional findings

Additional pulmonary findings

Ⓑ Effusion

Ⓒ Pneumothorax

Ⓓ Rib fractures

No flail chest

Flail chest

THORACENTESIS

Observe

Consider: Intubation
and mechanical ventilation

Large

Small

Hemothorax

Chest Tube Drainage

No hemothorax

Infiltrate occurring
within 12 hrs of injury

Infiltrate occurring
12 hrs or more after injury

Consider:
Infection or pulmonary embolism

Ⓔ Probable lung contusion

Arterial blood gas analysis

Mild hypoxemia

Severe hypoxemia

Observation

Ⓕ Intubation and Mechanical Ventilation

KYPHOSCOLIOSIS

Kyphoscoliosis is an abnormal increase in the curvature of the spine caused by defects in the vertebral bodies or vertebral connective tissue, or by neuromuscular disease. Specific etiologies of kyphoscoliosis are usually not found. Cobb's method is the most common system used to assess the degree of spinal curvature. (Cobb's angle is formed by the intersection of two lines made on a lateral chest film: the first, a line drawn parallel to the upper border of the superior vertebra bounding the area of curvature; the second, a line drawn parallel to the lower border of the inferior vertebra bounding the area of curvature; perpendiculars drawn to both these lines intersect at Cobb's angle.) The most common respiratory problem resulting from severe kyphoscoliosis is respiratory failure, which is caused by both the kyphosis and the scoliosis acting in concert. A combination of kyphosis greater than 20 degrees and a moderate degree of scoliosis is usually required in order to cause respiratory symptoms.

A. Young individuals with severe kyphoscoliosis are usually asymptomatic. Middle-aged individuals complain of dyspnea on exertion and decreased exercise tolerance, and they develop repeated respiratory infections. Eventually they develop cor pulmonale and respiratory failure.

B. The physical examination reveals a thoracic cage abnormality and signs of cor pulmonale, if present. Individuals who smoke may have evidence of obstructive airway disease. A chest x-ray examination rules out the presence of parenchymal lung disease; evaluation of pulmonary function reveals the degree of restrictive respiratory impairment, and analysis of arterial blood gas (ABG) enables one to assess the degree of functional impairment. Pulmonary function testing demonstrates decreases in total lung capacity and vital capacity, and hypoxemia and hypercapnemia may also be present. These data indicate whether the individual is in respiratory failure. Special testing may be required to make a specific diagnosis of a neuromuscular or connective tissue disease and should be performed if a specific therapy is available.

C. A combination of the history, physical examination, and laboratory and radiographic examinations usually enables one to diagnose the specific etiology of kyphoscoliosis. The most common causes other than those that are idiopathic include muscular dystrophy, poliomyelitis, cerebral ataxia, osteoporosis, tuberculous spondylitis, neurofibromatosis, Marfan's syndrome, Ehler-Danlos syndrome, Morquio's syndrome, and previous thoracoplasty.

D. The degree of scoliosis should be accurately measured. Smoking should be discouraged, and antibiotics and bronchodilatory therapy should be instituted if bronchitis is present or if the patient has a component of reversible airway obstruction. If the degree of scoliosis is greater than 100 degrees and the patient is a child, consider surgical correction of the deformity. Harrington rods and spinal fusions do not improve pulmonary function and gas exchange and should not be done.

E. Evaluate all other patients (young adults or older) for the presence of ventilatory failure; ventilatory failure should be treated by controlled positive-pressure ventilators, allowing the thoracic musculature to rest. Prolonged failure with inability to wean necessitates a tracheostomy.

F. Once weaning has occurred, test patients to determine whether night-time ventilation using a negative-pressure device or continuous positive airway pressure mask with supplemental oxygen will maintain daytime blood gas levels.

G. Patients who cannot be maintained using one of the above techniques require night-time ventilation with a positive-pressure device and oxygen. Use of these devices at night improves daytime exercise tolerance and decreases right ventricle failure.

References

Bergofsky E, Turino G, Fishman A. Cardiorespiratory failure in kyphoscoliosis. Medicine 1959; 38:263.

Ellis ER, Grunstein RR, Chan S, Bye PT, Sullivan CE. Noninvasive ventilatory support during sleep improves respiratory failure in kyphoscoliosis. Chest 1988; 94:811.

Hill NS. Clinical applications of body ventilators. Chest 1986; 90:897.

Hoeppner VH, Cockcroft DW, Dosman JA, Cotton DJ. Nighttime ventilation improves respiratory failure in secondary kyphoscoliosis. Am Rev Respir Dis 1984; 129:240.

Lisboa C, Moreno R, Fava M, Ferretti R, Cruz E. Inspiratory muscle function in patients with severe kyphoscoliosis. Am Rev Respir Dis 1985; 132:48.

Marklund T. Scoliosis angle. Acta Radiol Diag 1978; 19:78.

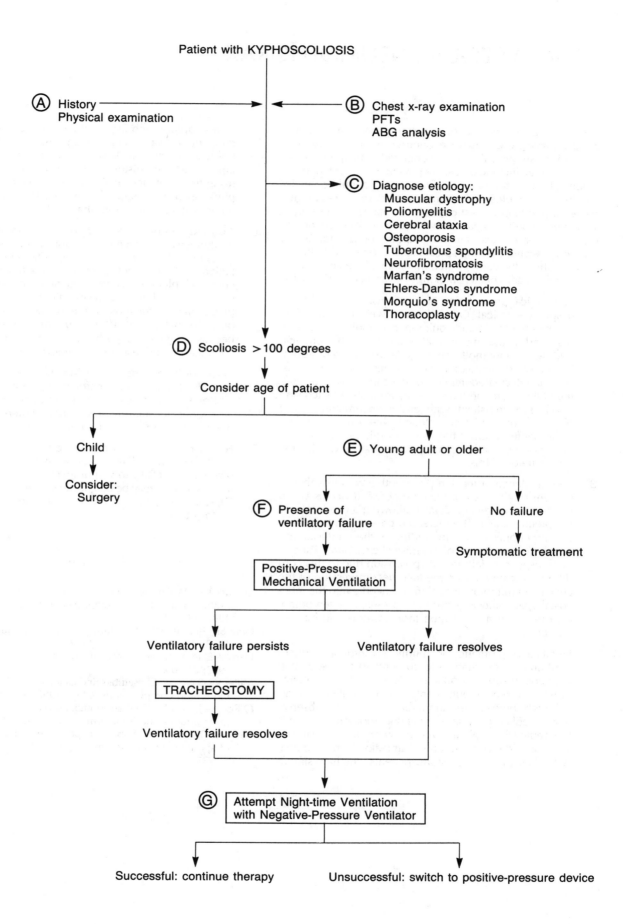

Patient with KYPHOSCOLIOSIS

Ⓐ History ——————→ ←—————— Ⓑ Chest x-ray examination
Physical examination   PFTs
                                        ABG analysis

Ⓒ Diagnose etiology:
   Muscular dystrophy
   Poliomyelitis
   Cerebral ataxia
   Osteoporosis
   Tuberculous spondylitis
   Neurofibromatosis
   Marfan's syndrome
   Ehlers-Danlos syndrome
   Morquio's syndrome
   Thoracoplasty

Ⓓ Scoliosis > 100 degrees

Consider age of patient

Child   Ⓔ Young adult or older

Consider:
Surgery

                         Ⓕ Presence of   No failure
                            ventilatory failure

                                                     Symptomatic treatment

                         Positive-Pressure
                         Mechanical Ventilation

Ventilatory failure persists   Ventilatory failure resolves

TRACHEOSTOMY

Ventilatory failure resolves

Ⓖ Attempt Night-time Ventilation
   with Negative-Pressure Ventilator

Successful: continue therapy   Unsuccessful: switch to positive-pressure device

SPONTANEOUS PNEUMOTHORAX

Spontaneous pneumothorax occurs in patients with underlying pulmonary diseases (secondary) or in their absence (primary or simple). Diseases associated with spontaneous pneumothorax include diffuse emphysema, primary lung carcinoma, lung metastases, sarcoidosis, asthma, pulmonary infarction, tuberculosis, *Pneumocystis carinii* pneumonia, bacterial pneumonia, histiocytosis X, catamenia, and interstitial pneumonitis. In patients without a prior history of pulmonary diseases, spontaneous rupture of pleural blebs, primarily located over the apical areas, is believed to be the etiology; this is the etiology predominantly in men in the third and fourth decades of life. Smoking is an additional risk factor.

A. The clinical presentation of acute-onset chest pain and dyspnea is typical. Other diseases with a similar clinical presentation include pulmonary embolism, pneumonia, and acute myocardial infarction. The physical findings of pneumothorax include decreased or absent breath sounds, increased or normal resonance to percussion, and decreased fremitus over the involved area. Shifting of the heart and trachea away from the affected side may be seen in patients with tension pneumothorax. The presence of a visceral pleural line on a standard posteroanterior chest film is diagnostic of pneumothorax; however, small pneumothoraces may be visible only on expiratory films.

B. The incidence of tension pneumothorax is less than 5 percent of all cases of pneumothorax. It occurs when there is a unidirectional valve allowing air to leak into the pleural space. The increased pressure in the affected hemithorax results in shifting of the mediastinum, which may result in a compromise of circulation. Patients with respiratory failure or hypotension due to this condition must undergo immediate decompression of the affected hemithorax. Insertion of a needle into the intercostal space allows pleural air to escape, a temporary measure until a chest tube thoracostomy can be performed.

C. Small asymptomatic or mildly symptomatic pneumothoraces (less than 15 to 20 percent) can be treated with cough suppression and analgesics. These patients may be followed as outpatients with frequent chest films, although some centers admit these patients for observation. Needle aspiration of small pneumothoraces speeds the removal of pleural air in symptomatic patients without evidence of continued air leaks. Admit and treat with chest tube thoracostomy patients who have significant symptoms and large pneumothoraces. Place chest tubes under water seal drainage. Apply suction in patients with active air leaks and/or significant lung collapse, and administer nasal oxygen to enhance the resorption of pleural air. Pulmonary edema is a rare complication of re-expanded lung, occurring primarily in lungs collapsed for more than 3 days.

D. Approximately one-third of spontaneous pneumothoraces recur on the same side; 10 percent may subsequently develop on the opposite side. Consider patients with recurrent spontaneous pneumothoraces for chemical pleurodesis or surgical obliteration of the pleural space. Pleural abrasion along with resection of pleural blebs is the most commonly used surgical procedure. For patients at risk for pulmonary complications because of general anesthesia or thoracotomy, perform chemical pleurodesis using tetracycline.

E. Place additional chest tubes in patients with continued air leaks. Consider thoracotomy in patients with recurrent pneumothoraces in whom this treatment fails for 7 days. Consider stapling or resection of blebs along with pleural abrasion, or total pleurectomy.

F. For all patients with a first episode of pneumothorax, there should be a diagnostic investigation into the etiology. The clinical history, sputum examinations, and routine chest films may be diagnostic in many patients; chest CT, spirometry, and flexible bronchoscopy may be needed for others.

References

DeCries WC, Wolfe WG. The management of spontaneous pneumothorax and bullous emphysema. Surg Clin North Am 1980; 60:851.

Getz SB, Beasley WE. Spontaneous pneumothorax. Am J Surg 1983; 145:823.

Harvey JE, Jeyasingham K. The difficult pneumothorax. Br J Chest 1987; 81:209.

Miller KS, Sahn SA. Chest tubes: indications, techniques, management, and complications. Chest 1987; 91:258.

O'Rourke JP, Yee ES. Civilian spontaneous pneumothorax: treatment options and long-term results. Chest 1989; 96:1302.

Weeden D, Smith GH. Surgical experience in the management of spontaneous pneumothorax, 1972–1982. Thorax 1983; 38:737.

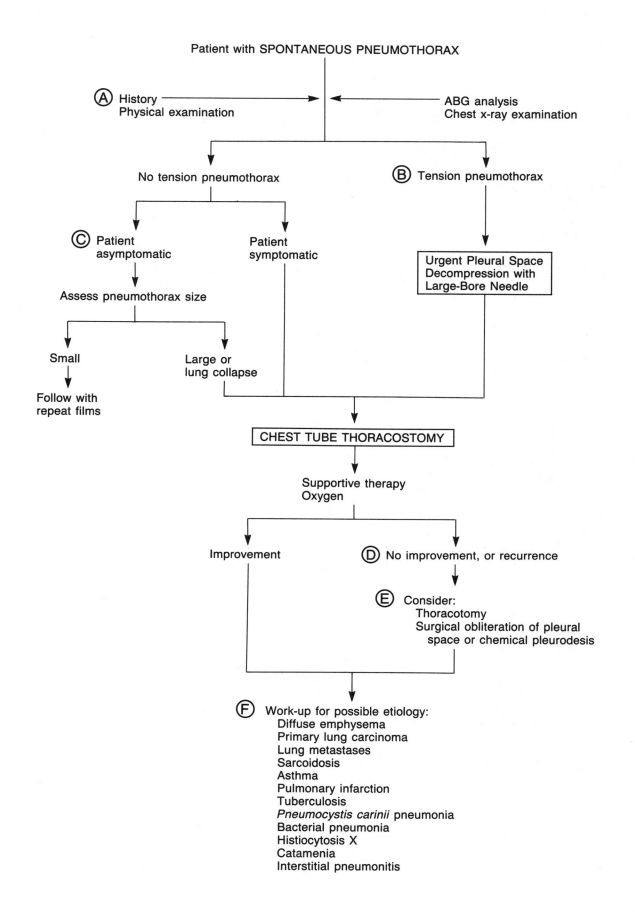

Patient with SPONTANEOUS PNEUMOTHORAX

(A) History
Physical examination

ABG analysis
Chest x-ray examination

No tension pneumothorax

(B) Tension pneumothorax

(C) Patient asymptomatic

Patient symptomatic

Urgent Pleural Space Decompression with Large-Bore Needle

Assess pneumothorax size

Small

Large or lung collapse

Follow with repeat films

CHEST TUBE THORACOSTOMY

Supportive therapy
Oxygen

Improvement

(D) No improvement, or recurrence

(E) Consider:
Thoracotomy
Surgical obliteration of pleural space or chemical pleurodesis

(F) Work-up for possible etiology:
Diffuse emphysema
Primary lung carcinoma
Lung metastases
Sarcoidosis
Asthma
Pulmonary infarction
Tuberculosis
Pneumocystis carinii pneumonia
Bacterial pneumonia
Histiocytosis X
Catamenia
Interstitial pneumonitis

OCCUPATIONAL LUNG DISEASE

Asbestos-Related Pulmonary Syndromes
Irritant Gas Exposure
Smoke Inhalation
Silicosis

ASBESTOS-RELATED PULMONARY SYNDROMES

Asbestos particles are mixtures of mineral silicates that occur in bundles of parallel, radiating, or interwoven fibers. They produce lung disease based on exposure characteristics, the ability of the lung to clear the fiber, and the type of fiber that is inhaled. In general, fibers that are long and thin produce asbestos-related pleural disease, both nonmalignant and malignant; fibers that are relatively short and thick produce interstitial lung disease. Dose-response curves indicate that the likelihood of developing lung or pleural disease increases with increasing exposure.

A. Individuals give a history of direct asbestos exposure working with asbestos in the following areas: cement products, insulation, fireproofing, friction materials, textiles, rubber or plastic fillers, or insulation. They may give a history of indirect exposure through a family member or may relate small or cursory exposures. Patients may have no complaints or may complain of mild cough, sputum production, or dyspnea on exertion.

B. The physical examination may be entirely within normal limits. The only specific finding may be that of "dry" inspiratory rales heard at the lung bases. Nonspecific findings include clubbing and those consistent with pleural effusion. Patients usually appear well.

C. The chest film demonstrates either no findings or pleural-based masses, calcified plaques, pleural effusion, or interstitial lung disease.

D. Pleural thickening is either diffuse or localized and may occur without parenchymal evidence of asbestosis. It usually is found incidentally on films obtained for other clinical reasons since these patients are usually asymptomatic. If it is generalized and severe, it can result in lung restriction, which will eventually produce dyspnea on exertion.

E. Isolated pleural masses are either benign fibrous or malignant mesotheliomas or are due to primary bronchogenic carcinomas or other metastatic lung disease.

F. Calcified pleural plaques are commonly seen on the rib margins and diaphragm on the chest film. Lungs of individuals with plaques usually contain amphibole fibers. Symptoms are uncommon in these individuals, and function is usually not impaired.

G. Asbestos-related pleural effusions rarely occur less than 10 years after exposure and are most common in young men. Effusions may be associated with pleuritis and cause pain and rubs, fever, and dyspnea. They are usually small.

H. Perform thoracentesis and pleural biopsy in all patients with effusions to rule out other causes of pleural effusions (e.g., tuberculosis and other infectious etiologies) and to make a diagnosis of neoplastic disease of either primary pleural or other origin. If the cytologies and/or histologies are neoplastic, perform a work-up for primary lung carcinoma, metastatic lung cancer, and mesothelioma.

I. If the cytology and histology are not diagnostic of infectious or neoplastic disease, perform a repeat thoracentesis to remove all pleural fluid in preparation for repeat imaging studies. After removing all fluid, obtain a repeat chest film to determine if a pleural-based mass is present. If a mass is seen, institute a work-up for mesothelioma or other forms of neoplastic disease.

J. If a mass is not seen on a chest film, obtain a CT scan of the chest to completely rule out the presence of a mass. Small pleural-based masses or those that are extremely flat and lying against the posterior pleura may not be seen on a routine chest film but will be visualized on CT. If a mass is noted, perform a neoplastic work-up.

K. Benign asbestos effusions have no distinguishing diagnostic characteristics. They may be bloody, contain a preponderance of lymphocytes, and also be albumin-rich. They also disappear without treatment and may recur. This diagnosis is one of exclusion; asbestos-related pulmonary syndromes should be ruled out.

References

Craighead JE, Abraham JL, Churg A, et al. The pathology of asbestos-associated diseases of the lung and pleural cavities: diagnostic criteria and proposed grading system. Arch Pathol Lab Med 1982; 106:544.

Craighead JE, Mossman BT. The pathogenesis of asbestos-related diseases. N Engl J Med 1982; 306:1446.

Gale ME, Karlinsky JB. Computed tomography of the chest: a teaching file. Chicago: Yearbook Medical Publishers, 1988, 57:191.

Selikoff IJ, Lee DHK. Asbestos and disease. New York: Academic Press, 1978:1–549.

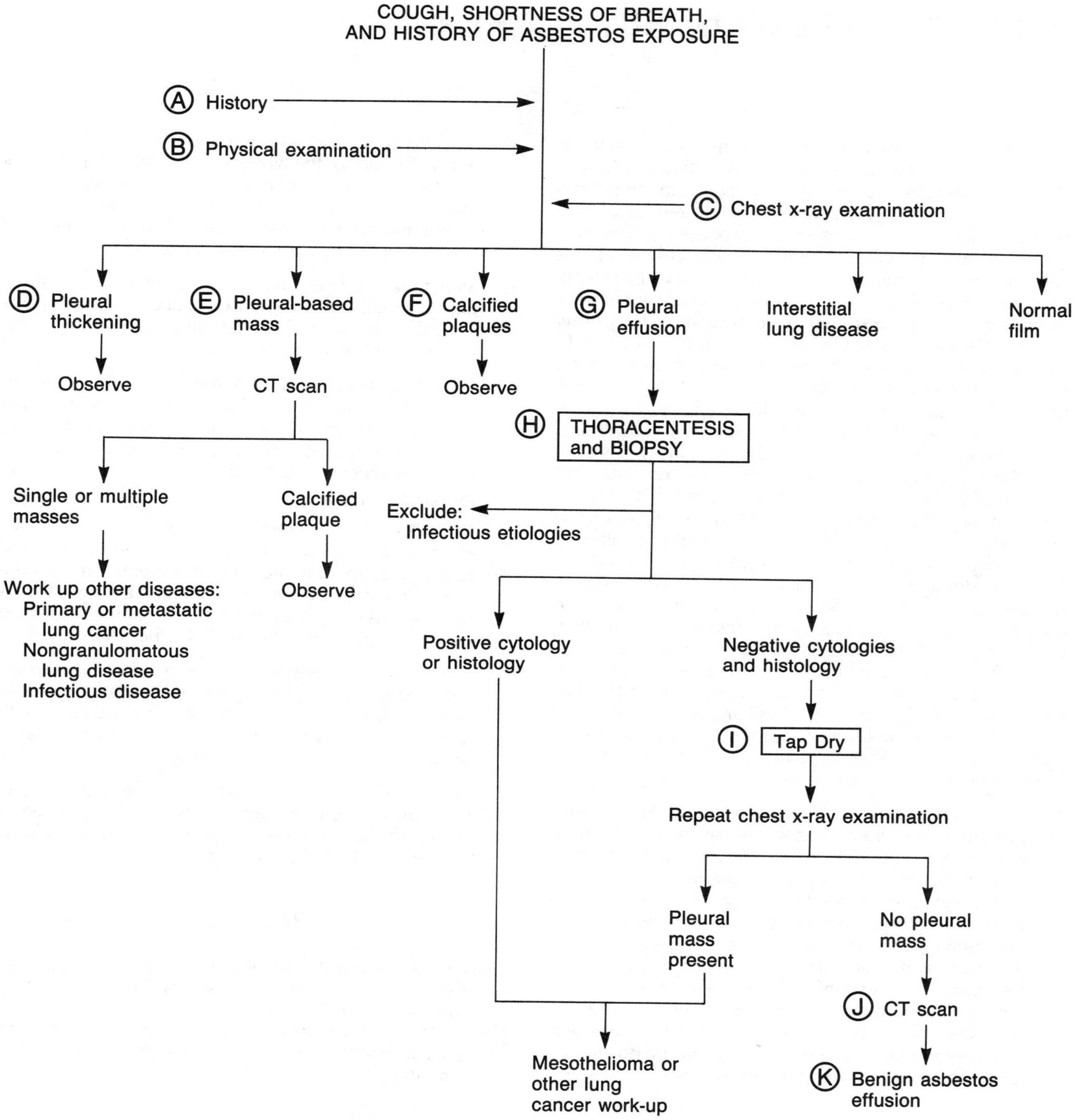

COUGH, SHORTNESS OF BREATH,
AND HISTORY OF ASBESTOS EXPOSURE

(A) History

(B) Physical examination

(C) Chest x-ray examination

(D) Pleural thickening

(E) Pleural-based mass

(F) Calcified plaques

(G) Pleural effusion

Interstitial lung disease

Normal film

Observe

CT scan

Observe

Single or multiple masses

Calcified plaque

(H) THORACENTESIS and BIOPSY

Work up other diseases:
Primary or metastatic lung cancer
Nongranulomatous lung disease
Infectious disease

Observe

Exclude:
Infectious etiologies

Positive cytology or histology

Negative cytologies and histology

(I) Tap Dry

Repeat chest x-ray examination

Pleural mass present

No pleural mass

(J) CT scan

(K) Benign asbestos effusion

Mesothelioma or other lung cancer work-up

181

IRRITANT GAS EXPOSURE

Most irritant gases produce injury to the mucosa of the lower airways; severe injury extends the alveolar surfaces and results in a clinical picture resembling acute permeability pulmonary edema and the adult respiratory distress syndrome (ARDS). Relatively common gases that produce injury include ammonia, hydrogen chloride, sulfur dioxide, chlorine, phosgene, and nitrogen dioxide. Ammonia is used in the synthesis of fertilizers, plastics, and explosives. Since ammonia is extremely irritating to exposed mucosal surfaces (eyes, nose, throat), toleration of amounts necessary to produce significant pulmonary injury cannot occur unless escape from the gas is impossible. Hydrogen chloride is liberated during plastic and insulation fires. Sulfur dioxide is a byproduct of the burning of coal and has widespread industrial uses. Chlorine, which is used in the chemical and plastics industry, has been spilled during transport. It is dangerous at low concentrations and can be hydrated to hydrochloric acid in the respiratory tree. Phosgene was used extensively as a poison gas during World War I, but now is used in the production of plastics. It is formed when chlorinated hydrocarbons are burned. It has little odor and is poorly soluble in upper airway mucosa, and thus it is able to penetrate to the alveoli. Nitrogen dioxide is formed during electric and acetylene arc welding, but is dangerous only when welding is done in enclosed areas, and is also formed by the action of nitric acid on organic materials. Since it is produced in silos, respiratory disease in this setting is termed silo-filler's disease. Nitrogen dioxide is poorly soluble and can produce injury (pulmonary edema) hours after exposure, and may result in obliterative bronchiolar damage weeks later.

A. The history establishes the type of injury. Patients complain of burning eyes, nose, and throat and may be dyspneic. Those exposed to agents that are soluble in water have primarily upper airway symptoms of cough and wheezing; those exposed to poorly soluble agents have lower respiratory symptoms of chest tightness. Nausea and vomiting may occur in all patients. Physical findings are nonspecific and include tachycardia, cyanosis, wheezing, rales, and inflammation of exposed mucous membranes. Arrhythmias due to hypoxemia may occur after severe exposures. Fever may be present. Hypotension after nitrogen dioxide exposure may be due to systemic absorption of nitrates and nitrites.

B. The arterial blood gas analysis and chest x-ray examination will establish the type and extent of injury. Patients will be hypoxemic and the chest film will demonstrate infiltrates compatible with pulmonary edema. Severe hypoxemia may be present in patients who are minimally symptomatic. The cardiac silhouette may be normal.

C. Start oxygen immediately after presentation and stabilize vital signs. Patients exposed to poorly soluble agents should be admitted for observation since these agents can have delayed effects.

D. Patients with signs and symptoms primarily of the airway who are medically stable may be treated as outpatients with bronchodilators, if necessary. There is no evidence that corticosteroids are of direct benefit in the setting of acute injury, but they may be used if the patient is wheezing.

E. Patients who are not medically stable or who have lower respiratory symptoms or signs should be admitted and receive care in a monitored unit. Patients with respiratory failure may require intubation and assisted ventilatory support for a brief period. Other routine supportive care including antibiotics will also be necessary.

F. Patients with methemoglobinemia require management with methylene blue (50 mg given intravenously over 10 minutes, repeated dosages given for concentrations >30 percent). Carboxyhemoglobinemia should be treated with high concentrations of oxygen.

G. Patients with NO_2 exposures may have recurrence of symptoms 2 to 6 weeks after exposure, which may result from bronchiolitis obliterans. These patients should be treated with high-dose steroids.

References

Jones RN. Acute and accidental exposures to irritant gases. In: Fishman AP, ed. Pulmonary diseases and disorders. New York: McGraw-Hill, 1980:793.

Sheppard D. Chemical agents. In: Murray JF, Nadel JA, eds. Textbook of respiratory medicine. Philadelphia: WB Saunders, 1988:1631.

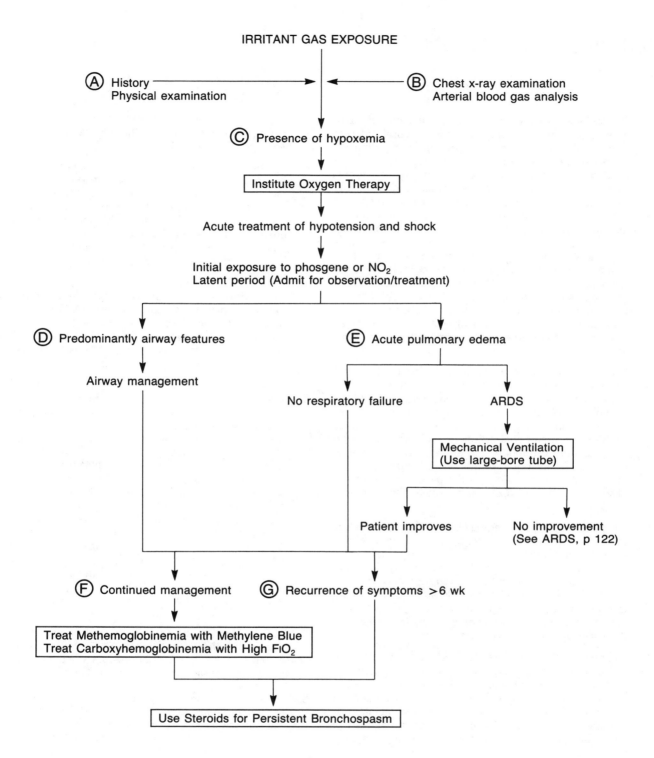

IRRITANT GAS EXPOSURE

(A) History
Physical examination

(B) Chest x-ray examination
Arterial blood gas analysis

(C) Presence of hypoxemia

Institute Oxygen Therapy

Acute treatment of hypotension and shock

Initial exposure to phosgene or NO₂
Latent period (Admit for observation/treatment)

(D) Predominantly airway features

Airway management

(E) Acute pulmonary edema

No respiratory failure

ARDS

Mechanical Ventilation
(Use large-bore tube)

Patient improves

No improvement
(See ARDS, p 122)

(F) Continued management

(G) Recurrence of symptoms >6 wk

Treat Methemoglobinemia with Methylene Blue
Treat Carboxyhemoglobinemia with High FiO₂

Use Steroids for Persistent Bronchospasm

SMOKE INHALATION

A. Smoke inhalation causes damage by inhalation of toxic gases and by thermal burns to exposed mucosal surfaces. Toxic gas inhalation produces significant pharyngeal, laryngeal, and airway edema and can result in airway obstruction. Patients therefore present with laryngeal symptoms such as cough, hoarseness, or mild stridor. Patients may also have common lower airway symptoms such as chest tightness, cough, or wheezing. Upper airway edema can progress rapidly within hours to complete airway obstruction. It is therefore necessary to exclude upper airway edema prior to discharging any patient exposed to smoke from the emergency room. Physical examination should include direct visualization of the pharyngeal structures and may include indirect laryngoscopy, depending on the history and pharyngeal findings. Obtain chest films on all patients not only as baselines, but also to exclude permeability pulmonary edema.

B. The initial examination includes a room-air arterial blood gas analysis and pulmonary function tests including a flow-volume loop. Measure carboxyhemoglobin levels; a level exceeding 15 percent, irrespective of any other findings, mandates care in an intensive care unit (ICU) setting. Spirometry enables one to estimate the degree of expiratory obstruction, and a flow-volume loop aids in making the diagnosis of inspiratory obstruction. Spirometric tests are of less help if the patient has a history of smoking or known obstructive airways disease, unless baseline tests are available.

C. If patients have carboxyhemoglobin (COHb) levels of less than 15 percent and are asymptomatic, further diagnostic distinctions are based on the presence or absence of pulmonary function abnormalities, respiratory signs, and hypoxemia. If the patient is not wheezing but has evidence of airway obstruction by PFTs, admission to a ward is required. In patients who are wheezing, the presence of hypoxemia determines whether the patient goes to an ICU or to a ward for management.

D. If carboxyhemoglobin levels are less than 15 percent but respiratory symptoms are present, consider emergency fiberoptic laryngoscopy to estimate the degree of upper airway edema. Fiberoptic laryngoscopy may be difficult to perform since burned patients often have facial burns and are in considerable pain. However, a diagnosis of severe laryngeal edema may signal impending complete upper airway obstruction. Patients with edema or frank obstruction must receive further management in an ICU setting.

E. Symptomatic patients with normal upper airway mucosa by laryngoscopy who wheeze or have low flow rates also require management in an ICU setting. However, if these patients are not wheezing or have normal flow rates, perform an arterial blood gas analysis to ensure that hypoxemia is not present. Hypoxemic patients should be admitted to the ICU; patients who do not have these findings but who are symptomatic may receive care in a medical ward.

F. Chest films are necessary to exclude the development of adult respiratory disease syndrome (ARDS) due to inhalation of toxic gases and to exclude the presence of secondary infectious problems. Patients who are admitted require close supervision because rapid changes may take place in their respiratory status.

G. Patients may slough airway mucosa or develop copious secretions, severe bronchoconstriction, pulmonary edema, and/or bacterial pneumonias. Patients who have high carboxyhemoglobin levels or who are hypoxemic need oxygen therapy, and positive airway pressure may be necessary. Inhaled or systemic bronchodilators and corticosteroids may also be used. However, there is no direct convincing evidence that corticosteroids prevent severe lower respiratory injury. Fluid management is of prime importance in patients who incur severe burns to the skin and/or respiratory tract. These patients require large amounts of fluid, which may worsen cardiogenic or noncardiogenic pulmonary edema. Antibiotics may be required, since hospitalized patients with respiratory burn injuries develop nosocomial infections.

References

Cahalane M, Demling RH. Early respiratory abnormalities from smoke inhalation. JAMA 1984; 251:771.

Fein A, Leff A, Hopewell PC. Pathophysiology and management of complications resulting from fire and the inhaled products of combustion. Crit Care Med 1980; 8:94.

Sammons JH, Coleman RL. Firefighters' occupational exposure to carbon monoxide. J Occup Med 1974; 16:543.

Waymack JP, Law E, Park R, et al. Acute upper airway obstruction in the postburn period. Arch Surg 1985; 120:1042.

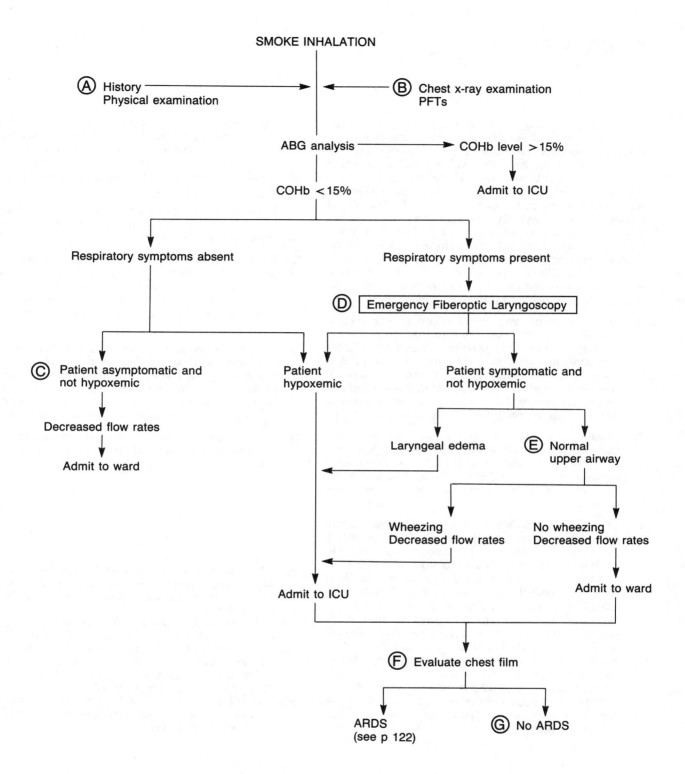

SMOKE INHALATION

(A) History — Physical examination

(B) Chest x-ray examination — PFTs

ABG analysis ————→ COHb level >15%

COHb <15%   Admit to ICU

Respiratory symptoms absent   Respiratory symptoms present

(D) Emergency Fiberoptic Laryngoscopy

(C) Patient asymptomatic and not hypoxemic   Patient hypoxemic   Patient symptomatic and not hypoxemic

Decreased flow rates   Laryngeal edema   (E) Normal upper airway

Admit to ward

Wheezing Decreased flow rates   No wheezing Decreased flow rates

Admit to ICU   Admit to ward

(F) Evaluate chest film

ARDS (see p 122)   (G) No ARDS

SILICOSIS

Silicosis may arise and progress years after exposure to silica dust. Silica particles cannot be degraded by lung phagocytic cells, and their presence initiates a cycle of events within pulmonary parenchyma, beginning with macrophage autolysis and ending with fibrosis. Immunocyte responses to these events have also been described. Although foundries are the most common source of quartz dust (silica), abrasive and ceramic workers, glass makers, dental technicians, and many other workers are also exposed. The risk of developing silicosis is directly related to the intensity and duration of the exposure with large, intense exposures producing an acute silicotic illness. Silicosis may follow a slow, chronic course or rapidly progress to death. Patients with this condition are particularly susceptible to pulmonary tuberculosis.

A. There may be no symptoms, and patients may present because of an abnormal chest film. The most common initial symptom is dyspnea on exertion, which indicates substantial lung involvement. Patients may complain of cough, but chest pain, wheezing, and constitutional symptoms are usually not reported unless another disease is also present. The physical examination is usually unremarkable unless hypoxemia is severe.

B. Clubbing is not a feature of the disease. Pulmonary function testing will reveal a restrictive defect; diffusing capacity will be unaffected initially but will eventually decrease. Arterial blood gas (ABG) analysis will reveal the presence of gas exchange abnormalities with hypoxemia.

C. Uncomplicated silicosis is characterized by small, rounded densities on the chest radiograph. The chest film is classified according to the ILO (International Labor Organization) criteria on the basis of nodular size and distribution. These tend to appear initially in upper lung zones but eventually involve all parts of the lung and may calcify. Hilar nodes may also be enlarged and may display calcification in the classic eggshell pattern. Complicated silicosis referred to as progressive massive fibrosis (PMF) is characterized by large lesions usually confined to the upper lung zones that retract, resulting in surrounding hyperlucent zones. Acute silicosis is characterized by rapidly expanding nodules and large lesions. Cavitation of nodules suggests the presence of tuberculosis. The diagnosis may be made with the appropriate history and chest film findings.

D. Acute silicosis may present as an alveolar proteinosis-like syndrome, and bronchoalveolar lavage (BAL), which has been used as treatment, is not often successful. Acute tuberculosis may accompany this presentation and should be ruled out. Lung transplantation has been performed in several cases.

E. In uncomplicated silicosis, bronchoscopy and transbronchial biopsy may be done to rule out metastatic cancer if the exposure history is unclear.

F. Bronchoscopy with transbronchial biopsy should also be performed in patients with PMF to rule out carcinoma and/or tuberculosis. Material should always be submitted for dust analysis. Increased lymphocyte counts in the bronchial washings may indicate acute, inflammatory silicosis.

G. The presence of arthritis in association with silicosis (or other pneumoconiosis) is designated Caplan's syndrome. The arthritis may precede the development of silicotic nodules in the lung and should be treated accordingly with standard therapies. Successful treatment of arthritis will not necessarily produce pulmonary improvement.

H. The treatment of PMF is supportive in nature and consists of oxygen therapy and treatment of cor pulmonale and infections.

References

Begin R, Cantin A, Masse S. Recent advances in the pathogenesis and clinical assessment of mineral dust pneumoconioses: asbestosis, silicosis and coal pneumoconiosis. Eur Respir J 1989; 2:988.

Galietti F, Giorgis GE, Oliaro A, et al. Lung diseases associated with silicosis: study of 618 cases. Minerva Med 1989; 80:987.

Nugent KM, Dodson RF, Idell S, Devillier JR. The utility of bronchoalveolar lavage and transbronchial lung biopsy combined with energy-dispersive x-ray analysis in the diagnosis of silicosis. Am Rev Respir Dis 1989; 140:1438.

Teculescu DB, Stanescu DC, Pilat L. Pulmonary mechanics in silicosis. Correlations with radiological stages. Arch Environ Health 1967; 14:461.

Patient with SILICOSIS

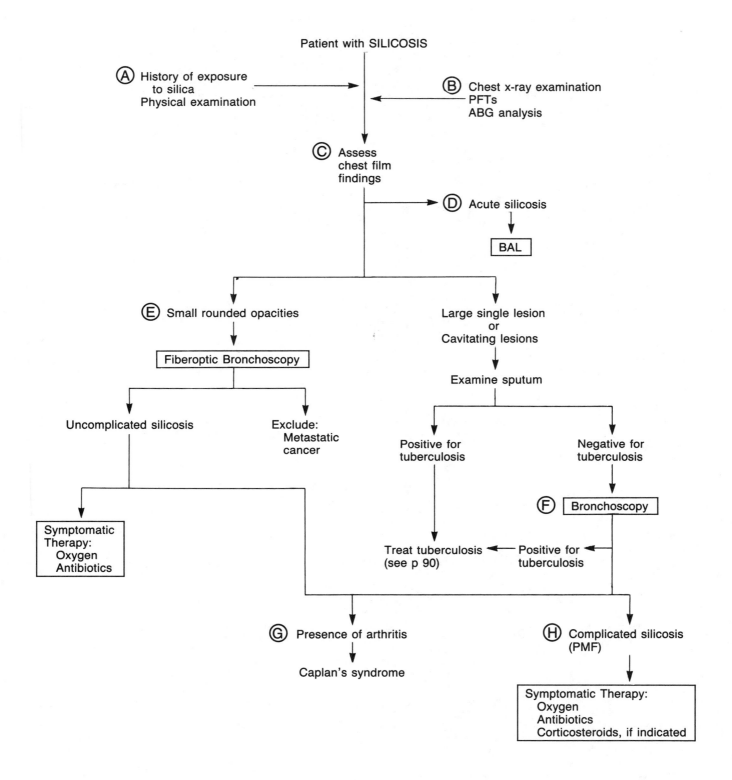

Ⓐ History of exposure
   to silica
   Physical examination

Ⓑ Chest x-ray examination
   PFTs
   ABG analysis

Ⓒ Assess
   chest film
   findings

Ⓓ Acute silicosis

BAL

Ⓔ Small rounded opacities

Fiberoptic Bronchoscopy

Uncomplicated silicosis

Exclude:
Metastatic
cancer

Symptomatic
Therapy:
Oxygen
Antibiotics

Large single lesion
or
Cavitating lesions

Examine sputum

Positive for
tuberculosis

Negative for
tuberculosis

Ⓕ Bronchoscopy

Treat tuberculosis
(see p 90)

Positive for
tuberculosis

Ⓖ Presence of arthritis

Caplan's syndrome

Ⓗ Complicated silicosis
   (PMF)

Symptomatic Therapy:
Oxygen
Antibiotics
Corticosteroids, if indicated

CHRONIC NONINFECTIOUS PARENCHYMAL DISEASE

Sarcoidosis
Chronic Eosinophilic Pneumonia
Pulmonary Eosinophilic Granuloma
Goodpasture's Syndrome
Wegener's Granulomatosis
Churg-Strauss Syndrome
Lymphomatoid Granulomatosis
Lymphocytic Interstitial Pneumonitis

Hypersensitivity Pneumonitis (Extrinsic Allergic Alveolitis)
Bronchiolitis Obliterans with Organizing Pneumonia
Pulmonary Involvement in Rheumatoid Arthritis
Drug-Induced Pulmonary Disease
Lipoid Pneumonia

SARCOIDOSIS

Sarcoidosis is a syndrome that is characterized by the presence of granuloma in multiple locations throughout the body. The disease frequently involves the lung, and non-caseating granuloma can often be demonstrated in lung parenchyma or airway wall by transbronchoscopic biopsy (TBB). The radiographic manifestations range from a fine reticulonodular pattern to large nodules. Cystic changes may be present. Sarcoidosis can also involve the larynx and pleura. The disease has a variable presentation and course. Initial work-up for pulmonary sarcoidosis consists of history, physical examination, chest x-ray examination, and PFTs. A tuberculin skin test and controls should be placed, although some patients with sarcoidosis are anergic. The subsequent work-up and treatment plans also vary from one medical institution to another.

A. The skin lesions, which are raised and nontender, provide an accessible site for biopsy and may preclude the need for more invasive procedures. Skin lesions often portend progressive disease.

B. Involvement of the larynx is a relatively uncommon manifestation of sarcoidosis (1 to 3 percent). It presents with hoarseness, cough, or dyspnea secondary to upper airway obstruction, and can occur early on or arise later in the course of the disease. A flow-volume loop may help to assess the patency of the upper airway. Laryngoscopy and biopsy provide the diagnosis.

C. The presence of bilateral hilar adenopathy and infiltrative disease on the chest film is highly suggestive of sarcoidosis. TBB reliably produces specimens containing granuloma. Approximately 3 to 4 biopsies are usually performed. Cultures should be obtained to exclude tuberculosis.

D. The evaluation of hilar adenopathy is controversial. Some believe that asymptomatic patients with bilateral hilar adenopathy should be observed. Others perform transbronchoscopic biopsies to make the diagnosis unequivocal. We employ transbronchoscopic biopsy if the PFTs indicate parenchymal involvement. In the absence of parenchymal involvement, we perform mediastinoscopy. Sarcoidosis can also present as unilateral hilar adenopathy; however, an alternate diagnosis, such as neoplasm or tuberculosis, should be considered.

E. If the initial transbronchoscopic biopsies are nondiagnostic, do either another transbronchoscopic procedure, mediastinoscopy, or an open-lung biopsy. Repeat the transbronchoscopic procedure, particularly if the specimens obtained from the first procedure did not contain alveolar structures.

F. The treatment for pulmonary sarcoidosis is controversial. Use steroids in patients with moderate pulmonary function abnormalities or in those with pulmonary symptoms, moderate interstitial abnormalities on the chest film, or evidence of progressive disease. After 1 month, switch to alternate-day steroids and slowly taper the dose as tolerated. The role of gallium scanning, serial measurements of angiotensin converting enzyme, and bronchoalveolar lavage with differential cell counts is uncertain, and we generally do not employ them. When endobronchial sarcoidosis presents with cough or wheezing, we use beta-agonists and inhalational steroids. Progressive disease occurs in approximately 10 to 15 percent of cases, and is indicated by increasing infiltrative disease and deteriorating pulmonary function. Over time, cystic structures may form which become colonized with *Aspergillus*. Recurrent pneumothoraces, hemoptysis, and respiratory failure may supervene in the final stages.

References

Bower JS, Belen JE, Weg JG, Dantzker DR. Manifestations and treatment of laryngeal sarcoidosis. Am Rev Respir Dis 1980; 122:325.

Gilman MJ, Wang KP. Transbronchial lung biopsy in sarcoidosis: an approach to determine the optimal number of biopsies. Am Rev Respir Dis 1980; 122:721.

Hollinger WM, Staton GW, Fajman WA, et al. Prediction of therapeutic response in steroid treated pulmonary sarcoidosis: evaluation of clinical parameters, bronchoalveolar lavage, gallium-67 lung scanning and serum angiotensin converting enzyme levels. Am Rev Respir Dis 1985; 132:65.

Hunninghake GW. Staging of pulmonary sarcoidosis. Chest 1987; 89:178S.

Kirks DR, McCormick VD, Greenspan RH. Pulmonary sarcoidosis: roentgenographic analysis of 150 patients. Am J Roentgenol 1973; 117:777.

Winterbauer RH, Belic N, Moores KD. A clinical interpretation of bilateral hilar adenopathy. Ann Intern Med 1973; 78:65.

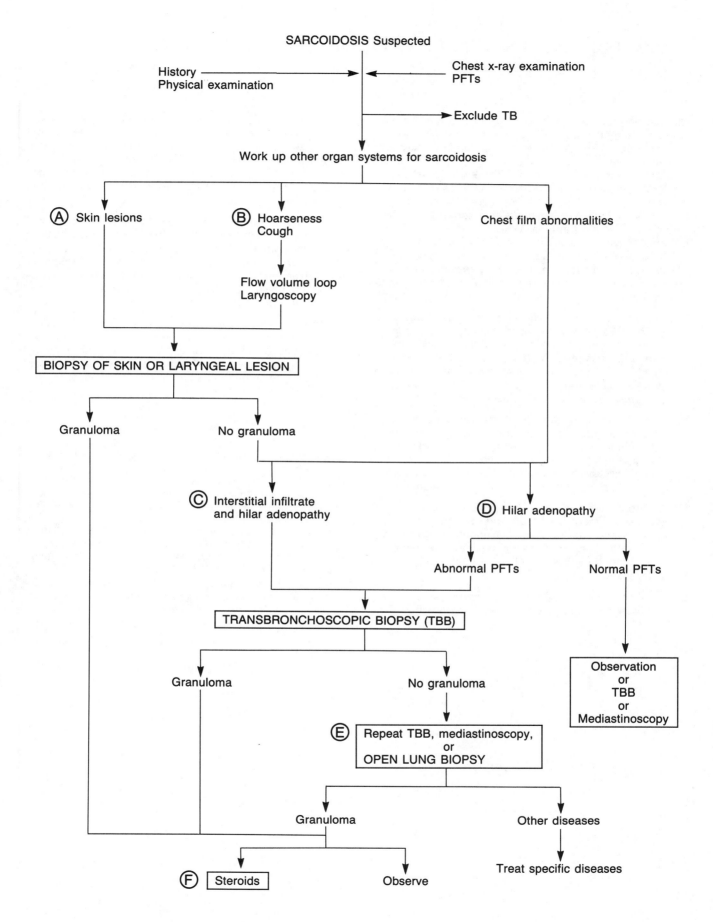

SARCOIDOSIS Suspected

History
Physical examination → ← Chest x-ray examination
PFTs

→ Exclude TB

Work up other organ systems for sarcoidosis

(A) Skin lesions   (B) Hoarseness
Cough   Chest film abnormalities

Flow volume loop
Laryngoscopy

BIOPSY OF SKIN OR LARYNGEAL LESION

Granuloma   No granuloma

(C) Interstitial infiltrate
and hilar adenopathy   (D) Hilar adenopathy

Abnormal PFTs   Normal PFTs

TRANSBRONCHOSCOPIC BIOPSY (TBB)

Granuloma   No granuloma

Observation
or
TBB
or
Mediastinoscopy

(E) Repeat TBB, mediastinoscopy,
or
OPEN LUNG BIOPSY

Granuloma   Other diseases

Treat specific diseases

(F) Steroids   Observe

CHRONIC EOSINOPHILIC PNEUMONIA

Chronic eosinophilic pneumonia (CEP) is a member of a group of disorders characterized by pulmonary infiltrates and eosinophilia. Although the classic picture presents little difficulty with regard to the diagnosis, the disease has a variable presentation. It can often be differentiated from other similar disorders by clinical criteria. CEP is associated with persistent peripheral infiltrates on chest radiographs and blood eosinophilia. Many patients are middle-aged women with a past history of asthma. Wheezing is more common in Loeffler's syndrome or allergic bronchopulmonary aspergillosis than in CEP. Constitutional signs consisting of fever, sweats, and weight loss are frequently present. Peripheral eosinophilia need not be present, and the infiltrates can be patchy and central.

A. The infiltrates are usually peripheral and involve the upper lobes. However, nonperipheral infiltrates or nodular infiltrates may also occur; the infiltrates may also cavitate. The diagnosis is suggested by the absence of infection or response to antibiotics. The presence of peripheral eosinophilia is helpful but does not occur in all cases. Tuberculosis must be excluded.

B. Symptoms and signs are usually present for a minimum of 2 weeks prior to presentation. In Loeffler's syndrome the infiltrates tend to be migratory, and the course of the illness is more benign. Tropical eosinophilia caused by filarial infection can be excluded by travel history, serum IgE levels, or by measurement of antifilarial antibodies.

C. Eosinophilic infiltration of extrapulmonic sites such as the heart, skin, or neurologic and vascular systems suggests the presence of another eosinophilic disorder. Patients with Churg-Strauss syndrome often have peripheral pulmonary infiltrates as well as vasculitis and extravascular granulomas.

D. In a few patients, the disorder may remit spontaneously, but most patients require treatment. Patients with chronic eosinophilic pneumonia often respond dramatically to high-dose daily steroid treatment. In the presence of classic clinical features and rapid response to prednisone therapy, histologic proof of eosinophilic pneumonia is not necessary. Rapid tapering of the medication may result in recurrence. Without treatment the disorder often persists or progresses.

E. A poor response to therapy or the presence of atypical clinical features requires further diagnostic evaluation. Some patients initially diagnosed as having chronic eosinophilic pneumonia may progress to multisystem involvement. The percentage of patients who do progress is unknown. Transbronchoscopic biopsy (TBB) is the usual initial procedure.

F. In some cases, open-lung biopsy is required for definitive diagnosis. Some patients require prolonged treatment (6 months) with every-other-day steroids, with intermittent trials of steroid withdrawal by slowly tapering the dose. The optimal duration of steroid treatment for the disorder is unknown.

References

Carrington CB, Addington WW, Goff AM, et al. Chronic eosinophilic pneumonia. N Engl J Med 1969; 280:787.

Divertie MB, Olsen AM. Pulmonary infiltration associated with blood eosinophilia (P.I.E.): A clinical study of Loeffler's syndrome and of periarteritis nodosa with P.I.E. syndrome. Dis Chest 1960; 37:340.

Fauci AS, Harley JB, Roberts WC, et al. The idiopathic hypereosinophilic syndrome. Ann Intern Med 1982; 97:78.

Jederlinic PJ, Sicilan L, Gaensler EA. Chronic eosinophilic pneumonia. Medicine 1988; 67:154.

Lanham JG, Elkon KB, Pusey CD, Hughes GR. Systemic vasculitis with asthma and eosinophilia: a clinical approach to the Churg-Strauss syndrome. Medicine 1984; 63:65.

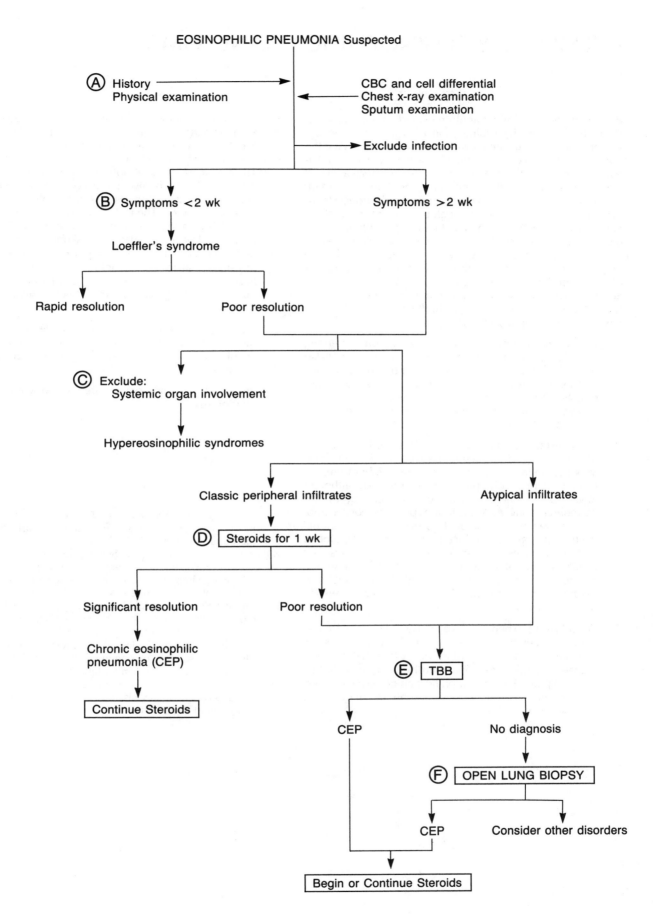

EOSINOPHILIC PNEUMONIA Suspected

(A) History
Physical examination

CBC and cell differential
Chest x-ray examination
Sputum examination

Exclude infection

(B) Symptoms <2 wk

Symptoms >2 wk

Loeffler's syndrome

Rapid resolution

Poor resolution

(C) Exclude:
Systemic organ involvement

Hypereosinophilic syndromes

Classic peripheral infiltrates

Atypical infiltrates

(D) Steroids for 1 wk

Significant resolution

Poor resolution

Chronic eosinophilic
pneumonia (CEP)

Continue Steroids

(E) TBB

CEP

No diagnosis

(F) OPEN LUNG BIOPSY

CEP

Consider other disorders

Begin or Continue Steroids

PULMONARY EOSINOPHILIC GRANULOMA

Pulmonary eosinophilic granuloma is a disorder characterized histologically by proliferation of histiocytes and eosinophils in the lung parenchyma. Histiocytes, which are the predominant cell type in the granuloma, resemble the epidermal Langerhans' cell. Granulomas are poorly demarcated and often centrally cavitated. Eosinophilic granuloma is a variant of the multisystem histiocytic proliferative disorder, Hand-Schüller-Christian disease. Although pulmonary eosinophilic granuloma is usually confined to the lung, patients with lung diseases and a few bony lesions or diabetes insipidus are also included in this group. Thus, there is a spectrum of disease ranging from primarily pulmonary disease (pulmonary eosinophilic granuloma) to a multisystem disorder (Hand-Schüller-Christian disease). These conditions are also related to the fulminant predominantly childhood variety, Letterer-Siwe disease, a rapidly fatal disorder.

A. Cough and dyspnea are the most common presenting complaints. Chest pain, fever, and hemoptysis may also occur. A few patients present with polyuria and polydypsia. Approximately one-third of patients are asymptomatic. Physical examination of the chest may reveal wheezing; rales are not usually present. Peripheral eosinophilia is absent.

B. The chest film is characterized by the presence of nodules that vary in diameter from 0.5 to 1.5 cm, have irregular stellate margins, and vary in number from few to many. Upper lobe predominance is seen, although lower lobes may be involved with sparing of the costophrenic angles. As the lesions progress, honeycombing may become the major abnormality. Hilar adenopathy is an uncommon finding in eosinophilic granuloma. Pneumothoraces occur in 5 to 10 percent of cases. The results of pulmonary function testing are variable and may reveal normal, obstructive, or restrictive alterations. Serum angiotensin-converting enzyme (ACE) levels are usually normal.

C. The relationship between localized and disseminated disease is uncertain. Hand-Schüller-Christian disease is characterized by lytic skull lesions, exophthalmos, and diabetes insipidus. Pulmonary involvement similar to that found in pulmonary eosinophilic granuloma also occurs. This condition occurs most commonly in children, but may be seen in all age groups.

D. The need for tissue confirmation of the diagnosis varies with the particular patient. A characteristic chest film in a patient with diabetes insipidus or with classic lytic bone lesions may not require histologic confirmation. The diagnosis can be established by transbronchoscopic biopsy and bronchoalveolar lavage. Biopsies reveal accumulations of histiocytes and eosinophils within the lung parenchyma. The histiocytes react with antibodies to the S-100 protein. Electron micrographs of cells derived from lung lavage or transbronchoscopic biopsy material reveal the presence of intracytoplasmic X-bodies. These rod-shaped structures are not found in normal lungs or in patients with sarcoidosis. They may be found in small numbers in lung biopsies of patients with interstitial fibrosis.

E. The prognosis in most cases is favorable without treatment. Although the efficacy of steroid therapy is not clearly defined, corticosteroids can be used to treat progressive disease.

F. Recurrent pneumothoraces are treated with surgical pleurodesis.

References

Friedman PJ, Liebow AA, Sokoloff J. Eosinophilic granuloma of lung: clinical aspects of primary pulmonary histiocytosis in the adult. Medicine 1981; 60:385.

Kullberg FC, Funahashi A, Siegesmund KA. Pulmonary eosinophilic granuloma: electron microscopic detection of X-bodies on lung lavage cells and transbronchoscopic biopsy in one patient. Ann Intern Med 1982; 96:188.

Lacronique J, Roth C, Battesti J-P, Basset F, Chretien J. Chest radiological features of pulmonary histiocytosis X: a report based on 50 adult cases. Thorax 1982; 37:104.

McDonnell TJ, Crouch EC, Gonzalez JG. Reactive eosinophilic pleuritis: a sequela of pneumothorax in pulmonary eosinophilic granuloma. Am J Clin Pathol 1989; 91:107.

Solar P, Chollet S, Jacque C, et al. Immunocytochemical characterization of pulmonary histiocytosis X cells in lung biopsies. Am J Pathol 1985; 118:439.

PULMONARY EOSINOPHILIC GRANULOMA Suspected

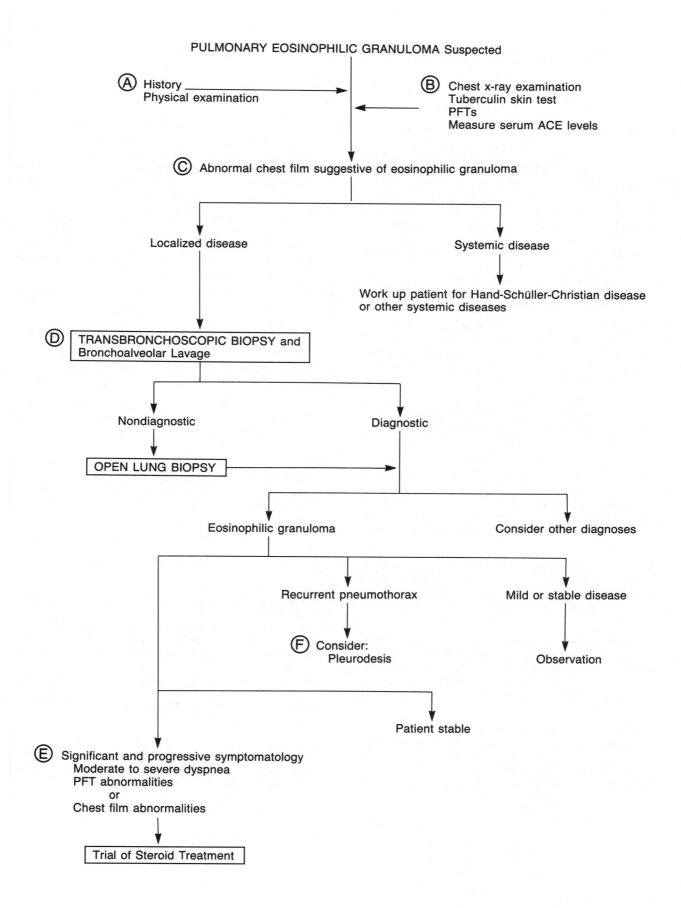

Ⓐ History
Physical examination

Ⓑ Chest x-ray examination
Tuberculin skin test
PFTs
Measure serum ACE levels

Ⓒ Abnormal chest film suggestive of eosinophilic granuloma

Localized disease

Systemic disease

Work up patient for Hand-Schüller-Christian disease
or other systemic diseases

Ⓓ TRANSBRONCHOSCOPIC BIOPSY and
Bronchoalveolar Lavage

Nondiagnostic

Diagnostic

OPEN LUNG BIOPSY

Eosinophilic granuloma

Consider other diagnoses

Recurrent pneumothorax

Mild or stable disease

Ⓕ Consider:
Pleurodesis

Observation

Patient stable

Ⓔ Significant and progressive symptomatology
Moderate to severe dyspnea
PFT abnormalities
or
Chest film abnormalities

Trial of Steroid Treatment

GOODPASTURE'S SYNDROME

A. Goodpasture's syndrome occurs most commonly in males in the second or third decades of life. These patients usually present with hemoptysis and may also have hematuria, anemia, lassitude, dyspnea, and cough. The diagnosis depends on the identification of positive linear immunofluorescent staining of IgG anti-GBM antibodies on glomerular basement membranes (GBM). Anti-GBM antibodies may also be found in serum. Hemoptysis may be mild or severe and may precede the renal disease by weeks to months. The physical examination may be within normal limits but may reveal evidence of anemia. Some patients have fine rales on examination of the chest; other nonspecific findings include clubbing, hepatosplenomegaly, and lymphadenopathy.

B. Findings on the chest film vary from normal to significant airspace disease. Opacities may be unilateral and are usually due to blood. Repeated episodes of intrapulmonic hemorrhage may lead to interstitial fibrosis, but individual episodes may resolve completely.

C. In patients who do not have renal disease at presentation, rule out other causes of hemoptysis. Assume that patients with hematuria or renal failure at presentation have Goodpasture's syndrome or another connective tissue disease until proven otherwise.

D. In patients with the appropriate clinical picture, perform a connective tissue screen (LE prep, complement levels, cryoglobulins, DIC screen). Assessment of serum levels of anti-GBM antibody must be performed by experienced, reliable laboratory personnel early in the work-up.

E. Other diagnoses that mimic Goodpasture's syndrome include those listed (see tree). They may be differentiated from Goodpasture's syndrome by the appropriate laboratory findings and the lack of renal immunofluorescent findings.

F. The diagnosis of Goodpasture's syndrome can be made by finding elevated levels of anti-GBM antibodies in serum or definitely, by positive direct immunofluorescent staining of linear antibodies on GBMs. Renal biopsies should be performed if there is any doubt regarding the diagnosis.

G. Goodpasture's syndrome has been known to remit spontaneously; however, since these patients have no special distinguishing characteristics, most patients will receive treatment. Current therapies include corticosteroids and cytotoxic agents, alone or in combination, which do suppress disease activity in some patients, and bilateral nephrectomy accompanied by dialysis or transplantation as a last resort in unresponsive individuals. If transplantation is to be considered, serum levels of anti-GBM antibodies must be zero prior to surgery, which usually requires repeated plasmapheresis.

H. In patients with the appropriate clinical syndrome but inconclusive laboratory values, a renal biopsy should be performed to confirm the diagnosis. Histologic examination of the tissue enables a firm diagnosis to be made more than 90 percent of the time.

I. When the diagnosis is not forthcoming after renal biopsy, a bronchoscopy with transbronchoscopic biopsies should be performed. This procedure may have already been done in some patients but should be repeated if the diagnosis remains uncertain.

J. Some patients must be observed and the tests repeated until a specific diagnosis is forthcoming.

K. In patients with hemoptysis but without evidence of renal disease, rule out the diagnoses of bronchitis, other inflammatory disease, and/or malignancy with sputum examination and bronchoscopy.

L. Other diagnoses of hemoptysis include malignancy, bronchitis, other inflammatory or infectious diseases, and rarer conditions such as mycetomas, pulmonary alveolar proteinosis, and noninfectious granulomatous diseases.

References

Goodpasture EW. The significance of certain pulmonary lesions in relation to the etiology of influenza. Am J Med Sci 1919; 158:863.

Johnson JP, Whitman W, Briggs WA, et al. Plasmapheresis and immunosuppressive agents in antibasement membrane antibody-induced Goodpasture's syndrome. Am J Med 1978; 64:354.

Soergel J, Sommers HC. Idiopathic pulmonary hemosiderosis and related syndromes. Am J Med 1962; 32:499.

Vanhille P, Raviart B, Morel-Maroger L, et al. Circulating immune complexes appearing in Goodpasture's syndrome. Br Med J 1980; 280:1166.

Walker RG, Scheinkestel L, Becher GJ, et al. Clinical and morphological aspects of the management of crescentic anti-glomerular basement membrane antibody (anti-GBM) nephritis/Goodpasture's syndrome. Clin J Med 1985; 54:75.

GOODPASTURE'S SYNDROME Suspected

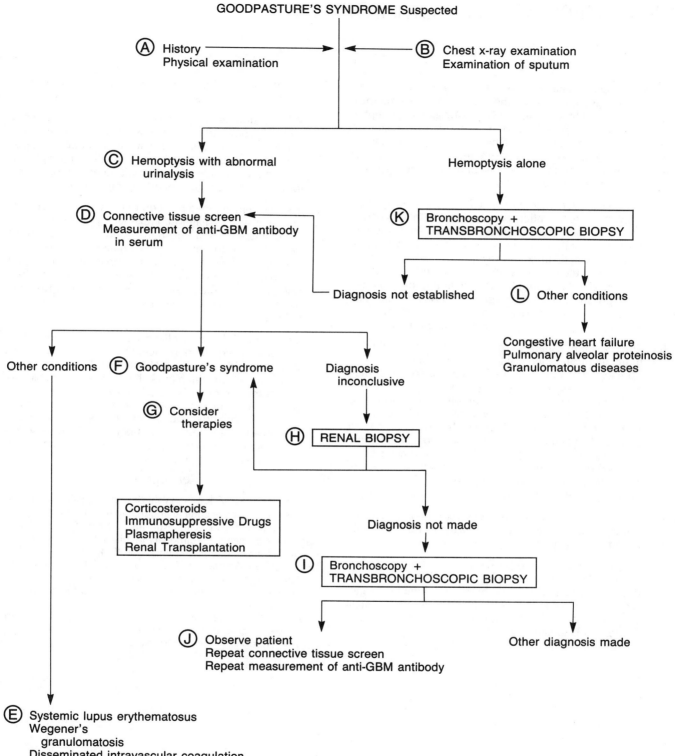

(A) History
Physical examination

(B) Chest x-ray examination
Examination of sputum

(C) Hemoptysis with abnormal
urinalysis

Hemoptysis alone

(D) Connective tissue screen
Measurement of anti-GBM antibody
in serum

(K) Bronchoscopy +
TRANSBRONCHOSCOPIC BIOPSY

Diagnosis not established

(L) Other conditions

Congestive heart failure
Pulmonary alveolar proteinosis
Granulomatous diseases

Other conditions

(F) Goodpasture's syndrome

Diagnosis
inconclusive

(G) Consider
therapies

(H) RENAL BIOPSY

Corticosteroids
Immunosuppressive Drugs
Plasmapheresis
Renal Transplantation

Diagnosis not made

(I) Bronchoscopy +
TRANSBRONCHOSCOPIC BIOPSY

(J) Observe patient
Repeat connective tissue screen
Repeat measurement of anti-GBM antibody

Other diagnosis made

(E) Systemic lupus erythematosus
Wegener's
granulomatosis
Disseminated intravascular coagulation
Drug reaction

WEGENER'S GRANULOMATOSIS

Wegener's granulomatosis presents with a triad of findings: necrotizing granulomata of the respiratory system, focal necrotizing vasculitis, and focal necrotizing glomerulonephritis. The disease may be limited to the respiratory tract. Current information suggests pathogenetic involvement by lymphoid T cells. Recently, measurement of anticytoplasmic antibodies has been found to assist in making the diagnosis and following results of therapy.

A. Since any organ system may be involved with necrotizing granulomata, patients may present with a myriad of symptoms, but major respiratory symptoms include intractable cough, hemoptysis, pleuritic pain, and rhinorrhea. The classic upper airway lesion, "saddle nose" or nasal septal ulceration, is commonly found. Ulcerations may be found in multiple sites including the orbit, ear passages, and sinuses. Skin lesions are also common, and patients may have cardiac, rheumatologic, or neurologic symptoms, as well as fever and weight loss.

B. The chest film usually demonstrates evenly distributed, multiple, thick-walled cavitating nodules ranging in size from less than 1 cm to 9 cm in diameter. The inner margins of cavities may be shaggy and ragged. Ill-defined infiltration may also be seen, and pleural effusions may be present. Secondary bacterial infection is common. Urinalysis may reveal red blood cells and red blood cell casts, and renal function may be impaired. Complement levels may be increased, but neutrophilia is not present unless the cavities in the lungs are secondarily infected. The sedimentation rate is high, eosinophilia may be present, and the patient may have a hemolytic anemia.

C. Patients with upper airway tract symptoms and signs require an ENT evaluation. The diagnosis may be established by biopsy of upper airway lesions.

D. If glomerulonephritis is present, biopsy the kidney first. Immunofluorescent staining of renal tissue reveals deposits of IgG with or without complement on glomeruli. Renal problems rarely bring patients to clinical attention. Measure the levels of anticytoplasmic antibodies; titers greater than 1:128 are highly specific and sensitive for active Wegener's granulomatosis.

E. In patients with lower respiratory tract signs and symptoms, a CT scan may localize nodular lesions.

F. When lesions are large and centrally located, fiberoptic bronchoscopy and transbronchial biopsy performed under fluoroscopic guidance may yield enough material to make a diagnosis. If lesions are small and peripherally located, consider transthoracic needle biopsy performed under CT guidance to obtain tissue.

G. The above-mentioned procedures usually do not provide enough tissue to diagnose Wegener's granulomatosis. If the diagnosis is still uncertain, open lung biopsy must be performed to obtain enough material for histologic diagnosis. Absence of IgG and complement staining on alveolar walls by immunofluorescent examination does not rule out the diagnosis. The levels of anticytoplasmic antibodies may be measured to provide confirming evidence.

H. Treatment of the generalized form of the disease with combined chemotherapy, including cytotoxic agents and corticosteroids, is generally beneficial. The limited form of the disease in which the kidneys are not involved has an improved prognosis. Renal transplantation has been performed in some cases, with no evidence of recurrent glomerulonephritis. Decreases in the levels of anticytoplasmic antibodies are associated with disease improvement. Conversely, relapses are associated with increased antibody titers.

References

Fauci AS, Haynes BF, Katz P, Wolff SM. Wegener's granulomatosis: prospective clinical and therapeutic experience with 85 patients for 21 years. Ann Intern Med 1983; 98:76.

Landman S, Burgener F. Pulmonary manifestations in Wegener's granulomatosis. Am J Roentgenol 1974; 122:750.

Rosenberg DM, Weinberger SE, Fulmer JD, et al. Functional correlates of lung involvement in Wegener's granulomatosis: use of pulmonary function tests in staging and follow-up. Am J Med 1980; 69:387.

Tervaert JWC, van der Woude FJ, Fauci AS, et al. Association between active Wegener's granulomatosis and anticytoplasmic antibodies. Arch Intern Med 1989; 149:2461.

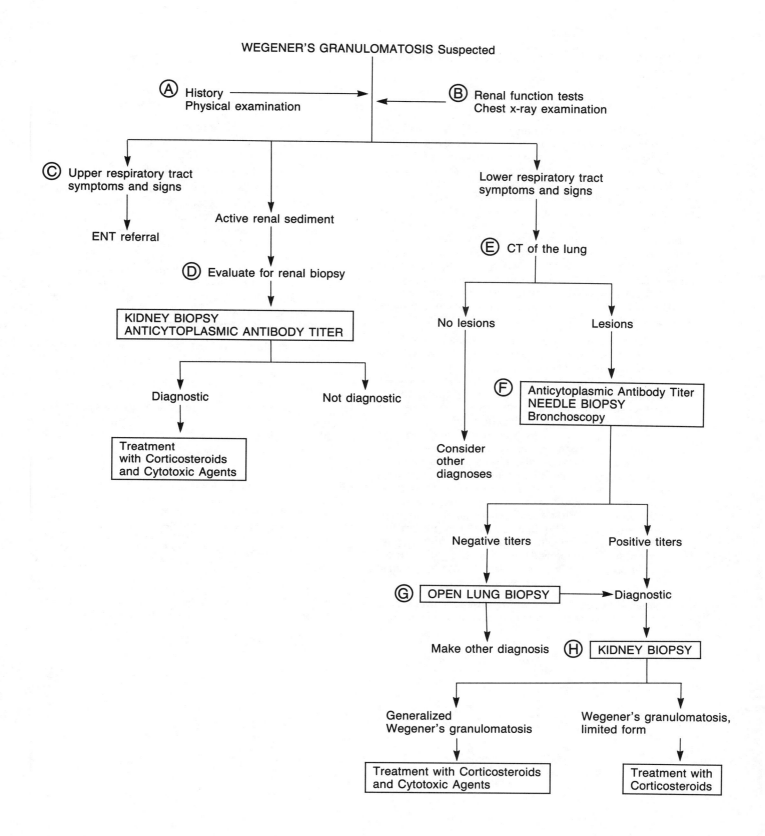

WEGENER'S GRANULOMATOSIS Suspected

(A) History
Physical examination

(B) Renal function tests
Chest x-ray examination

(C) Upper respiratory tract symptoms and signs

ENT referral

Active renal sediment

(D) Evaluate for renal biopsy

KIDNEY BIOPSY
ANTICYTOPLASMIC ANTIBODY TITER

Diagnostic

Not diagnostic

Treatment
with Corticosteroids
and Cytotoxic Agents

Lower respiratory tract symptoms and signs

(E) CT of the lung

No lesions

Lesions

(F) Anticytoplasmic Antibody Titer
NEEDLE BIOPSY
Bronchoscopy

Consider
other
diagnoses

Negative titers

Positive titers

(G) OPEN LUNG BIOPSY → Diagnostic

Make other diagnosis

(H) KIDNEY BIOPSY

Generalized
Wegener's granulomatosis

Wegener's granulomatosis,
limited form

Treatment with Corticosteroids
and Cytotoxic Agents

Treatment with
Corticosteroids

CHURG-STRAUSS SYNDROME

Churg-Strauss syndrome is a multisystem disorder consisting of necrotizing vasculitis, eosinophilia, and extravascular granulomas. Vasculitis is an essential component of the disorder, but whether extravascular granulomas are required to establish this diagnosis is controversial. Peripheral eosinophilia is usually present, and in some cases, the eosinophilia is confined to tissues. The Churg-Strauss syndrome is similar to Wegener's granulomatosis and polyarteritis nodosa, but these disorders usually can be differentiated on clinical grounds. Wegener's granulomatosis often causes upper airway pain and ulcerative lesions, whereas Churg-Strauss syndrome is associated with allergic rhinitis. Polyarteritis nodosa is not usually associated with eosinophilic infiltration or granuloma. In some cases, symptoms and signs may not permit a clear-cut diagnosis of any of these disorders.

A. Asthma or asthmatic bronchitis is a characteristic component of Churg-Strauss syndrome. The asthma may antedate the development of the vasculitis by many years. In some cases the onset of vasculitis is associated with a decrease in asthmatic symptomatology. Pulmonary infiltrates are common and are similar to those of eosinophilic pneumonia on the chest radiograph. They are generally patchy, nonlobar, and transient, although a variety of other patterns have been described including nodular or interstitial infiltrates. Pleural effusions may occur in approximately 30 percent of cases. Cardiac disease consisting of pericarditis, hypertension, myocardial infarction, or congestive heart failure is common in Churg-Strauss syndrome and may be fatal. Kidney involvement is less severe than that seen in polyarteritis nodosa. Both disorders can involve the gastrointestinal tract, producing abdominal pain, bleeding, and diarrhea. Perforation, peritonitis, or intestinal obstruction may occur.

B. Vasculitis is suspected if there is multisystem involvement and constitutional symptoms consisting of weight loss, fatigue, and fever. Common clinical features include a vasculitic skin rash (purpura, erythema, or nodules) and mononeuritis multiplex. The erythrocyte sedimentation rate is usually elevated, and the patient may have anemia.

C. Biopsy of the involved tissue usually shows evidence of necrotizing vasculitis. Small vessels are usually involved, but medium-sized vessels can also be affected. Granulomas may be found in approximately 40 percent of patients. An angiogram of an involved organ may show vessel irregularities, tortuosity, and small aneurysms. In polyarteritis nodosa, a necrotizing vasculitis is found in the small and medium-sized muscular arteries. Renal involvement occurs in approximately 70 percent of cases of polyarteritis nodosa. Renal involvement is less common in Churg-Strauss syndrome.

D. Unlike polyarteritis nodosa, the Churg-Strauss syndrome responds to treatment with steroids. High-dose steroids are given for at least several weeks or until symptoms remit. A rapid response is usually evident.

E. Some patients who fail to respond to steroids require immunosuppressive therapy (azathioprine or cyclophosphamide).

References

Chumbley LC, Harrison EG Jr, DeRemee RA. Allergic granulomatosis and angiitis (Churg-Strauss syndrome): report and analysis of 30 cases. Mayo Clin Proc 1977; 52:477.

Churg J, Strauss L. Allergic granulomatosis, allergic angiitis, and periarteritis nodosa. Am J Pathol 1951; 27:277.

Fauci AS, Katz P, Haynes BF, Wolff SM. Cyclophosphamide therapy of severe systemic necrotizing vasculitis. N Engl J Med 1979; 301:235.

Lanham JG, Elkon KB, Pusey CD, Hughes GR. Systemic vasculitis with asthma and eosinophilia: a clinical approach to the Churg-Strauss syndrome. Medicine 1984; 63:65.

CHURG-STRAUSS SYNDROME Suspected

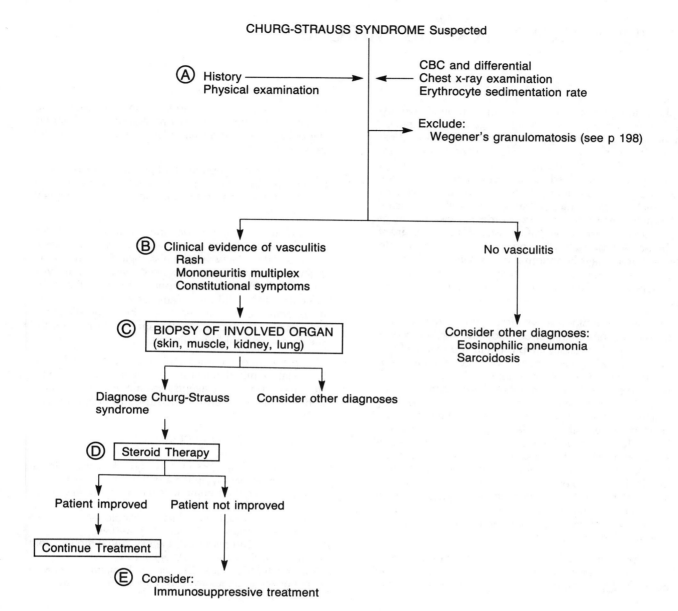

A History ——————→ CBC and differential
  Physical examination   Chest x-ray examination
                              Erythrocyte sedimentation rate

                              Exclude:
                                  Wegener's granulomatosis (see p 198)

B Clinical evidence of vasculitis   No vasculitis
  Rash
  Mononeuritis multiplex
  Constitutional symptoms

C BIOPSY OF INVOLVED ORGAN   Consider other diagnoses:
  (skin, muscle, kidney, lung)   Eosinophilic pneumonia
                                               Sarcoidosis

Diagnose Churg-Strauss   Consider other diagnoses
syndrome

D Steroid Therapy

Patient improved   Patient not improved

Continue Treatment

                      E Consider:
                          Immunosuppressive treatment

LYMPHOMATOID GRANULOMATOSIS

Lymphomatoid granulomatosis is a lymphoproliferative disease that involves the lung and other organs. It is characterized by an angiocentric infiltrate of normal and atypical lymphocytes, plasma cells, histiocytes, and necrosis. It commonly affects the lung, skin, and central nervous system, but any organ may be involved. Lymphocytic infiltration of the kidneys occurs in 40 percent of cases, but unlike Wegener's granulomatosis, glomerulonephritis and clinically significant renal impairment are absent. The disorder is viewed as either a premalignant lymphoproliferative disease or as a malignant lymphoma. Approximately 10 percent of cases develop into a clear-cut malignant lymphoma; in a small percentage of cases, the lesions regress without treatment. Usually lesions progress, however, resulting in death from respiratory insufficiency.

A. Patients are symptomatic with fever, cough, dyspnea, and chest pain. The cough may be productive and hemoptysis may occur. Skin lesions are present in approximately 40 percent of patients and include raised erythematous or macular lesions or, less commonly, subcutaneous nodules, which may be tender. Although skin manifestations may precede the onset of pulmonary problems, they usually occur concurrently. Physical examination of the chest may reveal bibasilar rales. Hepatomegaly is present in 5 to 10 percent of cases and is a sign of poor prognosis. Lymphocytic infiltration of the central nervous system occurs in approximately 30 percent of cases and usually indicates a poor prognosis. Several cases of CNS involvement have been reported in patients with acquired immunodeficiency syndrome (AIDS). Focal mass lesions in the CNS can result in major neurologic problems, including hemiparesis and aphasia.

B. The chest film usually reveals bilateral abnormalities. A variety of patterns may be found, the most common being multiple rounded peripheral densities that are often bilateral and basilar in location and may cavitate. Alveolar infiltrates, a reticular nodular pattern, hilar nodal enlargement, and small pleural effusions may also be seen.

C. The diagnosis of lymphomatoid granulomatosis can be established by skin biopsy. However, the pulmonary lesions should also be biopsied to exclude malignant lymphoma.

D. Examination of material obtained from transbronchoscopic lung biopsy may suggest lymphomatoid granulomatosis. However, the histologic distinction from other similar lymphoproliferative diseases such as lymphocytic interstitial pneumonia can sometimes be difficult with small biopsy samples. Open lung biopsy is generally recommended to establish the diagnosis definitively and exclude malignant lymphoma. All tissue samples should be cultured.

E. The treatment of lymphomatoid granulomatosis is controversial. Limited success has been reported with steroids and cytotoxic agents used alone or in combination. Radiation therapy is often used to treat localized lesions.

References

Anders KH, Latta H, Chang BS, et al. Lymphomatoid granulomatosis and malignant lymphoma of the central nervous system in the acquired immunodeficiency syndrome. Hum Pathol 1989; 20:326.

Jenkins TR, Zaloznik AJ. Lymphomatoid granulomatosis, a case for aggressive therapy. Cancer 1989; 64:1362.

Katzenstein ALA, Carrington CB, Liebow AA. Lymphomatoid granulomatosis. Cancer 1979; 43:360.

Nair BD, Joseph MG, Catton GE, Lach B. Radiation therapy in lymphomatoid granulomatosis. Cancer 1989; 64:821.

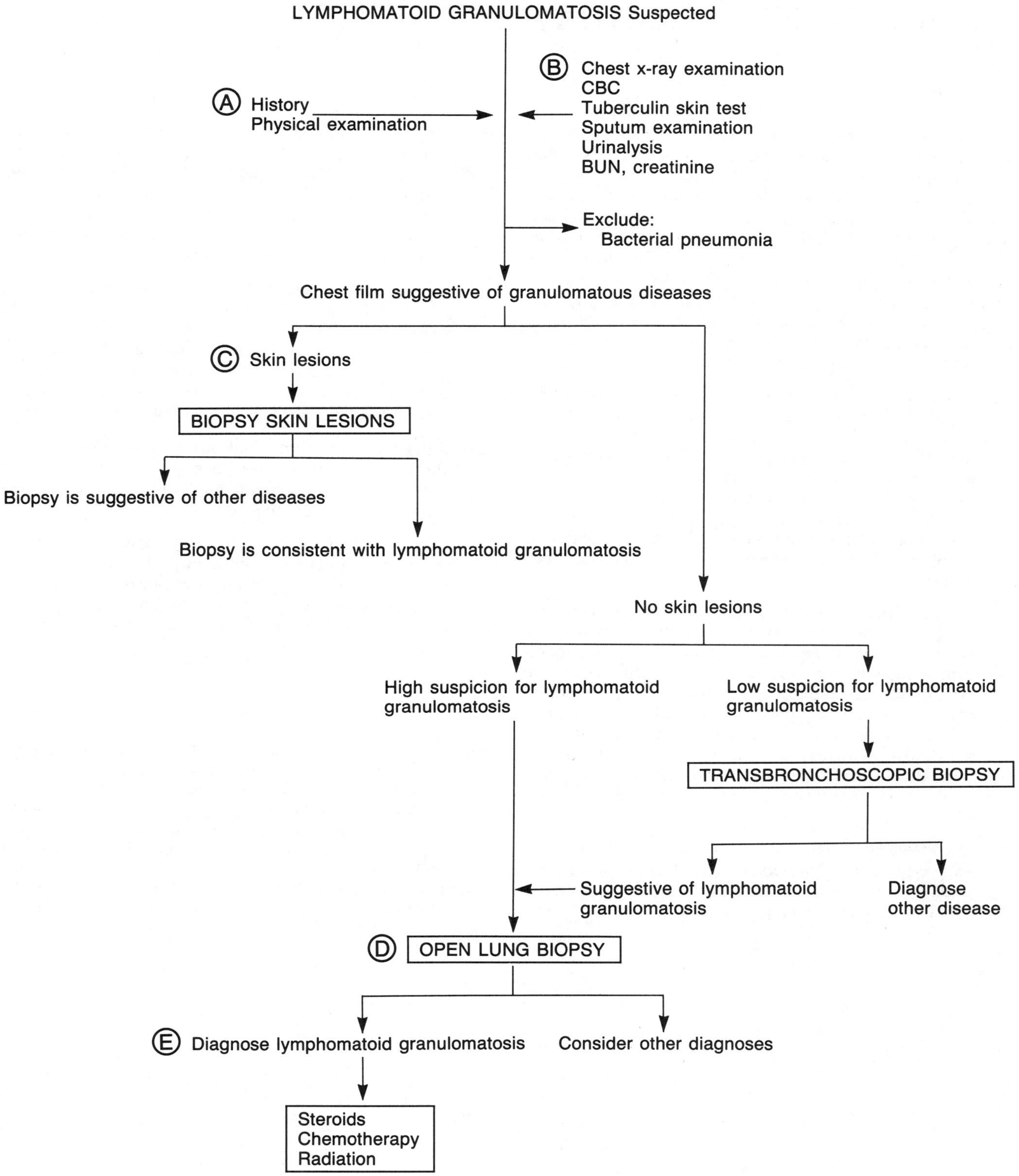

LYMPHOMATOID GRANULOMATOSIS Suspected

Ⓐ History
Physical examination

Ⓑ Chest x-ray examination
CBC
Tuberculin skin test
Sputum examination
Urinalysis
BUN, creatinine

Exclude:
    Bacterial pneumonia

Chest film suggestive of granulomatous diseases

Ⓒ Skin lesions

BIOPSY SKIN LESIONS

Biopsy is suggestive of other diseases

Biopsy is consistent with lymphomatoid granulomatosis

No skin lesions

High suspicion for lymphomatoid granulomatosis

Low suspicion for lymphomatoid granulomatosis

TRANSBRONCHOSCOPIC BIOPSY

Suggestive of lymphomatoid granulomatosis

Diagnose other disease

Ⓓ OPEN LUNG BIOPSY

Ⓔ Diagnose lymphomatoid granulomatosis

Consider other diagnoses

Steroids
Chemotherapy
Radiation

LYMPHOCYTIC INTERSTITIAL PNEUMONITIS

Lymphocytic interstitial pneumonitis (LIP) is characterized by infiltration of polyclonal lymphocytes and plasma cells within the lung interstitium. Vascular involvement may occur, but necrosis is absent. Chronic LIP is frequently associated with a dysproteinemia, involving a polyclonal increase in IgG and IgM and evidence of B-cell and T-cell dysfunction in approximately 75 percent of cases. One-third of all cases are associated with Sjögren's syndrome. Patients with human immunodeficiency virus (HIV) infection are at risk for developing LIP. LIP is also associated with chronic active hepatitis, myasthenia gravis, and other autoimmune diseases. The etiology of the disorder is unknown.

A. Most patients are symptomatic with nonproductive cough, low-grade fever, dyspnea, and weight loss, and may have pleuritic chest pain and fatigue. Physical examination reveals basilar rales, and digital clubbing may be evident. Symptoms associated with the sicca complex of Sjögren's syndrome include xerostomia, xerophthalmia, and keratoconjunctivitis sicca. Other diseases associated with Sjögren's syndrome include diffuse pulmonary fibrosis, amyloidosis, lymphoma, and bronchopneumonia.

B. Chest films reveal interstitial infiltrates that are predominantly basilar in location. The infiltrates may have a nodular component. Unlike sarcoidosis, mediastinal and hilar adenopathies are uncommon unless the patient has an additional disorder such as acquired immunodeficiency syndrome (AIDS). Pulmonary function tests reveal a restrictive disease with decreases in the diffusing capacity for carbon monoxide. Sputum examination should indicate normal flora, and serum angiotensin-converting enzyme levels will be within normal limits.

C. Because LIP is usually a chronic disorder that progresses slowly, the need for rapid diagnostic evaluation is not urgent. However, in patients with HIV infection, interstitial infiltrates require rapid evaluation to exclude *Pneumocystis carinii*, tuberculosis, or other opportunistic infections. In patients with normal immunity, acute viral pneumonia may also produce a similar clinical syndrome and interstitial pattern on the chest film. Viral pneumonitis usually resolves without specific therapy. However, some cases of viral pneumonia cause severe illness and require aggressive management.

D. The diagnosis can be made by transbronchoscopic biopsy. CT should be performed prior to the biopsy to detect any cystic areas and assess the mediastinum for nodal enlargement. When the HIV status is positive or unknown, bronchoalveolar lavage should also be performed at the same time. All material should be cultured to exclude the presence of opportunistic infections.

E. If the initial transbronchial biopsy is nondiagnostic, it should be repeated. Alternatively, an open lung biopsy can be performed, providing enough material to make the diagnosis unequivocally.

F. In symptomatic patients with progressive disease, a trial of corticosteroids is warranted. A variable number of patients respond favorably, including those who are HIV positive. Advanced age and evidence of honeycombing on the chest film are predictors of a poor prognosis.

References

Morris JC, Rosen MJ, Marchevsky A, Teirstein AS. Lymphocytic interstitial pneumonia in patients at risk for the acquired immune deficiency syndrome. Chest 1987; 91:63.

Oldham SAA, Castillo M, Jacobson FL, Mones JM, Saldana MJ. HIV-associated lymphocytic interstitial pneumonia: radiologic manifestations and pathologic correlation. Radiology 1989; 170:83.

Strimlan CV, Rosenow EC, Weiland HL, Brown LR. Lymphocytic interstitial pneumonitis. Ann Intern Med 1978; 88:616.

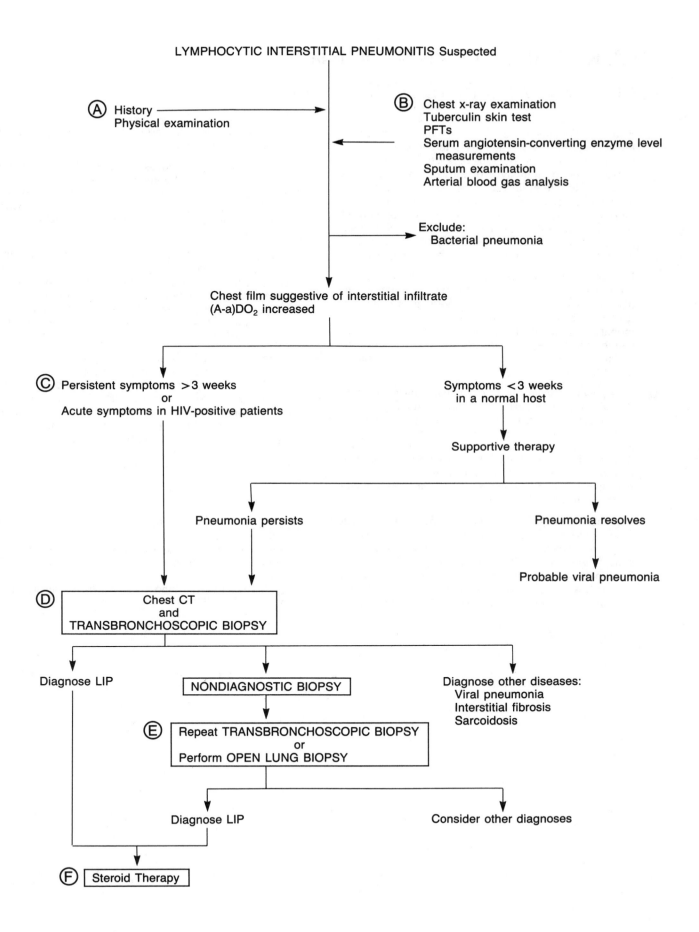

LYMPHOCYTIC INTERSTITIAL PNEUMONITIS Suspected

(A) History
Physical examination

(B) Chest x-ray examination
Tuberculin skin test
PFTs
Serum angiotensin-converting enzyme level
measurements
Sputum examination
Arterial blood gas analysis

Exclude:
Bacterial pneumonia

Chest film suggestive of interstitial infiltrate
(A-a)DO₂ increased

(C) Persistent symptoms >3 weeks
or
Acute symptoms in HIV-positive patients

Symptoms <3 weeks
in a normal host

Supportive therapy

Pneumonia persists

Pneumonia resolves

Probable viral pneumonia

(D) Chest CT
and
TRANSBRONCHOSCOPIC BIOPSY

Diagnose LIP

NONDIAGNOSTIC BIOPSY

Diagnose other diseases:
Viral pneumonia
Interstitial fibrosis
Sarcoidosis

(E) Repeat TRANSBRONCHOSCOPIC BIOPSY
or
Perform OPEN LUNG BIOPSY

Diagnose LIP

Consider other diagnoses

(F) Steroid Therapy

HYPERSENSITIVITY PNEUMONITIS (EXTRINSIC ALLERGIC ALVEOLITIS)

A. A variety of organic materials (animal or vegetable) may incite hypersensitivity reactions in the airways and pulmonary parenchyma. The type of reaction and extent of disease depend on the type of antigen inhaled and the quantity and rate of dosing of the antigen. The smaller the particle size and the greater the quantity and rapidity of exposure, the more likely is the development of pneumonitis. Patients usually give a history of dust exposure and complain of dyspnea, dry cough, fever, and weakness occurring some hours after the exposure.

B. Physical examination of the chest usually reveals the presence of diffuse, bibasilar dry rales. The chest film displays a diffuse nodular, reticulonodular, or interstitial pattern, and an airspace component may be present. Pulmonary function testing is consistent with a restrictive pattern, the single breath diffusing capacity is reduced, and the patient is hypoxemic at rest. Routine laboratory tests are usually not helpful.

C. If the patient is acutely ill, rule out viral or bacterial pneumonitis by sputum examination and culture. Given the proper history and lack of infectious findings, a presumptive diagnosis of hypersensitivity pneumonitis may be made. Prior to treatment of acute disease with corticosteroids, serum should be collected for evaluation of precipitin levels against the presumed antigen. Levels may be remeasured when the patient improves and will be found to have decreased.

D. If the patient does not have acute disease and is without fever or blood or sputum eosinophilia, then interstitial lung disease resulting from many other etiologies is possible. Sputum should still be examined, but PFTs should be done to confirm the presence of restrictive disease. Airway obstruction may be present as well since bronchiolitis with or without granulomata formation is common if the patient has had many repeated episodes of hypersensitivity pneumonitis.

E. If a hypersensitivity process is suspected, the patient should be challenged with small doses of the antigen by inhalation. Measure pulmonary function and arterial blood gases after exposure to antigen to indicate worsening obstruction and restriction. A physician should be present during testing.

F. A positive test establishes the diagnosis. Treat patients with corticosteroids and encourage them to discontinue exposure to the antigen. Most patients will improve after these measures have been taken. If the provocational test is negative, measure precipitin levels. If no contraindication to steroid use is present, begin therapy while waiting for levels to be measured.

G. If a patient whose likely diagnosis is hypersensitivity does not improve with treatment with steroids and antigen avoidance, consider open lung biopsy. Specific characteristics of hypersensitivity such as alveolitis, bronchiolitis, lymphocytic infiltration, and granuloma formation will be found on histologic examination of lung tissue. Treat these patients with high-dose corticosteroids by mouth as well as inhaled steroids until pulmonary function and the chest film pattern improve.

References

Pepys J. Pulmonary hypersensitivity disease due to inhaled organic antigens. Ann Intern Med 1966; 64:943.

Reynolds HY. Concepts of the pathogenesis and lung reactivity in hypersensitivity pneumonitis. Ann NY Acad Sci 1986; 465:287.

Salvaggio JE, deShazo RD. Pathogenesis of hypersensitivity pneumonitis. Chest 1986; 89:1905.

HYPERSENSITIVITY PNEUMONITIS Suspected

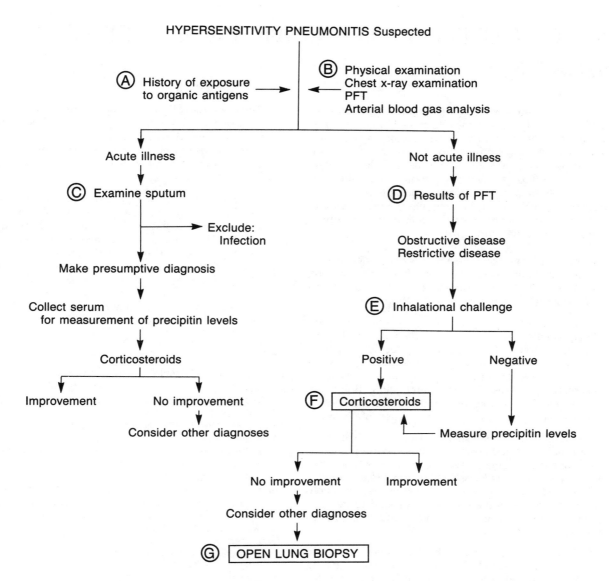

BRONCHIOLITIS OBLITERANS WITH ORGANIZING PNEUMONIA

Bronchiolitis obliterans with organizing pneumonia (BOOP) is usually classified as one of the interstitial fibrotic diseases. Bronchiolitis obliterans with or without organizing pneumonia is associated with exposures to certain toxic fumes, infections, drugs, and connective tissue diseases. Bronchiolitis obliterans without organizing pneumonia occurs after certain viral or *Mycoplasma* infections, especially in children. Penicillamine can also cause bronchiolitis obliterans without organizing pneumonia. Idiopathic BOOP results in respiratory and constitutional symptoms.

A. Patients usually present with a history of dyspnea, cough, or flu-like illness associated with fever, malaise, and weight loss. The chest examination is nonspecific and may show rales or wheezes or no abnormalities.

B. The chest film often reveals patchy densities, but interstitial infiltrates may also occur. Cavitation and effusions are uncommon. PFTs usually reveal a restrictive pattern with reductions in total lung capacity and diffusing capacity. However, the PFTs may be normal or show some obstructive changes. Sputum examination should not contain evidence of infection, and antibiotics do not influence the symptoms or the progression of disease.

C. Interstitial lung diseases such as usual interstitial pneumonia (UIP) or sarcoidosis often present with a reticular nodular pattern on the chest film. This is usually associated with a restrictive PFT pattern, but obstructive airways disease also occurs rarely in patients with this radiographic picture. Some of these patients respond to steroids. Whether this subgroup is a variant of BOOP is still uncertain.

D. BOOP is often mistaken for a bacterial pneumonia that fails to respond to antibiotics. Transbronchoscopic lung biopsy may be performed to rule this out; however, this approach is controversial.

E. The diagnosis of BOOP can be made definitively by open lung biopsy. The histologic picture consists of granulation tissue involving the bronchioles and alveolar ducts, with extension of the process into the alveoli. A mononuclear infiltrate may be present, and destruction of small airways may be seen.

F. Treatment consists of high-dose oral steroids. Patients usually respond within 2 to 6 weeks. By contrast, patients with chronic eosinophilic pneumonia respond more rapidly. The duration of treatment is not well defined. Usually patients receive 2 to 4 months of high-dose steroid therapy. If significant symptomatic, functional, and radiographic resolution has occurred, a careful steroid taper is begun. Some patients may have residual disease, and in a small minority of patients, the disease progresses to death despite therapy.

References

Chandler PW, Shin MS, Friedman SE, Myers JL, Katzenstein AL. Radiographic manifestations of bronchiolitis obliterans with organizing pneumonia vs usual interstitial pneumonia. Am J Radiol 1986; 147:899.

Epler GR, Colby TV. The spectrum of bronchiolitis obliterans. Chest 1983; 83:161.

Epler GR, Colby TV, McLoud TC, Carrington CB, Gaensler EA. Bronchiolitis obliterans organizing pneumonia. N Engl J Med 1985; 312:152.

Guerry-Force ML, Muller NL, Wright JL, et al. A comparison of bronchiolitis obliterans with organizing pneumonia, usual interstitial pneumonia, and small airways disease. Am Rev Respir Dis 1987; 135:705.

Katzenstein ALA, Myers JL, Prophet WD, Corley LS, Shin MS. Bronchiolitis obliterans and usual interstitial pneumonia. Am J Surg Path 1986; 10:373.

McLoud TC, Epler GR, Colby TV, Gaensler EA, Carrington CB. Bronchiolitis obliterans. Radiology 1986; 159:1.

BRONCHIOLITIS OBLITERANS AND ORGANIZING PNEUMONIA Suspected

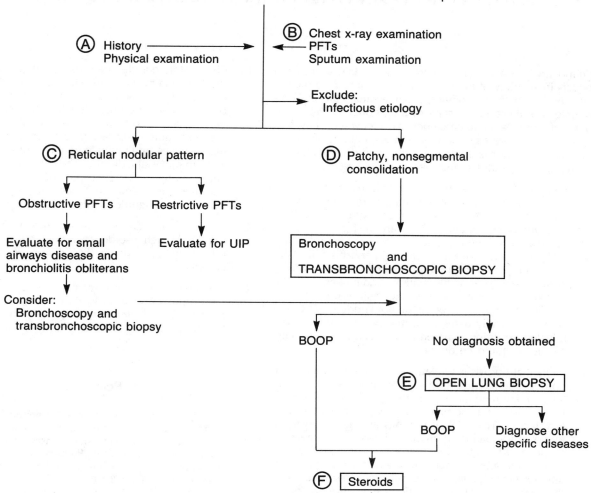

PULMONARY INVOLVEMENT IN RHEUMATOID ARTHRITIS

Pulmonary involvement is frequent in rheumatoid arthritis and occurs in a variety of forms. The most common are pleural effusion, parenchymal nodules, and interstitial fibrosis. Combinations of these manifestations are frequently seen. The onset of pulmonary manifestations may precede the development of the arthritis by months or years. Other pulmonary manifestations of rheumatoid arthritis include bronchiolitis obliterans, amyloidosis, and vasculitis.

A. Pleural effusions in rheumatoid arthritis are very common. The effusions are exudates, with a low glucose (<20 mg%), high LDH, and either neutrophilic or lymphocytic predominance. They vary in size and may be associated with pleuritic pain and dyspnea. Leukocytes with inclusion bodies ("rheumatoid arthritis cells") are frequently found in the fluid. Pleural biopsy is usually performed to exclude tuberculosis and malignancy. The biopsy usually reveals nonspecific pleuritis but may contain lesions suggestive of rheumatoid nodules. The effusions are usually benign but may become secondarily infected, resulting in an empyema. Large symptomatic effusions should be drained.

B. Interstitial fibrosis is a relatively uncommon manifestation of rheumatoid arthritis. The initial lesion is an interstitial infiltrate that may partially resolve. The course is variable and, in some cases, may progress to respiratory failure. The clinical findings are similar to those found in idiopathic pulmonary fibrosis and consist of dyspnea and cough. Gold therapy, which is used to treat rheumatoid arthritis, may cause an interstitial pneumonitis, resembling interstitial fibrosis weeks to months after the medication is started. Patients may develop cough, dyspnea, fever, and eosinophilia. Other signs of gold toxicity are dermatitis, bone-marrow suppression, and proteinuria. Discontinuing the gold treatment usually results in partial or complete resolution of the infiltrates.

C. Rheumatoid nodules are usually multiple, subpleural in location, and may cavitate. Histologically, there is a central area of acellular necrosis surrounded by epithelioid cells. In patients exposed to silica, the nodules may be massive and frequently cavitate (Caplan's syndrome). Solitary nodules must be differentiated from primary lung malignancies, and multiple nodules must be differentiated from metastatic disease. The extent of evaluation depends on the index of suspicion. A solitary, enlarging nodule requires a diagnostic work-up, particularly in patients with a significant history of smoking.

D. Atypical interstitial processes require further evaluation to exclude such disorders as bronchiolitis obliterans and organizing pneumonia (BOOP) or alveolar cell carcinoma.

E. The progression of the disease can be followed with serial chest films or serial PFTs. As in idiopathic pulmonary fibrosis, steroids and cytotoxic agents have been used to treat progressive disease with mixed results.

References

Petterson T, Klockars M, Hellstrom P-E. Chemical and immunological features of pleural effusions: comparison between rheumatoid arthritis and other diseases. Thorax 1981; 37:35.

Roschmann RA, Rothenberg RJ. Pulmonary fibrosis in rheumatoid arthritis: a review of clinical features and therapy. Semin Arthritis Rheum 1987; 16:174.

Scott DL, Bradby GVH, Aitman TJ, Zaphiropoulos GC, Hawkins CF. Relationship of gold and penicillamine therapy to diffuse interstitial lung disease. Ann Rheum Dis 1981; 40:136.

Steinberg DL, Webb WR. CT appearances of rheumatoid lung. J Comput Assist Tomogr 1984; 8:881.

PULMONARY INVOLVEMENT IN RHEUMATOID ARTHRITIS

History
Physical examination

Chest x-ray examination
Arterial blood gas analysis
PFTs
Chest CT scan

Rheumatoid arthritis and abnormal chest film

(A) Pleural effusion

(B) Interstitial fibrosis

(C) Pulmonary nodules

Typical
Multiple
Subpleural

Atypical
Solitary
Enlarging

Probable rheumatoid nodules

Exclude metastatic
lung disease

Observation

**THORACENTESIS
PLEURAL BIOPSY**

Exclude:
Heart failure

Stop gold therapy if used

Chest film
typical for
usual interstitial
pneumonia

(D) Chest film shows atypical pattern

TRANSBRONCHOSCOPIC OR OPEN LUNG BIOPSY

Usual interstitial pneumonia

Consider other diagnoses

Asymptomatic

(E) Symptomatic or progressive disease

Observation

Start Steroids

Consider other diagnoses

Rheumatoid pleural effusion

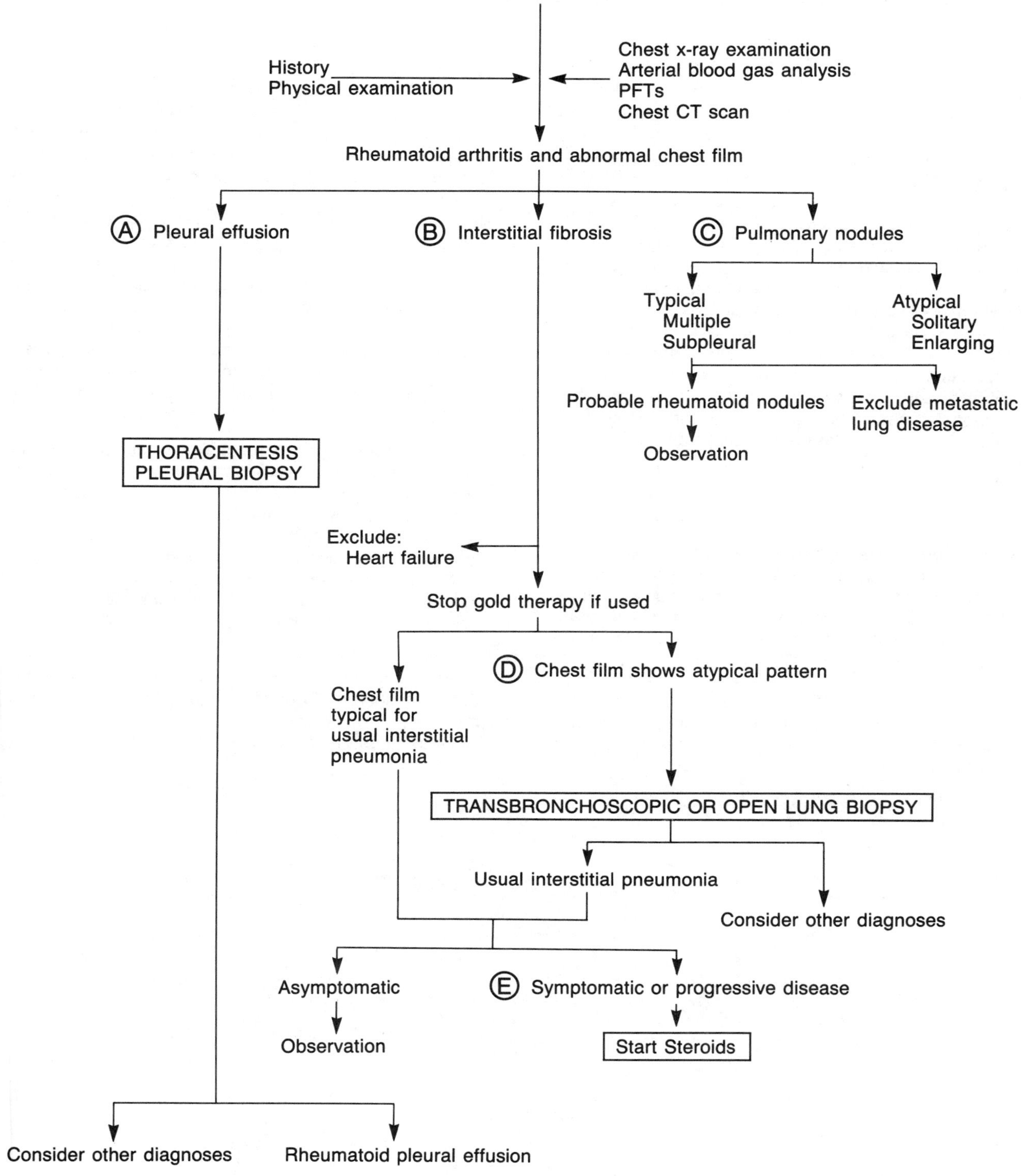

DRUG-INDUCED PULMONARY DISEASE

Drug reactions may be classified into six categories: overdosage, intolerance, idiosyncratic reactions, side effects, secondary effects, and allergic or hypersensitivity reactions. Drugs produce damage by one or more of the following mechanisms: oxidant injury, direct cytotoxic damage to capillary endothelium, accumulation of phospholipids within cells, and immunologically mediated injury. Injury may not be dose-related. Although the exact mechanism by which any particular drug exerts its untoward effect may not be known, the algorithm for diagnosis and treatment is similar for all drugs. Any drug suspected of causing a reaction should be immediately discontinued unless it is absolutely necessary to the therapeutic regimen. In those few cases where drugs are absolutely required, it is necessary to acquire proof that a pulmonary response to the drug has occurred. More than 75 drugs are known to cause pulmonary problems in many different ways. Table 1 provides a list of the most common of these drugs.

A. These patients are taking medications and usually present with constitutional symptoms alone along with breathlessness and interstitial or lobar infiltrates, or with acute pulmonary edema. Physical examination of the chest may be within normal limits or may reveal either rales or decreased breath sounds.

B. Pulmonary function testing may reveal restrictive lung disease along with a diffusion defect, and patients are usually hypoxemic. The chest film confirms the presence of pulmonary disease.

C. If the patient is taking one of the drugs known to produce pulmonary disease, a drug-related illness is suspected at the outset. If the clinical course is not consistent with infection, and if analysis of sputum does not reveal any specific pathogens, any drug suspected of producing pulmonary disease should be discontinued and the patient closely observed for improvement. Even if the pulmonary injury was caused by the drug in question, improvement may not occur; for example, injury due to alkylating agents is idiosyncratic and does not remit with drug withdrawal. If the question of drug-induced pulmonary toxicity remains open, or if the drug in question is required for patient maintenance, further diagnostic work-up will be necessary to confirm that the drug is producing disease.

D. Patients presenting with acute pulmonary edema who do not have cardiac disease may have narcotic-induced pulmonary edema. If the patient is young and is known to use narcotics, this would be the most likely diagnosis. The pulmonary capillary wedge pressure will be within normal limits and the syndrome may occur with the first intravenous use of the drug. Naloxone and oxygen therapy should be used. Mechanical ventilation may be necessary until the edema resolves.

E. Patients presenting with lobar and/or interstitial infiltrates should be worked up for either bacterial or viral infection with sputum Gram stain and culture. It will often be difficult to make the diagnosis of a viral illness, especially in immunocompromised patients on multiple-drug regimens.

(Continued on page 214).

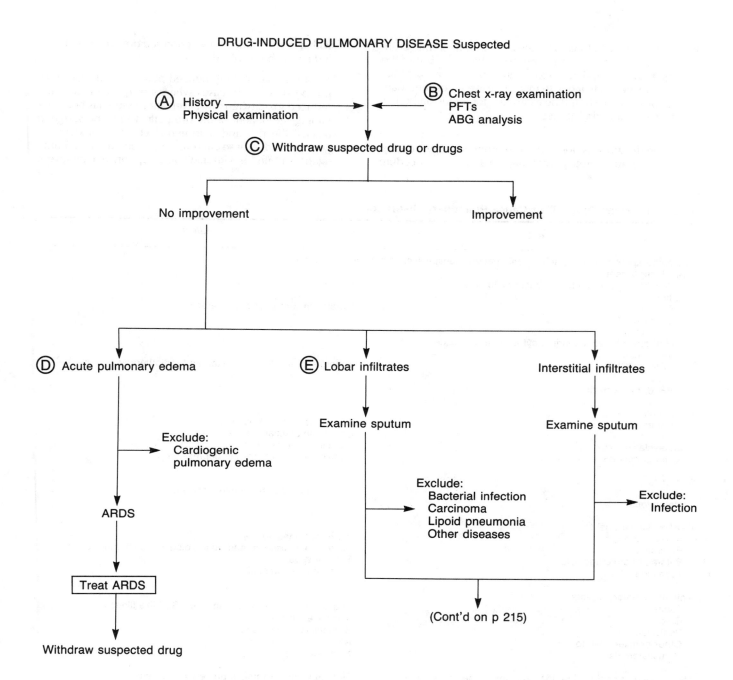

DRUG-INDUCED PULMONARY DISEASE Suspected

Ⓐ History
Physical examination

Ⓑ Chest x-ray examination
PFTs
ABG analysis

Ⓒ Withdraw suspected drug or drugs

No improvement

Improvement

Ⓓ Acute pulmonary edema

Exclude:
Cardiogenic
pulmonary edema

ARDS

Treat ARDS

Withdraw suspected drug

Ⓔ Lobar infiltrates

Examine sputum

Exclude:
Bacterial infection
Carcinoma
Lipoid pneumonia
Other diseases

Interstitial infiltrates

Examine sputum

Exclude:
Infection

(Cont'd on p 215)

F. In patients with lobar infiltrates, perform fiberoptic bronchoscopy with transbronchoscopic biopsy (TBB) of the lung early on during hospitalization before gas exchange deteriorates sufficiently to make invasive procedures dangerous. Tissue should be examined for inclusion bodies that indicate viral illness.

G. If the diagnosis is not clear from bronchoscopy, perform an open lung biopsy. This may be a limited procedure with a small thoracotomy performed over an area of lung judged to be involved.

H. The histology of drug-induced pulmonary disease may not be specific. In cases where the question of drug-induced toxicity remains, even after tissue has been obtained, the benefit of the drug effect must be weighed against the risk and detrimental effects of toxicity. In general, under these circumstances, potential offending agents should be withdrawn and supportive care given.

TABLE 1 Some Drugs That Cause Pulmonary Disorders

Drug	Effect
Chemotherapeutic agents (radiographic pattern nonspecific, alveolar-interstitial pattern)	
Alkylating Agents	
Busulfan, cytoxan, chlorambucil, melphalan	
Antibiotics	
Bleomycin	Synergism with prior radiotherapy
Mitomycin C	
Antimetabolites	
Methotrexate, azathioprine, cytosine, arabinoside	
Nitrosoureas	
BCNU, CCNU	Synergistic effect with cytoxan and radiotherapy
Others	
VP16, procarbazine	
Antibiotics	
Nitrofurantoin	Acute pneumonic reactions
	Chronic interstitial fibrosis
Sulfasalazine	? Eosinophilic pneumonitis
Aminoglycosides	Respiratory weakness and depression
Narcotics	
Heroin	Acute noncardiogenic pulmonary edema
Methadone	
Cardiovascular agents	
Amiodarone	Interstitial pneumonitis
Protamine	Acute bronchospasm and noncardiogenic pulmonary edema
Beta-adrenergic agonists	Bronchospasm
Tocainide	Interstitial pneumonitis
Anti-inflammatory agents	
Aspirin	Acute, severe bronchospasm, PIE, SLE-like illness
Gold	Interstitial fibrosis
Penicillamine	Bronchiolitis obliterans
Other nonsteroidal agents	Aspirin-like syndromes
Corticosteroids	Mediastinal fat
Hydralazine, procainamide, INH, hydantoin, penicillamine, and others	Drug-induced systemic lupus erythematosus
Inhalants	
Oil	Lobar infiltrates, lipoid pneumonia
Oxygen	ARDS, interstitial fibrosis
Blood transfusions	Leukoagglutinin-mediated pulmonary edema
Radiographic contrast media	Noncardiogenic pulmonary edema
Nitrofurantoin, penicillins, sulfonamides, naproxen, salicylates, methotrexate	PIE (pulmonary infiltrates with eosinophilia)
Miscellaneous	
Hydrochlorothiazide	Diffuse pulmonary infiltrates
Oral contraceptives	Deep venous thrombosis and pulmonary embolic disease
Dantrolene	Chronic pleural effusion

(Cont'd from p 213)

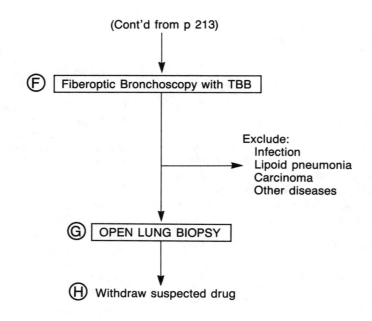

(F) Fiberoptic Bronchoscopy with TBB

Exclude:
Infection
Lipoid pneumonia
Carcinoma
Other diseases

(G) OPEN LUNG BIOPSY

(H) Withdraw suspected drug

Reference

Kilburn KH. Pulmonary disease induced by drugs. In: Fishman AP, ed. Pulmonary diseases and disorders. New York: McGraw-Hill, 1980: 707.

LIPOID PNEUMONIA

Lipoid pneumonia is an uncommon disease that is a chronic inflammatory reaction of the lung to the aspiration of exogenous animal, vegetable, or mineral oils. Mineral oil is the most common etiologic agent, as it is used widely in commercial products such as baby oil and laxatives. Oil aspiration may occur in patients with depressed gag reflex or esophageal motility abnormalities. The chronic use of oily nose drops or those that contain liquid paraffin is also associated with the development of this disease. Lipoid pneumonia has also been reported to develop in automobile mechanics because of the inhalation of mineral oil mists.

A. Because less than half of the patients with lipoid pneumonia are symptomatic, most cases of lipoid pneumonia are discovered incidentally on chest films. Symptoms may be episodic and include cough, pleuritic chest pain, dyspnea, wheezing, chills, hemoptysis, and low-grade fever. Careful questioning may be necessary to reveal a history of occupational exposure to oil or of the ingestion or inhalation of oily medications. The physical examination is not specific and may be normal or demonstrate findings compatible with the diagnosis of bacterial pneumonia. Patients frequently receive repeated courses of empiric antibiotics for the treatment of presumed nonresolving bacterial pneumonia; indeed, some patients may have a complicating bacterial process. Because mineral oil is nonirritative to the trachea, most patients do not associate the use of oil with their symptoms. Symptomatic lipoid pneumonia may not occur for many years, and symptoms may develop only after repeated aspirations.

B. Routine laboratory blood tests are generally unremarkable. Bacterial pneumonia and tuberculosis must be excluded with appropriate sputum examinations and tuberculin skin testing. Hypoxemia is a common finding. Patients with mild disease may have normal arterial blood gases while at rest but may become hypoxemic with exercise. The finding of oil droplets contained within macrophages in sputum along with a history of exposure to oil suggests the diagnosis, although this finding is not specific. Macrophages containing lipid may be present in normal subjects without pulmonary disease.

C. The radiographic appearance of lipoid pneumonia is highly variable; multiple lung segments are frequently involved. The pattern seen depends on the duration and amount of oil aspirated or inhaled and on the resultant inflammatory response. Early radiographic appearances include local or diffuse alveolar consolidation, usually localized to the lower lobes. Interstitial disease may develop with progression to fibrosis and nodule formation. Tuberculosis and bronchogenic carcinoma are two of the major diseases in the differential diagnosis.

D. Because the radiographic appearance of lipoid pneumonia is not diagnostic of the disease, CT helps establish the diagnosis. Fat has a low attenuation value (a bottle of mineral oil has a CT number of −132 Hounsfield units [HU]). Pulmonary lesions associated with lipoid pneumonia have values ranging from −30 HU to −140 HU. The range of CT attenuation is due to variable amounts of fat mixed with the surrounding inflammatory exudates and tissues.

E. The diagnostic likelihood of lipoid pneumonia is increased by the identification of lipid-laden macrophages in pulmonary specimens. The occurrence of alveolar cell carcinoma and other primary lung carcinomas has been reported as a long-term complication of lipoid pneumonia. Fiberoptic bronchoscopy with transbronchoscopic biopsy and bronchoalveolar lavage may be required to obtain specimens for lipid staining as well as to exclude other diagnoses.

F. The use of oil or any exposure to oil must be stopped. Since expectoration is the only mechanism for removing mineral oil from the lung, patients must be instructed in coughing exercises that should be performed daily. Oral expectorants have not been found to be helpful. Precautions against aspiration should be taken. Administration of systemic corticosteroids (prednisone dosages of 40 to 60 mg daily) has been recommended for patients with progressive infiltrates or significant symptoms. Resolution of the disease is generally slow. Rarely, the condition of some patients may deteriorate with the development of cor pulmonale.

References

Genereux GP. Lipids in the lungs: radiologic-pathologic correlation. J Can Assoc Radiol 1970; 21:2.

Kennedy JD, Costello P, Balikian JP, Herman PG. Exogenous lipoid pneumonia. AJR 1981; 136:1145.

Lipinski LK, Weisbrod GL, Sanders DE. Exogenous lipoid pneumonitis: pulmonary patterns. AJR 1981; 136:931.

Scully RE, Galdabini JJ, McNeely BU. Case records of the Massachusetts General Hospital, case 19-1977. N Engl J Med 1977; 296:1105.

LIPOID PNEUMONIA Suspecte

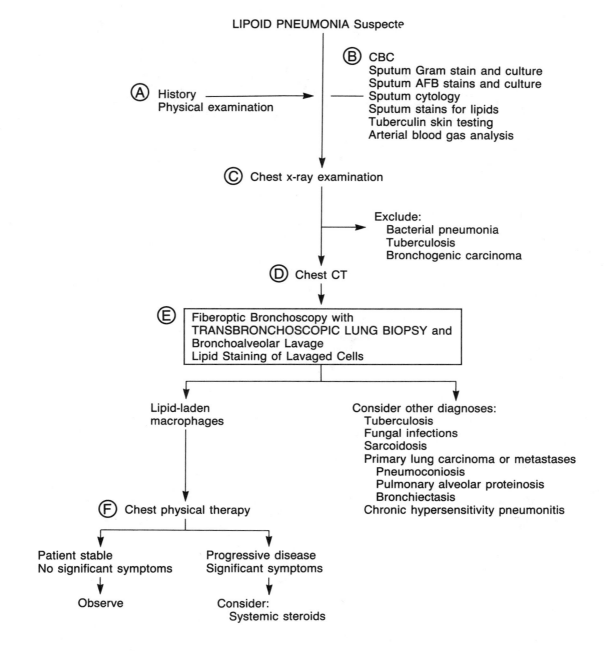

Ⓐ History ⟶ Ⓑ CBC
Physical examination   Sputum Gram stain and culture
                           Sputum AFB stains and culture
                           Sputum cytology
                           Sputum stains for lipids
                           Tuberculin skin testing
                           Arterial blood gas analysis

Ⓒ Chest x-ray examination

Exclude:
  Bacterial pneumonia
  Tuberculosis
  Bronchogenic carcinoma

Ⓓ Chest CT

Ⓔ Fiberoptic Bronchoscopy with
   TRANSBRONCHOSCOPIC LUNG BIOPSY and
   Bronchoalveolar Lavage
   Lipid Staining of Lavaged Cells

Lipid-laden   Consider other diagnoses:
macrophages   Tuberculosis
                             Fungal infections
                             Sarcoidosis
                             Primary lung carcinoma or metastases
                               Pneumoconiosis
                               Pulmonary alveolar proteinosis
                               Bronchiectasis
                             Chronic hypersensitivity pneumonitis

Ⓕ Chest physical therapy

Patient stable   Progressive disease
No significant symptoms   Significant symptoms

Observe   Consider:
                              Systemic steroids

MISCELLANEOUS LUNG DISEASE

Foreign Body Aspiration
Pulmonary Alveolar Proteinosis
Bronchopleural Fistula
Tracheoesophageal Fistula

FOREIGN BODY ASPIRATION

Aspiration of particulate substances usually results in severe coughing and varying degrees of respiratory distress. This occurs more commonly in children, with peanuts as the most commonly aspirated object; in adults aspiration of a bolus of partially chewed meat during an evening meal is the most common circumstance. Obesity and alcohol use increase the risk of this event. However, aspiration of small objects may occur, which produces only minimal cough and may be clinically inapparent for months or years. Late complications of foreign-body aspiration include recurrent pneumonia, lung abscess formation, and bronchiectasis. These complications often result in a medical evaluation, which detects the presence of the unsuspected foreign body.

A. Aspiration of large objects is readily diagnosed on clinical grounds and presents as a medical emergency. Aspiration of small objects may be recalled as a bout of severe coughing or wheezing during a meal. Determining the nature of the object suggests the best approach for its removal.

B. Most foreign bodies are radiolucent. Some, such as an aspirated tooth, are radiopaque and can be seen on the chest film. Most radiolucent objects are detected by bronchoscopy that is performed as part of a evaluation of possible bronchial obstruction. The foreign body is usually located in the right lung. The indications for bronchoscopy are recurrent pneumonia in a particular lobe, atelectasis, localized persistent wheezing, or recurrent hemoptysis. In certain cases, removal of the foreign body can be accomplished through the flexible bronchoscope.

C. Large proximal foreign bodies are best removed with a rigid bronchoscope, which permits more careful control of the airway and the use of larger forceps.

D. Distal foreign bodies can be removed with a flexible fiberoptic bronchoscope placed through a cuffed endotracheal tube. Either a modified forceps or basket arrangement may be used. Zavala et al recommended the use of a Fogarty balloon catheter to dislodge impacted objects. However, considerable caution must be exercised since the objects may break during removal or bleeding may result when the object is dislodged. Surgical intervention is rarely needed.

References

Berger P, Kuhn JP, Kuhns LR. Computed tomography and occult tracheobronchial foreign body. Radiology 1980; 134:133.

Linton JS. Long standing intratracheal foreign bodies. Thorax 1957; 12:164.

Schloss MD, Pham-Dang H, Rosales JK. Foreign bodies in the tracheobronchial tree—a retrospective study of 217 cases. J Otolaryngol 1983; 12:212.

Workove N, Kreisman H, Cohen C, Frank H. Occult foreign-body aspiration in adults. JAMA 1982; 248:1350.

Zavala DC, Rhodes ML. Foreign body removal: a new role for the fiberoptic bronchoscope. Ann Otolaryngol 1975; 84:650.

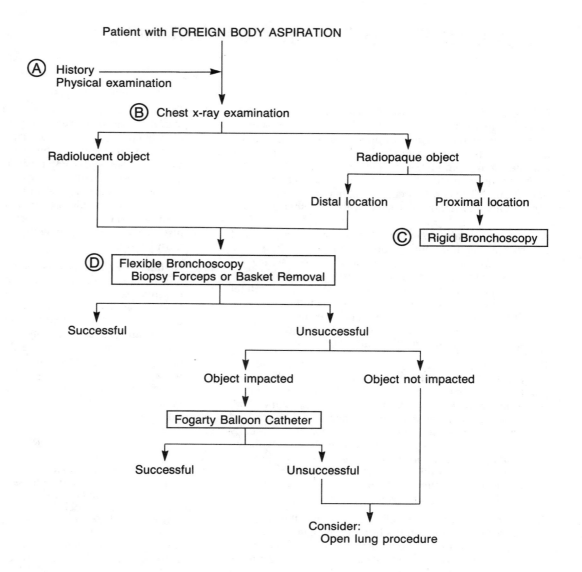

Patient with FOREIGN BODY ASPIRATION

Ⓐ History ———————→
   Physical examination

Ⓑ Chest x-ray examination

Radiolucent object   Radiopaque object

                              Distal location   Proximal location

                                                      Ⓒ Rigid Bronchoscopy

Ⓓ Flexible Bronchoscopy
   Biopsy Forceps or Basket Removal

Successful   Unsuccessful

                    Object impacted   Object not impacted

                    Fogarty Balloon Catheter

              Successful   Unsuccessful

                              Consider:
                              Open lung procedure

PULMONARY ALVEOLAR PROTEINOSIS

Pulmonary alveolar proteinosis (PAP) is a disease of unknown etiology in which alveoli become filled with an insoluble, proteinaceous material rich in phospholipid. This material appears to be derived from sloughed type II pneumocytes and their major product, surfactant. Macrophages are commonly found in the filled alveolar spaces. Alveolar walls are not inflamed. The condition usually affects young to middle-aged adults and is not associated with any other diseases.

A. Patients usually complain of dyspnea on exertion and have a mild unremitting cough. Sputum may be chalky white in appearance and "gummy" in consistency. Fatigue and weight loss are common. Physical findings are few and limited to cyanosis, clubbing, and retinal petechial hemorrhages in severely affected individuals. Breath sounds are decreased, and rales are not always present since inhaled gas may not traverse filled airspaces. The lungs may be dull to percussion.

B. The chest film demonstrates perihilar "bat wing" infiltrates that resemble those of pulmonary edema, but the cardiac silhouette is usually normal. The laboratory examination is within normal limits except for the LDH, which is usually elevated. PFTs reveal normal-to-reduced lung volumes, and the diffusing capacity is usually reduced. These patients are hypoxemic and hypocapnemic at rest. Patients who are normoxic at rest become hypoxic with mild-to-moderate exercise. The history, physical examination, and laboratory examination usually allow other diagnoses to be excluded.

C. Sputum should be examined to rule out the presence of *Nocardia* prior to bronchoscopy. Nocardial pneumonia occurs with high frequency in this group of patients, and other opportunistic infections may also be more common. Nocardial infection should be treated with sulfonamides prior to any invasive pulmonary procedure.

D. The diagnosis may be made by histologic examination of bronchoalveolar lavage fluid obtained during fiberoptic bronchoscopy. This material has a beige color and a high specific gravity. When viewed by light microscopy, large quantities of PAS-positive material are seen filling air spaces. This finding is characteristic of PAP. Alveolar walls are normal in structure, fibrosis is not a part of the histologic picture, and cultures of fluid are usually sterile. When the absence of the appropriate histology rules out the diagnosis of PAP, other diagnoses must be sought.

E. No definitive therapy is available. Patients who have significant airway filling and are hypoxemic at rest or with minimal exercise (PaO_2 < 55 mm Hg) require whole-lung lavage. Each lung is treated separately. Lungs are degassed and lavaged with large quantities of physiologic saline (20 to 50 L) heated to 37 °C. This procedure removes the material from the alveoli and improves the gas exchange function of the lungs but is not curative. It may be necessary to repeat the lavage depending on the rate at which refilling of alveolar spaces occurs. Some patients may experience spontaneous remissions for unknown reasons.

References

Gale ME, Karlinsky JB, Robins AG. Bronchopulmonary lavage in pulmonary alveolar proteinosis: chest film observations. Am J Roentgenol 1986; 146:91.

Kariman K, Klystra JA, Spock A. Pulmonary alveolar proteinosis: prospective clinical experience in 23 patients for 15 years. Lung 1984; 162:223.

Ramirez RJ, Keffer RF Jr, Ball D Jr. Bronchopulmonary lavage in man. Ann Intern Med 1965; 63:819.

Rosen SH, Castleman B, Liebow AA. Pulmonary alveolar proteinosis. N Engl J Med 1958; 258:1123.

PULMONARY ALVEOLAR PROTEINOSIS Suspected

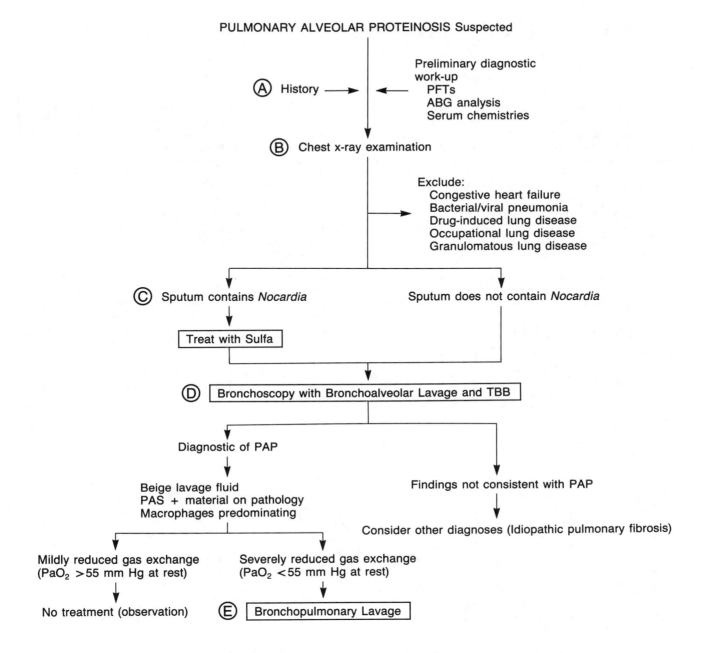

(A) History ⟶ ⟵ Preliminary diagnostic
work-up
PFTs
ABG analysis
Serum chemistries

(B) Chest x-ray examination

Exclude:
Congestive heart failure
Bacterial/viral pneumonia
Drug-induced lung disease
Occupational lung disease
Granulomatous lung disease

(C) Sputum contains *Nocardia*   Sputum does not contain *Nocardia*

Treat with Sulfa

(D) Bronchoscopy with Bronchoalveolar Lavage and TBB

Diagnostic of PAP   Findings not consistent with PAP

Beige lavage fluid
PAS + material on pathology   Consider other diagnoses (Idiopathic pulmonary fibrosis)
Macrophages predominating

Mildly reduced gas exchange   Severely reduced gas exchange
(PaO$_2$ >55 mm Hg at rest)   (PaO$_2$ <55 mm Hg at rest)

No treatment (observation)   (E) Bronchopulmonary Lavage

BRONCHOPLEURAL FISTULA

A bronchopleural fistula is a communication between an airway and the pleural space. This may result from a variety of causes. Bronchopleural fistulae may follow pulmonary resection or the rupture of a bleb. In the past, tuberculosis was a frequent cause. Bronchopleural fistula may also result from a necrotizing pneumonia such as that caused by anaerobic organisms or it may be iatrogenically induced following a diagnostic or therapeutic thoracentesis. The mortality and morbidity depend in part on the etiology. When bronchopleural fistula follows pneumonectomy, the mortality and morbidity rates are very high; in this case the fistula results from stump failure or infection.

A. The diagnosis is suggested by a pneumothorax but is confirmed by a persistent air leak after placement of a chest tube. Ordinarily a chest tube is inserted if the pneumothorax exceeds 20 percent of the hemithorax or when the respiratory status is significantly compromised.

B. Obtain a CT scan to assess the state of the underlying lung and to verify the position of the tube. A bronchopleural fistula can be created by incorrect placement of a chest tube. This usually occurs when the tube is inserted into lung parenchyma that had been previously damaged by a necrotizing pneumonia.

C. Our initial approach is to follow the patient conservatively for a period of 2 to 4 weeks. Treat infections aggressively, if present. In many cases, the fistula seals spontaneously. A major goal of chest tube drainage is to allow the lung to expand to fill the pleural space. When the lung is not completely expanded, connect the chest tube to high suction. If the lung fails to expand, the fistula often remains patent and a second procedure is required to obliterate the space. If the lung is fully expanded and the bronchopleural fistula persists, the chest tube is connected to low suction or to underwater seal only. The treatment of large fistulae in ventilated patients who require PEEP is a special problem. Approaches used in this situation involve high-frequency ventilation, continuous positive intrapleural pressure, and others.

D. When initial conservative treatment fails and the air leak persists, the choice of therapy depends on whether empyema is present as well as the state of the lung parenchyma. In the absence of infection, certain fistulae such as those resulting from a ruptured bleb can be closed surgically. Attempts have been made to occlude the airway leading to the fistula by the fiberoptic placement of a material such as lead shot. This is performed in patients who have little expectation of prolonged survival. The precise location of the fistula can be identified by scanning with xenon-133. When an empyema is also present, open drainage with rib resection is performed. The exact timing of this procedure is a difficult clinical decision. The patient's failure to improve while receiving antibiotics and chest tube drainage suggests the need for surgery.

E. The best surgical approach to persistent bronchopleural fistulae is controversial and varies from center to center. We ordinarily employ rib resection and open drainage, which allows for slow recovery by ingrowth of granulation tissue. This can be followed by a sinogram to evaluate the size of the residual cavity. Other centers use other approaches such as obliteration of the space with muscle flaps (myoplasty). Decortication is used when the CT scan reveals a markedly thickened pleura and otherwise normal lung parenchyma.

References

Chicarilli ZN, Ariyan S, Glenn WWL, Seashore JH. Management of recalcitrant bronchopleural fistulas with muscle flap obliteration. Plast Reconstr Surg 1984; 75:882.

Downs JB, Chapman RL. Treatment of bronchopleural fistula during continuous positive pressure ventilation. Chest 1976; 69:363.

Hankins JR, Miller JE, Attar S, Satterfield JR, Mclaughlin JS. Bronchopleural fistula. J Thorac Cardiovasc Surg 1978; 76:755.

Hoier-Madsen K, Schulze S, Pedersen VM, Halkier E. Management of bronchopleural fistula following pneumonectomy. Scand J Thorac Cardiovasc Surg 1984; 18:263.

Lillington GA. Bronchoscopic localization of bronchopleural fistula with xenon-133. J Nucl Med 1982; 23:322.

Ratliff JL, Hill JD, Tucher H, Fallat R. Endobronchial control of bronchopleural fistulae. Chest 1977; 71:98.

Weissberg D. Empyema and bronchopleural fistula. Chest 1982; 82:447.

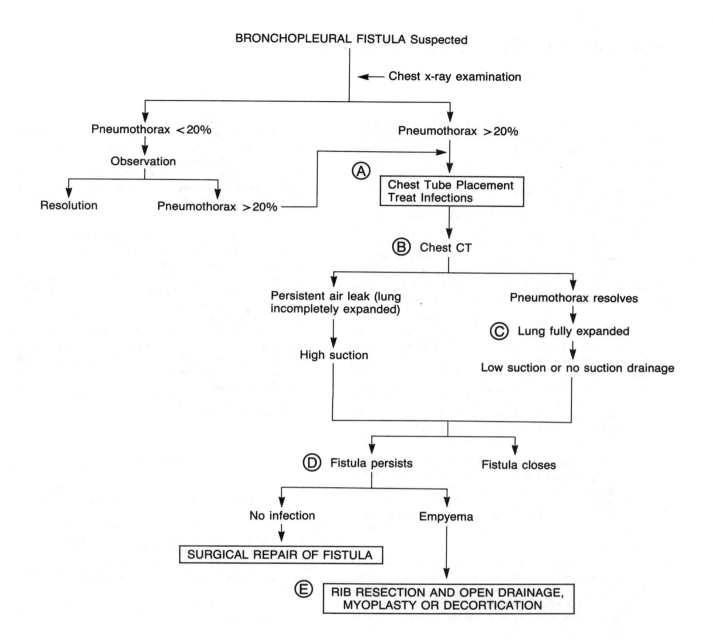

BRONCHOPLEURAL FISTULA Suspected

← Chest x-ray examination

Pneumothorax <20%

Observation

Resolution

Pneumothorax >20%

Pneumothorax >20%

(A)

Chest Tube Placement
Treat Infections

(B) Chest CT

Persistent air leak (lung
incompletely expanded)

High suction

Pneumothorax resolves

(C) Lung fully expanded

Low suction or no suction drainage

(D) Fistula persists

Fistula closes

No infection

Empyema

SURGICAL REPAIR OF FISTULA

(E) RIB RESECTION AND OPEN DRAINAGE,
MYOPLASTY OR DECORTICATION

TRACHEOESOPHAGEAL FISTULA

A tracheoesophageal fistula in adults is usually an acquired lesion that may result from a variety of causes including malignancy, trauma, infections such as tuberculosis or actinomycosis, or may follow tracheotomy. A malignancy originating in either the trachea or the esophagus can erode into the adjacent lumen, causing a fistula. The most common cause of tracheoesophageal fistulae is malignancy (60 percent) involving the trachea or the esophagus. Traumatic injuries account for another large group, particularly those resulting from steering wheel injuries in automobile accidents. The incidence of tracheoesophageal fistulae resulting from prolonged use of endotracheal tubes has declined since the advent of low-pressure cuffs. Among patients with tracheoesophageal fistula, pneumonia is the most common cause of death.

A. The presenting symptoms often involve spasms of cough after the ingestion of liquids and solid foods. Intermittent symptoms suggest aspiration, although small fistulae may become intermittently occluded with food or other materials. When the fistula results from traumatic injuries, associated injuries such as rib fractures or pneumothorax are usually present. Subcutaneous emphysema is seen in approximately half of these cases. The onset of symptoms is often delayed 3 to 5 days after injury because the fistula is initially occluded by edema or blood.

B. Patients with evidence of swallowing dysfunction should be initially evaluated with a barium swallow. This procedure detects the presence of diverticulum or esophageal abnormalities, including the possibility of a tracheoesophageal fistula. If a fistula is suspected, use a water-soluble contrast material to minimize the dangers of aspiration.

C. In patients who are intubated, a tracheoesophageal fistula can be detected by instillation of methylene blue into the trachea. A positive methylene blue test supports the diagnosis of tracheoesophageal fistula but does not clearly rule out aspiration as a possibility. The presence of cough independent of body position favors a fistula.

D. The chest CT scan offers a noninvasive approach to the evaluation of possible tracheoesophageal fistulae. Esophago-airway communications can be visualized. In the case of esophageal malignancy, suggestive evidence for fistula includes obscuration of the mediastinal fat by a soft-tissue density. Large fistulae are readily identified due to the free passage of air between the trachea and the esophagus.

E. Barium swallows are frequently used to establish the diagnosis of swallowing dysfunction. However, they must be used with caution because of the possibility of passage of a large quantity of barium into the airway. Bronchoscopy has been used successfully in many cases to document the presence of a fistula and to determine the etiology if unknown. The bronchoscopic findings consist of marked posterior tracheal wall impingement and mucosal inflammation. Esophagoscopy is an alternate approach to confirming the presence of a fistula. The particular diagnostic approach selected depends on the facilities available and the individual patient. In patients with severe respiratory problems, esophagoscopy is the preferred approach.

References

Berkmen YM, Auh Y-H CT. Diagnosis of acquired tracheoesophageal fistula in adults. J Comput Assist Tomogr 1985; 9:302.

Ghazi A, Nussbaum M. A new approach to the management of malignant esophageal obstruction and esophagorespiratory fistula. Ann Thorac Surg 1986; 41:531.

Leeds WM, Morley TF, Zappasodi SJ, Giudice JC. Computed tomography for diagnosis of tracheoesophageal fistula. Crit Care Med 1986; 14:591.

Spalding AB, Burney DP, Richie PE. Acquired benign tracheoesophageal fistulas in adults. Ann Thorac Surg 1979; 28:378.

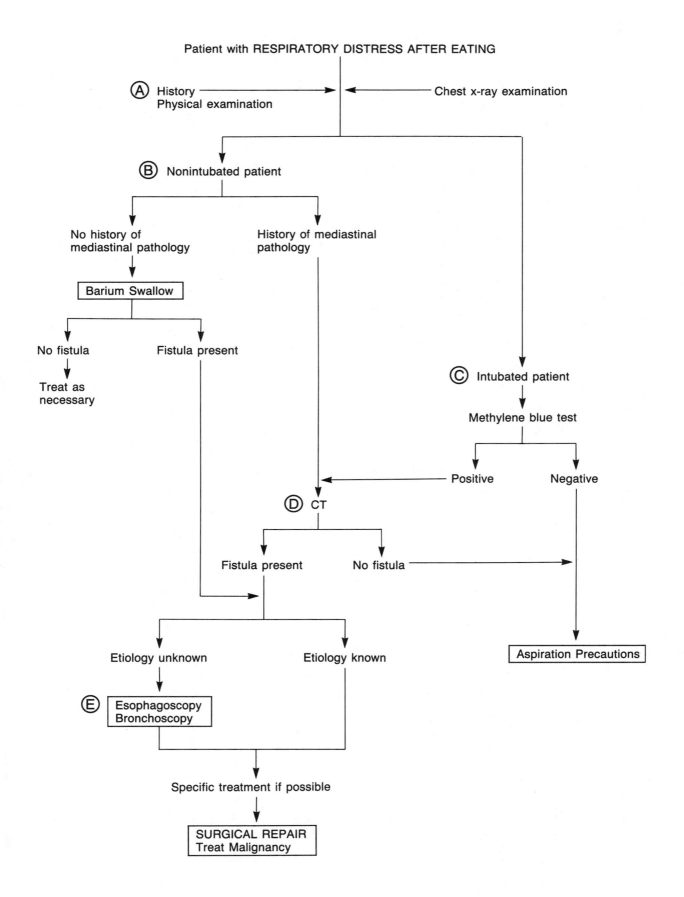

Patient with RESPIRATORY DISTRESS AFTER EATING

(A) History —————→ ←————— Chest x-ray examination
Physical examination

(B) Nonintubated patient

No history of   History of mediastinal
mediastinal pathology   pathology

Barium Swallow

No fistula   Fistula present

Treat as
necessary

(C) Intubated patient

Methylene blue test

Positive   Negative

(D) CT

Fistula present   No fistula

Etiology unknown   Etiology known

(E) Esophagoscopy
Bronchoscopy

Aspiration Precautions

Specific treatment if possible

SURGICAL REPAIR
Treat Malignancy

INDEX